Comprehensive Virology 4

Comprehensive Virology

Edited by Heinz Fraenkel-Conrat
University of California at Berkeley

and Robert R. Wagner
University of Virginia

Editorial Board

Comprehensive

Edited by

Heinz Fraenkel-Conrat

Department of Molecular Biology and Virus Laboratory
University of California, Berkeley, California

and

Robert R. Wagner

Department of Microbiology
University of Virginia, Charlottesville, Virginia

Virology

4

Reproduction
Large RNA Viruses

PLENUM PRESS · NEW YORK AND LONDON

Library of Congress Cataloging in Publication Data

Fraenkel-Conrat, Heinz, 1910-
  Reproduction, large RNA viruses.

  (Their Comprehensive virology; v. 4)
  Includes bibliographies and index.
  1. Viruses—Reproduction. I. Wagner, Robert R., 1923-   joint author. II.
Title. III Series: Fraenkel-Conrat, Heinz, 1910-   Comprehensive virology; v. 4.
QR357.F72 vol. 4 [QR470]   576'.64'08s   [576'.64]
ISBN 0-306-35144-7   74-20501

© 1975 Plenum Press, New York
A Division of Plenum Publishing Corporation
227 West 17th Street, New York, N.Y. 10011

United Kingdom edition published by Plenum Press, London
A Division of Plenum Publishing Company, Ltd.
4a Lower John Street, London W1R 3PD, England

Printed in the United States of America

Foreword

The time seems ripe for a critical compendium of that segment of the biological universe we call viruses. Virology, as a science, having only recently passed through its descriptive phase of naming and numbering, has probably reached that stage at which relatively few new—truly new—viruses will be discovered. Triggered by the intellectual probes and techniques of molecular biology, genetics, biochemical cytology, and high-resolution microscopy and spectroscopy, the field has experienced a genuine information explosion.

Few serious attempts have so far been made to chronicle these events. This comprehensive series, which will comprise some 6000 pages in a total of about 22 volumes, represents a commitment by a large group of active investigators to analyze, digest, and expostulate on the great mass of data relating to viruses, much of which is now amorphous and disjointed and scattered throughout a wide literature. In this way, we hope to place the entire field in perspective as well as to develop an invaluable reference and sourcebook for researchers and students at all levels. This series is designed as a continuum that can be entered anywhere but which also provides a logical progression of developing facts and integrated concepts.

The first volume contains an alphabetical catalogue of almost all viruses of vertebrates, insects, plants, and protists, describing them in general terms. Volumes 2–5 deal primarily, though not exclusively, with the processes of infection and reproduction of the major groups of viruses in their hosts. Volume 2 deals with the simple RNA viruses of bacteria, plants, and animals; the togaviruses (formerly called arboviruses), which share with these only the feature that the virion's RNA is able to act as messenger RNA in the host cell; and the reoviruses of animals and plants, which all share several structurally singular features, the most important being the double-strandedness of their multiple RNA molecules. This grouping, of course, has only slightly more in its favor than others that could have been or indeed were considered.

Volume 3 addresses itself to the reproduction of all DNA-containing viruses of vertebrates, a seemingly simple act of classification, even though the field encompasses the smallest and the largest viruses known.

The reproduction of the larger and more complex RNA viruses represents the subject matter of Volume 4. These share the property of lipid-rich envelopes with the togaviruses included in Volume 2. They share as a group, and with the reoviruses, the presence of enzymes in their virions and the need for their RNA to become transcribed before it can serve messenger functions.

Volume 5 attends to the reproduction of DNA viruses in bacteria, again ranging from small and simple to large and complex.

Aspects of virion structure and assembly of many of these viruses will be dealt with in the following series of volumes, while their genetics, the regulation of their development, viroids, and coviruses will be discussed in subsequently published series. The last volumes will concentrate on host–virus interactions, and on the effects of chemicals and radiation on viruses and their components. At this juncture in the planning of *Comprehensive Virology,* we cannot foresee whether certain topics will become important aspects of the field by the time the final volumes go to press. We envisage the possibility of including volumes on such topics if the need arises.

It is hoped to keep the series at all times up to date by prompt and rapid publication of all contributions, and by encouraging the authors to update their chapters by additions or corrections whenever a volume is reprinted.

Contents

Chapter 3

Reproduction of Myxoviruses

Richard W. Compans and Purnell W. Choppin

Chapter 4

Reproduction of RNA Tumor Viruses

John P. Bader

Reproduction of Rhabdoviruses

Robert R. Wagner

Department of Microbiology
The University of Virginia
Charlottesville, Virginia 22901

1. DESCRIPTIVE BIOLOGY

1.1. Definition

The rhabdoviruses are ubiquitous, highly infectious agents of animal and plant disease and are generally transmitted by arthropods. Assignment of viruses to the taxon rhabdoviruses (rod-shaped viruses) was originally based entirely on morphology. This classification has turned out to be fortuitously fortunate because later biochemical studies have revealed remarkable uniformity among these structurally similar viruses isolated from extremely diverse hosts. It is perhaps not farfetched to postulate a common ancestor for all the rhabdoviruses of plants, arthropods, and vertebrates. Classification of a virus as a rhabdovirus should be based on the following most important characteristics:

1. Rhabdoviruses are rod-shaped particles, varying considerably in length (60–400 nm) but of a reasonably consistent width (60–85 nm).

2. Animal rhabdoviruses tend to be bullet-shaped in appearance, flat at one end and a tapered sphere at the other. Plant rhabdoviruses are usually bacilliform in shape, quite elongated and with two round ends.

3. All rhabdoviruses appear to be surrounded by a membranous

envelope with protruding spikes. All these viruses probably contain lipids and are, therefore, susceptible to disruption by ether and detergents.

4. Wound inside the envelope of rhabdoviruses is a ribonucleocapsid (RNC) core which gives the appearance of striations when viewed by electron microscopy. All rhabdoviruses examined to date contain one molecule of single-stranded RNA, which is not by itself infectious and does not serve as messenger. Therefore, rhabdoviruses are generally classified along with the myxoviruses and paramyxoviruses as "negative-strand viruses," in contradistinction to the "positive-strand" picornaviruses and togaviruses (Baltimore, 1971).

5. Many, if not all, rhabdoviruses contain an RNA-dependent RNA polymerase (transcriptase) as part of the nucleocapsid which renders it infectious in the absence of the envelope.

6. A common characteristic of animal rhabdoviruses, conceivably also applicable to plant rhabdoviruses, is the frequent occurrence of defective truncated (T) virions which are noninfectious because a considerable segment (one-third to two-thirds) of the RNA genome is deleted.

A reliable overview of the rhabdoviruses is available in the then-topical review of Howatson (1970), which provides important information on the biology and morphology of these viruses and their distribution in nature. Much of the older literature on rabies is available in the review by Matsumoto (1970). The excellent, very recent review by Knudson (1973) is recommended reading for a true understanding of comparative rhabdovirology, as is the even more recent and more comprehensive review by Francki (1973). Some rhabdoviruses are important causative agents of human disease, particularly rabies, and others are of considerable economic importance as serious infectious agents of disease in animals, both livestock and wild animals. Probably the greatest economic impact is caused by the rhabdoviruses that infect a great variety of plants. The extensive literature on the pathogenesis of rhabdoviral infections will not be covered in this chapter. Highly recommended for the interested reader is the excellent article on the pathogenesis of infection with vesicular stomatitis virus by Miyoshi *et al.*, (1971), as is the review of the natural history of vesicular stomatitis by Hanson (1952). Very good articles and reviews of the literature on the comparative pathogenesis of rabies and rabieslike viruses have recently been written by Murphy *et al.* (1973*a,b*); also recommended is "Natural History of Rabies" edited by Baer (1973).

1.2. Morphology

1.2.1. Vesicular Stomatitis Virus

1.2.1a. Infectious B Virions

Vesicular stomatitis (VS) virus, the prototype of rhabdoviruses, has been examined by electron microscopy in many laboratories (Chow *et al.*, 1954; Reczko, 1960; Howatson and Whitmore, 1962; Bradish and Kirkham, 1966; McCombs *et al.*, 1966; Simpson and Hauser, 1966; Nakai and Howatson, 1968). Only minor variations can be discerned in the morphological characteristics of other rhabdoviruses, and they will not be described here in detail. The reader is referred to the reviews of Howatson (1970) and Knudson (1973) for comparative analyses of the electron microscopy of rhabdoviruses. Figures 1 and 2 illustrate the general structure of VS virus as viewed by negative staining and thin-section electron microscopy; Fig. 3 shows a schematic representation of the infectious virion. The typical infectious virion is a bullet-shaped (B particle) cylinder, 180 ± 10 nm in length and 65 ± 10 nm in diameter at the blunt end. Most intact virions are planar at one end and hemispheric at the other; occasional particles can be seen to be round at both ends, but they are rarely, if ever, flat at both ends, unless broken. The B-virion cylinder appears to have a hollow center that is penetrable by phosphotungstic acid (PTA) to a varying extent, up to almost its whole length in some virions. PTA almost invariably penetrates through the planar (blunt) end of the virion, a finding which has given rise to the concept that the virion envelope is weaker or structurally defective at the planar end. This structural weakness is consistent with the observation that the virion is invariably pinched off at the blunt end as it buds from the plasma membrane; the resealed membrane that forms the virion envelope is, therefore, presumed to be more permeable at the blunt end. A distended piece of membrane, often seen ballooning from the blunt end of the virion, is thought to be a distinctive feature by some investigators.

Any structural model of the VS virion must consider that the virion is composed of two separate and distinct components: (1) the RNC and (2) the envelope (see Fig. 3). When the envelope is stripped off completely with detergents such as deoxycholate, the RNC structure remains (Fig. 4). The RNC has a buoyant density in CsCl of about 1.31 g/ml and contains only RNA and protein (Wagner *et al.*, 1969*b*; Kang and Prevec, 1969). When viewed by PTA negative-

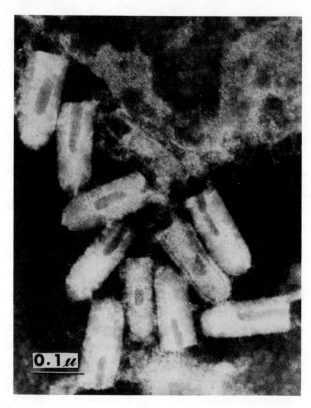

Fig. 1. Electron micrograph of unfixed L cells infected with VS virus and negatively-stained with phosphotungstic acid. Reprinted by permission from Printz and Wagner (1971).

staining electron microscopy, the RNC of infectious B virions appears as a partially or completely extended coil, about 3.5 μm in length. When the RNC is wound up in the virion envelope, it assumes a helical configuration of 35 ± 1 turns with a total of about 1000 subunits (undoubtedly protein) of dimensions $\sim 9 \times 3 \times 3$ nm; the long axis of the subunits appears to be oriented radially (Nakai and Howatson, 1968; Howatson, 1970). The intact RNC, completely devoid of envelope, is infectious, but at a considerably lower order of efficiency than the whole virion (Brown *et al.*, 1967*b*; Szilágyi and Uryvayev, 1973). The RNA without protein is not infectious (Huang and Wagner, 1966*b*).

The outer surface of the VS virion is composed of a lipoprotein membrane that surrounds and envelopes the nucleocapsid (Howatson, 1970; Nakai and Howatson, 1968; Cartwright *et al.*, 1972). Morphologically, the envelope comprises two distinct structural units. The more internal component is a membrane that has all the morphological

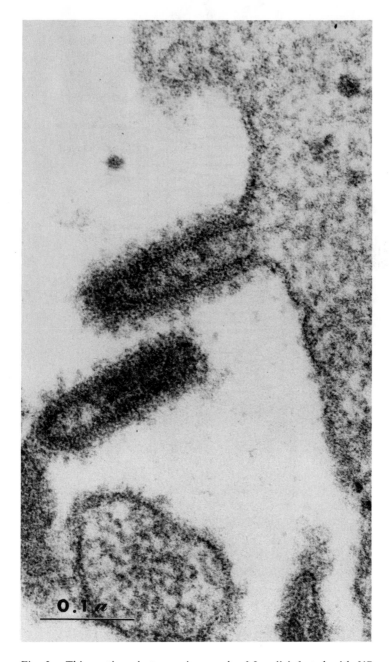

Fig. 2. Thin-section electron micrograph of L cell infected with VS virus, fixed with glutaraldehyde and OsO$_4$, and stained with uranyl acetate and lead.

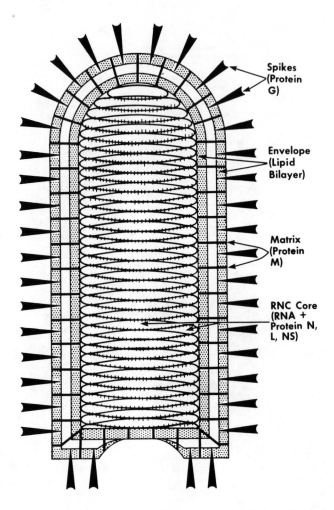

Fig. 3. Model of the idealized structure of VS virus showing
the ribonucleocapsid (RNC), the envelope, and the spikes with
their associated protein constituents.

characteristics of a unit membrane derived from plasma or other
smooth membranes of animal (or plant) cells (Knudson, 1973). Embed-
ded in the membranous envelope and surrounding the virion is an array
of radiating spikes which protrude from the surface and measure about
10 nm in length.

1.2.1b. Defective Truncated (T) Virions

The concept of defective rhabdovirus virions dates from the
observation of Cooper and Bellett (1959) of a transmissible (T)

component in VS viral preparations that interferes with VS viral infectivity. Hackett (1964) demonstrated a possible morphological basis
for this autointerference phenomenon which was subsequently proven
by definitive identification and purification of a truncated (T) particle
in undiluted-passage preparations of VS virus (Huang *et al.*, 1966;
Huang and Wagner, 1966*a*; Brown *et al.*, 1967*c*). When such preparations are examined by PTA negative-staining electron microscopy, the
predominant virions are about one-third the length (about 65 nm) of

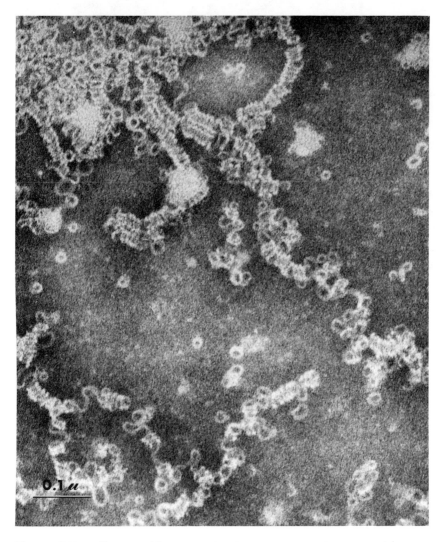

Fig. 4.   RNC coils released from VS virions by exposure to Triton X-100 in 0.74 M
NaCl and negatively stained with PTA. Reprinted by permission from Emerson
and Wagner, (1972).

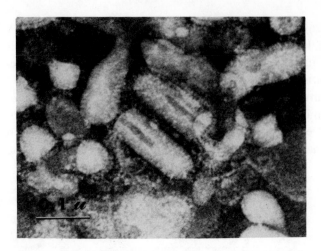

Fig. 5. Mixture of PTA negatively stained defective T and infective B virions obtained from cells infected under conditions of autointerference with undiluted passage of VS virus.

the infectious B virions (Fig. 5). In every other respect, the T virions are morphologically identical to the B virions. However, they contain RNA only one-third the length of infectious B-virion RNA (Huang and Wagner, 1966c), their extended RNC measures only 1.1 μm in length (Nakai and Howatson, 1968), and the intact T particle contains 8–10 cross-striations, as opposed to the 35 $\pm$ 1 in the infective virion.

T particles of varying lengths can also be found in different rhabdoviruses, suggesting that the truncated, defective form is a universal phenomenon for this group of viruses. Hackett (1964) described a longer T particle with 14 cross-striations in preparations of VS-New Jersey virus, and the HR (heat-resistant) variant of VS-Indiana virus gives rise to "long" T particles (Petric and Prevec, 1970), which contain a nucleocapsid strand 1.6 $\pm$ 0.2 μm in length, or almost half that of the B-virion nucleocapsid (Schincariol and Howatson, 1970). In addition, various temperature-sensitive (*ts*) mutants of VS-Indiana virus give rise, even at permissive temperatures, to a diversity of T particles of varying length, depending on the mutant (Reichmann *et al.*, 1971). Many of the data obtained by electron microscopy have been confirmed by the interesting new technique of laser light-scattering microscopy which has been used to determine the particle weights of VS virus and its defective particles (Ware *et al.*, 1973). The origin, chemistry and physiology of T particles will be discussed later.

1.3. Classification of Rhabdoviruses

No attempt will be made here to list or describe all the rhabdoviruses. A complete list of 62 known or suspected rhabdoviruses is provided in the comparative review by Knudson (1973). The rhabdoviruses are most conveniently and most realistically divided into two groups, those that infect animals and those that infect plants. Some additional help can be provided by using morphological criteria for classification, but quite obviously these will be superseded by physical and biochemical comparisons (Hummeler, 1971). The fact that most infectious animal rhabdoviruses are bullet-shaped and most plant rhabdoviruses are bacilliform may be of some help (Howatson, 1970). In my opinion the bacillary form of plant rhabdoviruses and the very long, aberrant forms of animal rhabdoviruses (Galasso, 1967; Hummeler *et al.*, 1967) are most likely artifacts or diploid bullets fused end-to-end.

1.3.1. Biological Properties

1.3.1a. Antigenicity

Cells infected with VS virus release into the medium four antigenic components that can be separated by rate zonal centrifugation into infective B virions, defective T virions, and two subviral constituents of 20 S and 6 S, each of which reacts with VS viral antiserum (Bradish *et al.*, 1956; Brown *et al.*, 1966; Brown and Cartwright, 1966). Kang and Prevec (1970) showed conclusively that the 20 S component is related antigenically to the major protein (now called N) of the RNC and that the 6 S component reacts specifically with viral envelope antibodies.

A quite valid approach and first approximation for relegating rhabdoviruses to subclasses is antigenic relatedness. Quite recent data have revealed the existence of two major specific antigens in those rhabdoviruses that have been studied. Each of these antigens can be readily separated from the other and each raises excellent, primarily monospecific, antibody in immunized animals. One of these antigens is the glycosylated (G) spike protein that protrudes from each rhabdovirus and can be readily solubilized in a pure state by nonionic detergents; the G protein gives rise to antibody which specifically neutralizes the infectivity of the VS virus or rabies virus from which it was obtained (Kelley *et al.*, 1972; Wiktor *et al.*, 1973). These G proteins

TABLE 1

Tentative Classification of Some Animal Rhabdoviruses[a]

Group	Members	Isolation	References
Vesicular stomatitis	VS-Indiana[b]	Horse	Federer et al. (1967)
	VS-Cocal[b]	Cattle	Cartwright and
	VS-Argentina[b]	Swine	Brown (1972b)
	VS-Brazil[b]	Insect	
	VS-New Jersey[c]		
Rabies and	Street and fixed	"Mammals"	Wiktor et al. (1973)
rabieslike	Lagos bat	Bat	Shope (1973)
	Mokola	Shrew	Shope et al. (1970)
	Kotonkan	Midge	Shope (1973)
	Obodhiang	Mosquito	Schneider et al. (1973)
"Amorphous"	Piry[d]	Opposum	Bergold and Munz (1970)
	Chandipura[d]	Human	Howatson (1970)
	Kern Canyon	Bat	Murphy and Fields (1967)
	bovine ephemeral	Cattle	Murphy et al. (1972)
	Flanders-Hart Park	Birds	Murphy et al. (1966)
	Mount Elgon bat	Bat	Murphy et al. (1970)
	Many others		Karabatsos et al. (1973)
"Fish"	Egtved	Trout	Zwillenberg et al. (1965)
	"Salmonid viruses" [e]	Salmon	Amend and Chambers (1970) Printz (1973)
"Ungrouped"	Sigma	Drosophila	Berkaloff et al. (1965)
	Marburg	Monkey-man	Almeida et al. (1971)

[a] General categories were suggested by R. E. Shope (1973, and personal communication). The list is far from complete: at least 27 distinguishable animal rhabdoviruses have been identified.
[b] Indiana serotype subgroup.
[c] Separate serotype.
[d] Piry and Chandipura viruses are not listed under the VSV group because Cartwright and Brown (1972b) failed to confirm even a minor antigenic cross-reaction with VS viruses.
[e] Includes hematopoetic necrosis of salmon, Oregon sockeye disease of salmon and Sacramento River Chinook disease of salmon.

react specifically with the same or closely related antisera and are designated type-specific antigens (Cartwright and Brown, 1972b). About 70% of the complement-fixing antibody produced by infection with VS virus reacts with the G-protein antigen; virtually all the remaining 30% of complement-fixing antibody reacts with the N protein of the RNC. Moreover, the RNC antibody made in response to one rhabdovirus may cross-react to varying degrees with the RNC antigen of a related rhabdovirus in the same group, but it will not neutralize the infectivity of the same fully enveloped rhabdovirus. By the same token, G-protein antibody will neutralize the infectivity of only the fully enveloped rhabdovirus but not of its infectious RNC (Cartwright and Brown, 1972b).

The type-specific G antigen should provide a useful tool for serotyping closely related rhabdoviruses, and the group-specific RNC antigen promises to provide a useful method for placing rhabdoviruses into larger groups. Dietzschold et al. (1974) have recently validated the antigenic specificity of the three major VS viral proteins; such pure protein antigens provide the basis for a tentative classification of animal rhabdoviruses attempted in Table 1.

1.3.1b. Hemagglutination

Rhabdoviruses also contain a hemagglutinin which appears to have activity only for goose erythrocytes (Halonen et al., 1968; Kuwert et al., 1968; Arstila et al., 1969). The hemagglutination reaction is extremely dependent on pH and ionic strength as well as the erythrocytes which vary from goose to goose. Tremendous amounts of virus are required to give even low titers, possibly because of the presence of inhibitors in all sera. In our experience (unpublished data) hemagglutination inhibition is of little value for comparing the antigenic relationships among rhabdoviruses.

1.3.1c. Interference

Crick and Brown (1973) have suggested a method for determining the relatedness of rhabdoviruses based on viral interference. As will be discussed later in greater detail, defective T particles produced by most, if not all, rhabdoviruses interfere with the growth of homologous infectious B virions (Huang and Wagner, 1966b). There are varying degrees of cross-interference by T virions of one rhabdovirus for B virions of another. The degree of this cross-interference appears to be a function of the antigenic relatedness of the two rhabdovirus types and, therefore, provides some basis, albeit a bit tedious, for confirming rhabdovirus classification based on group-specific and type-specific antigenicity. These relationships do not apply to the long T defective particle of the HR strain of VS virus, which gives rise to heterotypic interference (Prevec and Kang, 1970).

1.3.2. Animal Rhabdoviruses

At least 27 distinguishable animal rhabdoviruses have been
identified and the number will keep increasing at a rapid rate. A complete analysis of these viruses is outside the scope of this chapter, but a
general outline will indicate the magnitude of the problem. The classification shown in Table 1 is modified from one suggested by R. E.
Shope and is based primarily on information supplied by him and F.
A. Murphy. The responsibility for the interpretation is my own,
particularly in not paying much attention to morphological criteria for
subgrouping. The inevitable basis for accurate and meaningful classification is likely to be RNA homology, which should be a not-too-
distant reality. The base-sequence homology of antigenically related
and unrelated rhabdoviruses has been studied by Repik *et al.* (1974) by
hybridization of virion RNA with mRNA transcribed *in vitro* or *in
vivo*. They found 100% complementarity between each virion RNA
and its homologous messenger. However, less than 10% base-sequence
homology could be demonstrated between VS-Indiana virus and the
group-specific, antigenically related VS-New Jersey and the homotypic
VS-Cocal viruses as determined by resistance to RNases A and T_1.
Somewhat greater "inexact" homology among the RNAs of these
viruses could be demonstrated by resistance of hybridized RNA to
RNase A alone. Repik *et al.* (1974) interpret these data as indications
of evolution of the various antigenic types of VS viruses from a common ancestor. However, no RNA base-sequence homology could be
demonstrated between the VS viruses and the rhabdoviruses of rabies,
Piry, and Chandipura. Some degree of "genome" conservation has
been postulated by Chang *et al.* (1974) based on comparable 5′ nucleotide sequences for initiation of transcription in the genomes of five
different rhabdoviruses. Using *in vivo* and *in vitro* mRNA transcribed
from VS-Indiana virion RNA, Prevec (1974) also tested base-sequence
homology of antigenically related and unrelated rhabdoviruses. He
found as much as 14–23% resistance (above background) of VS-New
Jersey and Cocal RNA to pancreatic RNase after hybridization with
VS-Indiana mRNA, whereas no significant homology could be
demonstrated for Piry and Chandipura rhabdoviruses.

1.3.3. Rhabdoviruses of Plants

Rhabdoviruses are turning out to be extremely important
pathogens in plants. They have been isolated from a wide spectrum of

plant species; frequently, if not invariably, they are transmitted by insect vectors such as leafhoppers and aphids. Therefore, the vector–host relationships appear to be quite similar for animals and plants. This chapter is not the proper forum for dealing with rhabdovirus pathogenicity in plants; the reader is referred to the excellent reviews and summaries of Francki (1973) and Knudson (1973). However, it seems worthwhile to list some of the plant rhabdoviruses that have been implicated as the causative agents of disease in order to illustrate the enormous scope of the problem. Among these are the following viruses: maize mosaic virus, wheat striate mosaic virus, lettuce necrotic yellows virus, *Gomphrena* virus of globe amaranth, potato yellow dwarf virus, plaintain virus, sowthistle yellow vein virus, broccoli necrotic yellows virus, eggplant mottled dwarf virus, Northern cereal mosaic virus, rice transitory yellowing virus, and melitotis latent virus. Little research has been done on the antigenic relationships among the plant rhabdoviruses or between them and animal rhabdoviruses. However, Sylvester *et al.* (1968) could demonstrate no serologic cross-reactions between sowthistle yellow vein and VS viruses.

1.4. Some Genetic Considerations

Rhabdovirus genetics will be the subject of a detailed analysis in a later volume of this series. However, a brief description of strain variation and mutants of rhabdoviruses is essential for discussion of the many aspects of rhabdovirus reproduction. The search for mutants has been extensive, but it must be expanded further to provide probes in areas that have not yet yielded to available methods. This summary will be limited largely to the genetics of VS viruses simply because no other rhabdoviruses have been adequately studied to date.

1.4.1. VS-Indiana Virus Genetics

1.4.1a. Plaque Mutants

Wagner *et al.* (1963) were the first to describe a moderately stable, spontaneous mutant of VS virus that uniformly produced small plaques (*SP*) on chick embryo and mouse L cells. Compared to the wild-type (*wt*), large-plaque (*LP*) virus, the *SP* variant grew to considerably lower titer, particularly in L cells, caused less and delayed cytopathic effects, and tended to persist in continuous cell culture. The nature of the mutant lesion was never identified, but the *SP* mutant was more susceptible to the action of interferon than the *LP* form. Shechmeister *et al.* (1967) isolated a series of *SP* mutants induced by UV irradiation of VS-New Jersey virus. One of these mutants, *P-la*, plated with lower efficiency on HeLa cells than did the wild type and was less pathogenic for mice by intracerebral injection.

A similar small-plaque (S_2) mutant derived from L_1 VS-Indiana virus has been described in greater detail (Youngner and Wertz, 1968; Wertz and Youngner, 1970, 1972; Wertz and Levine, 1973). The S_2 mutant is 1000 times less lethal for mice, than L_1, despite the fact that S_2 and L_1 induced the formation of about the same amount of interferon. The yields of S_2 progeny virus were 97% lower in L cells and 85% lower in chick embryo cells than were yields of L_1 virus. The only consistent defect noted in cells infected with the S_2 mutant was considerable reduction in intracellular progeny 38 S RNA, suggesting that the S_2 lesion is located somewhere after transcription and before replication (Wertz and Levine, 1973).

1.4.1b. Temperature-Sensitive Mutants

Conditional, lethal, temperature-sensitive (*ts*) mutants of VS-Indiana virus have been extensively studied and characterized in three laboratories (Flamand, 1969, 1970; Pringle, 1970; Holloway *et al.*, 1970). Different wild-type (*wt, ts*$^+$) strains of VS virus were used in each laboratory, but a general agreement has been reached for classification of all these mutants. By convention, each mutant receives a number designation assigned by the laboratory in which it was isolated but prefixed by a letter to identify the city in which the laboratory is located. Therefore, all mutants (which are spontaneous) originating in Orsay are called *ts* O5, *ts* O100, etc.; those from Glasgow (most of which were induced by exposure to the mutagen 5-fluorouracil) are designated *ts* Gll, *ts* G44, etc.; and those mutants isolated in Winnipeg (which originated from a heat-resistant, HR, variant of VS virus) are called *ts* W16B, *ts* W10, etc. Different cell types have been used by each laboratory, but this does not seem to influence significantly the results of experiments done with the Orsay, Glasgow, and Winnipeg mutants. In addition, each laboratory has used permissive and restrictive temperatures that differ by about one degree. In this summary we shall consider the permissive temperature for relatively normal yield of mutant virus to be 31°C and the restrictive (nonpermissive) temperature to be 39°C. Excluded from consideration in this section are the host-range and temperature-sensitive VS-Indiana mutants of Simpson and Obijeski (1974), who described a series of amber-ochre mutants restricted in certain cell types, either independent of or dependent on temperature sensitivity at 35°C or 41°C. Another series of as yet unclassified *ts* mutants has been selected by Mudd *et al.* (1973) from persistently infected cell cultures of *Drosophila*, in which the virus acquires greater growth potential.

By means of reciprocal complementation crosses, Flamand and Pringle (1971) were able to assign 71 spontaneous Orsay *ts* mutants and 175 induced Glasgow *ts* mutants of VS-Indiana virus to 5 complementation groups. They are designated by Roman numerals as follows: I (209 mutants), II (19 mutants), III (6 mutants), IV (4 mutants), and V (2 mutants). The fact that 209 of the 246 randomly selected mutants are in complementation group I attests to the genetic instability and possibly also to the large size of the cistron represented by group I mutants. The Winnipeg *ts* mutants of the VS-Indiana HR strain, formerly designated groups A, B, and C, could be relegated to complementation groups I, III, and IV when tested in cross-complementation tests with prototype Glasgow and Orsay mutants (Cormack *et al.*, 1973). A small number of mutants from each laboratory could not be assigned definitely to any of the complementation groups, and these may be double mutants.

The reversion rate of VS-Indiana *ts* mutants is usually remarkably low; most of the mutants that have been studied carefully have a plating efficiency of $<10^{-8}$ at 39°C compared with that at 31°C and very few seem to have reversion frequencies $>10^{-5}$. Some of the mutants, in our experience, will produce numerous tiny plaques at the restrictive temperature of 39°C, presumably indicating a variable degree of leakiness. Suggestive evidence for genetic recombination of VS-Indiana mutants (Pringle, 1970) has subsequently been retracted (Pringle *et al.*, 1971) on the basis of evidence for complementation on the assay plate and invariable segregation of mutants on repeated cloning. Wong *et al.* (1971) also failed to detect recombination among three mutants of different complementation groups; they attributed increased plaque numbers at 38°C on plating a mixture of two complementing mutants to aggregates or heteroploid virions with two genomes.

At restrictive temperatures a variety of physiological defects have been attributed to VS-Indiana *ts* mutants. These will be discussed in greater detail under the appropriate heading for viral functions. Suffice it to say that attempts have been made, partly successfully, to divide *ts*

TABLE 2

**Temperature-Sensitive Mutants of VS Viruses: A Summary and
Comparison of the Genetics of Three Serotypes**

Complementation Groups			Phenotypes		
Indiana[a]	New Jersey[b]	Cocal[c]	RNA	Protein	T RNA[d]
I	A, B	α	−	L[e]	410 S, 280 S
II	E	δ	±	?G[f]	435 S
III	C	γ	+	?M[g]	150 S
IV	F	β	−	?N[h]	−
V	D	−	+	?G[i]	−

[a] Pringle (1970), Flamand and Pringle (1971).
[b] Pringle et al. (1971).
[c] Pringle and Wunner (1973).
[d] Reichmann et al. (1971). RNA of ts^+B = 610 S, RNA of ts^+T = 330 S.
[e] Hunt and Wagner (1974). VS-Indiana.
[f] Printz and Wagner (1971), Pringle and Wunner (1974).
[g] Lafay (1971), Printz and Wagner (1971).
[h] Combard et al. (1974).
[i] Deutsch and Berkaloff (1971), F. Lafay (1974).

mutants according to their altered capacity to synthesize RNA (Pringle
and Duncan, 1971; Wong et al., 1972), to synthesize or incorporate
several virion proteins (Printz and Wagner, 1971; Lafay, 1971), and to
produce defective virions (Reichmann et al., 1971). Classification of
VS virus mutants according to genetic complementation groups and
phenotypic expression of RNA synthesis, virion proteins, and defective
T RNA is summarized in Table 2.

1.4.2. Genetics of Other Rhabdoviruses

Pringle and his colleagues in Glasgow have been making a
systematic study of the genetics of many animal rhabdoviruses by inducing the formation of temperature-sensitive mutants with 5-
fluorouracil as a mutagen. Thus far, they have reported on the analysis
of 48 *ts* mutants of VS-New Jersey virus which can be divided into six
genetic complementation groups (Pringle et al., 1971), 49 *ts* mutants of
VS-Cocal virus which can be divided into four complementation
groups (Pringle and Wunner, 1973), and two complementing mutants
of the non-VS virus Chandipura rhabdovirus (Pringle and Wunner,

1973, 1974). Table 2 summarizes the complementation data and known phenotypes of three VS virus serotypes.

Of considerable interest is the report by Pringle *et al.* (1971) of absolutely no genetic overlap of VS-Indiana and VS-New Jersey viruses despite evidence of relatedness based on cross-reacting RNC group-specific antigens (Cartwright and Brown, 1972*b*) and a degree of cross-interference (Huang and Wagner, 1966*a*; Crick and Brown, 1973). None of the representative mutants of the 6 VS-New Jersey complementation groups were able to complement any of the representative mutants of the 5 VS-Indiana complementation groups. These convincing negative data require interpretation of the rather anomalous finding that VS-Indiana mRNA will hybridize with VS-New Jersey virion RNA to a moderate extent (Prevec, 1974) or to only a slight extent (Repik *et al.*, 1974). The genetic relatedness, if any, of VS-Indiana and VS-New Jersey viruses remains an unsolved question.

VS-Cocal virus is antigenically closely related to VS-Indiana virus by type-specific as well as group-specific antigens but shares only group-specific antigen with VS-New Jersey virus (Cartwright and Brown, 1972*b*). Therefore, one would anticipate a closer genetic relationship between VS-Cocal and VS-Indiana viruses than would be expected of either with the New Jersey serotype. Pringle and Wunner (1973) found no cross-complementation among any representatives of four complementation groups of VS-Cocal virus and the six complementation groups of VS-New Jersey virus. The data for cross-complementation of VS-Indiana and VS-Cocal mutants were not unambiguous but some degree of complementation was definitely evident when VS-Cocal mutants *ts* α1, *ts* β1 and *ts* δ1 were tested with VS-Indiana group III (*ts* G31) and group V (*ts* O45). The data suggest that VS-Indiana group III is analogous to VS-Cocal group γ.

Preliminary data indicated RNA phenotypes of the VS-Cocal mutants similar to those of VS-Indiana and VS-New Jersey. VS-Cocal groups α and β appear to be RNA$^-$ and presumably similar to VS-Indiana complementation groups I and IV. VS-Cocal group γ mutants synthesized greater than normal amounts of RNA at restrictive temperature, whereas one mutant of group δ was RNA$^-$ and another was RNA$^+$, not unlike the situation with VS-Indiana group II and VS-New Jersey group E (See Table 2).

Very preliminary data on two *ts* mutants of the Chandipura rhabdovirus indicate complete genetic unrelatedness to any of the VS viruses (Pringle and Wunner, 1974). Five mutagen-induced *ts* mutants of "fixed" rabies virus have been isolated by Clark and Koprowski

(1971). These mutants showed low reversion frequency and leakiness at the restrictive temperature of 40.5°C; two of them were characterized for thermolability and pathogenicity in mice.

2. STRUCTURAL COMPONENTS AND THEIR FUNCTIONS

2.1. Chemical Composition of Virions

VS-Indiana virus will serve as the prototype because it is, by far, the best studied and the easiest to study of all the rhabdoviruses. Many of the chemical characteristics of VS virus also apply to other rhabdoviruses; differences in chemical composition or structure of other rhabdoviruses will be noted, if known. Essential to any reliable chemical characterization is the homogeneity and purity of the virus stock. Rhabdoviruses such as rabies are difficult to purify but some success has been achieved by Sokol *et al.* (1968). McSharry and Wagner (1971*a*) have reported in detail methods for bulk production of VS virus and for purification of virions by precipitation with poly-ethylene glycol, DEAE-cellulose chromatography, rate zonal centrifugation in sucrose or tartrate gradients, and equilibrium centrifugation. Infective VS virions purified in this manner were found by chemical analysis to contain 3% RNA, 64% protein, 13% carbohydrate, and 20% lipid.

2.1.1. Virion RNA

2.1.1a. Infective VS Virions

The first evidence that VS virions contain single-stranded RNA as their genetic information was supplied by Prevec and Whitmore (1963), who analyzed alkaline and enzymatic digests chromatographically and found no effect on virus growth of 5-iodouridine-deoxyriboside. Huang and Wagner (1966*b*) extracted the RNA from infective VS B virions and estimated its molecular weight at $3.1–4.0 \times 10^6$ daltons based on a sedimentation coefficient of 42 S. Similar values, ranging from 38 S to 43 S, have been obtained subsequently by many investigators (Brown *et al.*, 1967*c*). Comparable values have also been obtained by poly-acrylamide gel electrophoresis; by this method the molecular weight of VS B-virion RNA was estimated to be 4.4×10^6 daltons at the upper extreme (Bishop and Roy, 1971*a*) and 3.2×10^6 daltons at the lower extreme (Kiley and Wagner, 1972). Schaffer and Soergel (1972) obtained an intermediate value of 4.0×10^6 daltons for B RNA of VS-Indiana strain L and VS-Cocal viruses, but values for B-virion RNA of VS-Indiana strain BT-78 and several strains of VS-New Jersey virus were estimated to be 4.5×10^6 daltons by electrophoresis on polyacrylamide gels. Repik and Bishop (1973) used a third, independent method to determine the molecular weight of RNA from VS B virions by specific base labeling, nuclease digestion, and computation of the minimum molecular weight from the number of oligonucleotides recovered from a mole of viral RNA; they came up with the value of $3.82 \pm 0.14 \times 10^6$ daltons for VS B-virion RNA. All these values are quite consistent with the measurements by Nakai and Howatson (1968) of 3.3–4.0 μm for the length of the B-virion nucleocapsid, which gives an equivalent molecular weight of $3.4–3.8 \times 10^6$ daltons for its RNA. It would seem that a reasonable average value for the VS B-virion RNA would be 3.6×10^6 daltons.

The molecular weight of VS B-virion RNA is not significantly altered by formaldehyde denaturation (Mudd and Summers, 1970b), by boiling (Kiley and Wagner, 1972), or in dimethyl sulfoxide gradients (Kiley and Wagner, unpublished results). These data indicate that VS B-virion RNA is single-stranded, without significant secondary structure or hydrogen-bonded regions. The base composition determined by Brown $et\ al.$ (1967c) of 29.3% A, 21.1% C, 20.9% G, and 28.7% U probably represents fortuitous base pairing. VS B-virion RNA is virtually devoid of complementary RNA, as shown by almost complete digestion by RNase even after attempted melting and reannealing (Bishop and Roy, 1971b). The RNAs of three strains of rabies virus were found to have nucleotide composition very similar to that of VS virus (Aaslestad and Urbano, 1971).

2.1.1b. Defective VS Virions

Huang and Wagner (1966b) originally estimated the molecular weight of purified VS T-virion RNA as $1.2–1.3 \times 10^6$ daltons, based on a sucrose gradient sedimentation coefficient of 23 S. Similar values for the molecular weight of short T-virion RNA have been reported by Brown $et\ al.$ (1967c) and Schaffer $et\ al.$ (1968). Bishop and Roy (1971a) and Kiley and Wagner (1972) came up with equivalent values for molecular weight determined by polyacrylamide gel electrophoresis. A careful study by Schaffer and Soergel (1972) showed comparative molecular weight values of 1.0×10^6, 0.7×10^6, and 1.2

$\times$ 10^6 daltons for RNAs of T virions of VS-Indiana (L strain), VS-Cocal, and VS-New Jersey (Ogden strain) viruses, respectively. The inability of T particles to replicate in the absence of B particles and their similarity in other respects led to an hypothesis, perhaps a bit prematurely, that T RNA was a fragment which was one-third of the infective B-virion RNA (Huang et al., 1966). Some evidence to support this hypothesis was lent by the finding of Nakai and Howatson (1968) that T RNA was present in truncated virions and nucleocapsids of approximately 1.1 μm in length, or roughly one-third the length of the B nucleocapsid. They also counted 310 protein subunits on the T nucleocapsid, compared with about 1000 on the B nucleocapsid.

Some doubt was cast on the postulated origin of T-virion RNA by the finding of Petric and Prevec (1970) that Howatson's HR variant of VS virus gives rise on undiluted passage to a defective virion, estimated to contain RNA of molecular weight 1.7–2.0 $\times$ 10^6 daltons. This HR defective virion was called long T (LT) and was thought to contain about half of the B genome. Moreover, Reichmann et al. (1971) found that infection of BHK cells with ts mutants of VS virus gave rise to defective T particles of widely varying lengths, including species which were much smaller than the now classical short T and long T virions. It is possible, therefore, that segmentation of the VS genome can be random or that the site of cleavage is genetically controlled.

Roy and Bishop (1972) showed quite conclusively that RNA from a standard preparation of short T particles is identical to one or more segments of B-virion RNA. This close relatedness of T and B RNA was demonstrated by showing complete hybridization to both T- and B-virion RNA by mRNA made in vitro on a B-virion template (see Sect. 2.2.1). Conclusive analysis is prevented by inability to transcribe short T virions in vitro (Bishop and Roy, 1971a; Emerson and Wagner, 1972) or in vivo (Huang and Manders, 1972) in order to obtain specific hybridizable mRNA. Another technical stumbling block to resolving the question of the origin of T RNA is inability to produce T RNA with enough radioactivity to analyze the 5′ and 3′ termini (Bishop, personal communication).

Further complicating a definitive attempt to determine the origin of T RNA is the finding by Roy et al. (1973) of considerable RNase-resistant RNA present in long T virions derived from the HR VS virus strain of Howatson. These studies reveal that 20% of the HR T RNA is RNase resistant aftr melting and self-annealing. Moreover, only 80% of HR T RNA, compared to 100% of the standard short T or B RNA, hybridizes to mRNA made *in vitro* on a standard wild-type B-virion template.

Despite all these obstacles, very recent data by Leamnson and Reichmann (1974) reveal by hybridization studies that the RNA from defective long T particles of the HR strain is complementary to all the VS viral 13–18 S mRNA species. In contrast, all RNA in short T virions of various strains contain exclusively or predominantly nucleotide sequences homologous to 28 S mRNA. Based on these data, models were proposed for the origin of T particles and for a cistronic map of the VS virion genome.

2.1.1c. Virion RNA of Other Rhabdoviruses

The relatedness of the rhabdoviruses is emphasized by the similarity of their RNA genomes, at least to the extent that they have been investigated. However, there are some potential differences that are worth noting. Early studies by Sokol *et al.* (1969) revealed a somewhat larger genome size for rabies virus, as judged by a sedimentation coefficient of 45 S for the RNA and a modal length of 4.2 μm of the extended nucleocapsid. Bishop *et al.* (1974), however, have reported virtually identical migration on polyacrylamide gels of the RNAs extracted from infectious virions of VS virus, rabies virus, and Kern Canyon virus. Crick and Brown (1974) arrived at figures of 43 S for infective-rabies-virion RNA and 18–20 S for defective-rabies-virion RNA; incidentally, the defective rabies T virions interfered with the growth of infectious rabies virus but defective VS T virions did not. RNA from a standard VS-New Jersey virion contained 41 S RNA of molecular weight $\simeq 4.5 \times 10^6$ daltons on polyacrylamide, about the same as VS-Indiana virions, but a mutant (*p-laH60*) New Jersey-serotype virion was found to contain 51 S RNA with a molecular weight estimated by gel electrophoresis as 6.3×10^6 daltons (Schaffer *et al.*, 1972). These are the highest values reported for any rhabdovirus RNA; confirmation of these data has not been forthcoming.

The virion RNA species of plant rhabdoviruses have only been studied in a preliminary way but they reveal considerable similarity to the virion RNAs of animal rhabdoviruses (Knudson, 1973). A preliminary report of Knudson and MacLeod (1972) states that the RNA of potato yellow dwarf virus (PYDV) has an $s_{20,w} \simeq 45.3$ S, equivalent to a molecular weight of 4.7×10^6 daltons (Reeder *et al.*, 1972). Francki and Randles (1974) made the very interesting

TABLE 3

Comparison of Rhabdovirion RNA and Protein Species

Virus	Mol. wt. B RNA, $\times 10^6$ daltons	Mol. wt. proteins, $\times 10^3$ daltons					Protein references
		L	G	N	NS	M	
VS-Indiana	3.6	190	69	50	45	29	Wagner et al. (1972)
		—	62	45	38	28	Wunner and Pringle (1972a)
		160	65	54	42	27	Obijeski et al. (1974)
VS-New Jersey	4.5	—	62	47	39	26	Wunner and Pringle (1971)
		161	64	52	42	24	Obijeski et al. (1974)[b]
VS-Cocal		—	64	45	38	26	Wunner and Pringle (1971)
Chandipura		162	68	53	—	24	Obijeski et al. (1974)[b]
Piry		160	75	54	—	23	Obijeski et al. (1974)[b]
Rabies	4.6	—	69[c]	60	45	29[c]	Sokol et al. (1971) Neurath et al. (1972)
LNYV[a]	4.0	>100	75	55	—	22	Francki and Randles (1974)
PYDV[a]	4.6	—	78	56	45	33	Knudson and MacLeod (1972)

[a] LNYV = lettuce necrotic yellows virus; PYDV = potato yellow dwarf virus.
[b] Average data of Obijeski et al. are only for continuous, not discontinuous gels.
[c] Estimates for rabies proteins G_1 and M_1. $G_2 = 60 \times 10^3$, $M_2 = 24 \times 10^3$.

observation that lettuce necrotic yellows (LNYV) rhabdovirus contains 43 S RNA, equivalent in molecular weight to 4×10^6 daltons. Since LNYV is about twice the length of animal rhabdoviruses and is bacilliform in shape with two hemispheric ends, it does not seem unlikely that each infectious LNYV unit consists of back-to-back bullets filled with two copies of the LNYV genome. Also of great interest, as noted below, is that the LNYV virion contains an RNA transcriptase and four proteins very similar in molecular weight to those of VS virus. The striking similarity in the base composition of the virion RNAs of VS-Indiana virus, rabies virus, and PYDV cited by Knudson (1973) is difficult to rationalize as being anything but fortuitous.

Table 3 presents a comparison of the virion RNA and protein species found in 8 different rhabdoviruses.

2.1.2. Virion Proteins

2.1.2a. VS-Indiana Virus Structural Proteins

Wagner et al. (1969a) and Kang and Prevec (1969) simultaneously first identified the three major structural proteins of the Indiana

serotype of VS virus by electrophoresis on neutral polyacrylamide gels
in the presence of sodium dodecyl sulfate (SDS), 2-mercaptoethanol,
and urea. All investigators missed a minor structural protein until it
was identified on gels with higher resolving power (Mudd and Summers, 1970a). In 1972, all investigators in this field agreed that five VS
virion proteins could be definitely identified and a standard nomenclature was adopted for VS virus and, with some modifications, for all
rhabdoviruses (Wagner et al., 1972). Other minor components, such as
the a and b proteins of Bishop and Roy (1972) and the NS_2 protein of
Wagner et al. (1971) have never been confirmed and are probably artifacts of the gel procedures. The five agreed-upon VS virion proteins
have an aggregate molecular weight of 383,000; this accounts for almost all the coding potential of the VS viral genome, estimated at 3.6
$\times 10^6$ daltons. It also seems likely that each of these five polypeptides
is translated individually from a single monocistronic messenger RNA
(see Sect. 3.2). No one has conclusively demonstrated post-translational
cleavage of VS viral proteins.

In their original studies, Wagner et al. (1969a) demonstrated quite
conclusively by coelectrophoresis that defective T particles have exactly
the same five proteins as fully infective B virions of VS virus. Identical
results with the B- and T-virion proteins of Chandipura and Piry
viruses were also obtained by Obijeski et al. (1974).

Figure 6 shows a representative electrophoretic pattern of ^{3}H-la-
beled proteins extracted with SDS and mercaptoethanol from purified
VS virions. This pattern on standard Maizel SDS gels is somewhat different from that obtained on Laemmli-Maizel supergels, which result
particularly in the relatively slower migration of the NS protein. The
proteins illustrated in the electropherogram are lettered L, G, N, NS,
and M, according to the convention adopted for nomenclature of these
individual virion polypeptides (Wagner et al., 1972). Listed below are
the salient features, as well as the rationale behind the designation, of

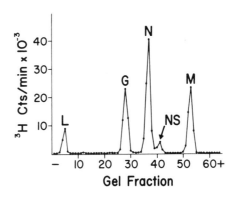

Fig. 6. Polyacrylamide gel electropherogram of VS virion proteins labeled
with ^{3}H-amino acids and extracted with
SDS and 2-mercaptoethanol. The letters
designate each of the 5 viral proteins.
Courtesy of R. L. Imblum.

each of the five proteins in decreasing order of molecular weights. Comparative data for the proteins and RNA of VS virus and seven other rhabdoviruses are shown in Table 3.

L protein. This was originally thought to be an aggregate or *large* uncleaved precursor of the other VS virion proteins. Recent evidence obtained by comparative analysis of tryptic peptides (Stampfer and Baltimore, 1973) and of cyanogen bromide peptides (Emerson and Wagner, 1973) reveals that the L protein shows peptide maps different from at least three of the other VS virion polypeptides. As noted below, the L protein has been found to be associated with VS viral nucleocapsid where it serves as the endogenous RNA-dependent RNA polymerase (Emerson and Wagner, 1973).

G protein. This protein is so designated because of ample evidence that it is the only identifiable VS virion protein which is glycosylated (Burge and Huang, 1970; Wagner *et al.*, 1970; Mudd and Summers, 1970*a*; Cohen *et al.*, 1971). Among all the VS viral proteins, there is somewhat less assurance that the G protein is a single polypeptide because it gives a less discrete band on neutral polyacrylamide gels. Another possible explanation for diffuse or notched peaks on gels might be attributable to lack of uniform glycosylation of the G protein.

N protein. N stands for nucleocapsid because the evidence is clear that this major component is the structural protein that is tightly complexed with virion RNA to form the RNC (Kang and Prevec, 1969; Wagner *et al.*, 1969*b*).

NS protein. This designation is the least satisfactory of those proposed for the VS viral proteins and will undoubtedly be superseded when more information becomes available concerning the function of this nucleocapsid protein. The original term NS_1 stood for non-structural protein number 1 because large amounts of this protein were found to be synthesized in VS virus-infected cells despite failure originally to detect it in released purified virions (Wagner *et al.*, 1970; Kang and Prevec, 1971). Mudd and Summers (1970*a*) identified on higher-resolution acrylamide gels a minor VS virion protein, now designated NS, which migrates to the same position as cytoplasmic NS_1 and slightly ahead of protein N (see Fig. 6). The relatedness of the soluble and structural NS proteins is suggested by the fact that they are both phosphoproteins (Sokol and Clark, 1973; Imblum and Wagner, 1974; Moyer and Summers, 1974*a*).

M protein. This protein is an integral nonglycosylated component of the VS viral membrane (Wagner *et al.*, 1970; Cohen *et al.*, 1971). Its designation also derives from the the fact that the M protein appears to serve as the matrix in close association with lipids to form the basic lipoprotein envelope.

2.1.2b.   Structural Proteins of Rhabdoviruses Other Than VS-Indiana Virus

The virion proteins of all rhabdoviruses studied to date are remarkably similar in number and molecular weight to those of VS-Indiana virus (Wagner *et al.*, 1972). In their original study of the VS virion proteins, Wagner *et al.* (1969*a*) could distinguish a difference in electrophoretic mobility of only one structural protein (M) of VS-New Jersey virions compared with the proteins of VS-Indiana virions. These data have been confirmed and additional minor differences in migration have been reported among corresponding proteins of various rhabdoviruses coelectrophoresed on high-resolution acrylamide gels (Wunner and Pringle, 1972*a*; Obijeski *et al.*, 1974). Table 3 lists the comparative molecular weights of similar polypeptides of widely different rhabdoviruses. A universal trait of all rhabdoviruses appears to be possession of L, G, N, and M proteins. The NS protein has not yet been identified in all rhabdoviruses due, almost undoubtedly, to the technical difficulty of detecting this minor component. The rabies virion has been reported to possess two additional minor components, an extra G protein (G_2) and an extra M protein (M_2) of lower molecular weight than the common G and M proteins (Sokol *et al.*, 1971). Two M proteins have also been identified in fish rhabdoviruses (de Kinkelin, personal communication; McAllister and Wagner, unpublished data).

2.1.3.   Lipids and Glycolipids

Prevec and Whitmore (1963) first reported a high content of phospholipid in VS virus, which was also found to be chloroform sensitive. McSharry and Wagner (1971*a*) reported a detailed analysis of the lipid composition of the Indiana and New Jersey serotypes of VS virus. Virions grown in L cells and purified 150-fold contained about 20% lipid; the molar ratio of cholesterol to phospholipid was 0.6 or greater. There were no unusual neutral lipids or fatty acids as determined by thin-layer and gas–liquid chromatography. The New Jersey serotype grown in L cells revealed the same lipid profile as did the Indian serotype, except for a somewhat greater proportion of neutral lipids, a finding which was less pronounced when VS-New Jersey virus was grown in primary chick embryo cells. The lipid composition of both viruses grown in L or chick embryo cells resembled more closely the lipid composition of the plasma membrane than of whole cells. The only consistent difference in virion lipids was the greater concentration of phosphatidylethanolamine and sphingomyelin and the relatively small amount of phosphatidylcholine in both types of VS virions compared with uninfected L and chick embryo cells or their plasma membranes.

Bates and Rothblat (1972) studied the incorporation of sterols into VS virus grown in L cells. Since L cells cannot synthesize cholesterol but can synthesize the precursor desmosterol (cholest-5,24-diene-3β-ol), VS virus grown in L cells in the absence of cholesterol will incorporate only desmosterol. When cholesterol is present in the medium, the virus will incorporate cholesterol in preference to the desmosterol, whose synthesis is inhibited in the presence of cholesterol. The sterol composition of VS virus does not influence its stability or infectivity.

Purified VS virions also contain glycolipids which can be readily detected by incorporation of radioactive glucosamine, galactosamine, and galactose during viral growth (McSharry and Wagner, 1971b). These small glycolipid molecules migrate very rapidly, almost with the marker dye front, on SDS-polyacrylamide gels. In the one cell system examined, Klenk and Choppin (1971) found that VS virions grown in BHK-F cells contained the same ganglioside, hematoside, neuraminosyl-galactosyl-glucosyl-ceramide, as did the plasma membrane of the host cell. Cartwright and Brown (1972a) also reported that cellular antigenic components are incorporated into budding VS virions and these cellular antigens migrate on polyacrylamide gels as do glycolipids.

The lipid composition of rabies rhabdovirus appears to be quite similar to that of VS virus (Blough and Tiffany, 1973; Schlesinger et al., 1973). Rabies virus grown in BHK21 cells contains 24% lipid, has a cholesterol-to-phospholipid molar ratio of 0.87, and the major phospholipid, as in the case of VS virus, is phosphotidylethanolamine. No significant differences could be found in the lipid composition of intracellular and extracellular rabies virus (Schlesinger et al., 1973), a finding which suggests no difference in the membrane maturation site of the two kinds of rabies virions. The presence of 1.5% sphingoglycolipids in rabies virus (Blough and Tiffany, 1973) also suggests some similarity to VS virus. Potato yellow dwarf virus contains 19% lipid, but the plant rhabdoviruses have not yet been thoroughly analyzed (Ahmed et al., 1964).

These data are quite scanty but they indicate that preformed lipids and glycolipids of the host cell are incorporated into the envelope of rhabdoviruses during their maturation and budding from the cell membrane. Some of the cellular phospholipids may be preferentially selected for complexing with VS virion envelope protein to form a more stable lipoprotein complex.

2.2. Structure–Function Relationships of Virion Components

2.2.1. The Nucleocapsid: Transcription

2.2.1a. Composition

The basic structure of the VS virus nucleocapsid is a single molecule of RNA associated with at least three viral proteins: N, L, and NS. Bishop and Roy (1972) have estimated that the VS nucleocapsid contains 60 molecules of L protein, 230 molecules of NS protein, and 2300 molecules of structural protein N, equivalent to 1 N-protein molecule per 6 nucleotides. Cartwright *et al.* (1972) estimate that the VS nucleocapsid has 1100 N-protein units. Additional studies revealed that N protein forms an extremely stable complex with virion RNA, whereas nucleocapsid proteins L and NS are more readily dissociable and are presumably more superficial or are complexed by more labile bonds. Experiments by Kiley and Wagner (1972) revealed that cytoplasm of infected cells contains VS viral nucleocapsids of varying length but that each contains RNA as well as proteins N, L, and NS, but the presence of 0.5 M NaCl stripped off all detectable L and NS proteins and left the RNA–N-protein complex intact. Similar studies with nucleocapsids isolated from VS virions were reported by Emerson and Wagner (1972) and by Szilágyi and Uryvayev (1974), who found that CsCl also removes L and NS proteins. Of considerable interest is the finding that the intact nucleocapsid, containing all three of its proteins, is infectious in the presence of DEAE-dextran, whereas the RNA–N-protein complex devoid of proteins L and NS is not infectious (Szylágyi and Uryvayev, 1973).

2.2.1b. The Transcriptase

The discovery by Baltimore, Huang, and Stampfer (1970) that VS virions contain an RNA-dependent RNA polymerase (transcriptase) opened up many avenues of investigation. The basic hypothesis that led Baltimore and Huang to do their original experiment was the finding some years previously (Huang and Wagner, 1966*b*) that the VS viral RNA devoid of protein was not infectious. In addition, the messenger

RNA made in infected cells was found to be complementary to virion RNA (Huang *et al.*, 1970); therefore, it was essential that the "negative-strand" RNA of VS virus be transcribed before translation could occur (Baltimore, 1971). An analysis of the kinetics and products of transcription will be presented in Sect. 3.2

Identification of the transcriptase protein was thwarted for some time because of lability of the transcription complex to temperature elevation and shear forces. Another obvious problem is that the specific enzyme as well as the template are both essential for transcription to occur; no other templates or enzymes have yet been found as substitutes. Emerson and Wagner (1972) finally solved the problem by proving that the transcriptase and template of VS virions could be separated by exposure to a high ionic environment into a supernatant fraction and a pellet fraction of nucleocapsid cores, neither of which contains much transcriptive activity. As shown in Fig. 7, when the pellet and supernatant fractions are recombined, most of the transcriptase activity is restored as evidenced by incorporation of ^{3}H-UTP into an acid-insoluble fraction complementary to VS virion RNA. The assumption can be made that the pellet, which contains nucleocapsid RNA and N protein, is the template and that the salt-released supernatant fraction contains the enzyme. Partial degradation of VS virions with Triton X-100 and lower salt concentrations results in virtually complete removal of envelope proteins G and M without significant reduction of transcriptase activity of the resulting nucleocapsid template (Emerson and Wagner, 1972; Bishop and Roy,

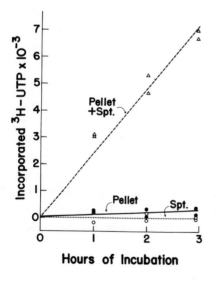

Fig. 7. Polymerase activity of supernatant fraction (Spt.), pellet, and reconstituted supernatant fraction plus pellet of VS virions fractionated by exposure to Triton X-100 and 0.74 M NaCl. The components were separated by centrifugation at 125,000 g and then adjusted in incorporation buffer with nucleoside triphosphates. Reprinted with permission from Emerson and Wagner (1972).

1972). Very recently, Szilágyi and Uryvayev (1974) reported that controlled degradation of VS nucleocapsids indicated that transcriptase activity is associated with L or L and NS proteins.

Even more recently, the reconstitution experiments of Emerson and Wagner were confirmed by Bishop *et al.* (1974*b*), who were also able to reconstitute the transcriptase activity and infectivity of dissociated VS-Indiana, VS-New Jersey, VS-Cocal, and Chandipura virions by recombining homologous enzyme and template. Cross-complementation of both transcriptase activity and infectivity could be demonstrated between VS-Indiana and VS-Cocal viruses, but VS-New Jersey and Chandipura soluble enzymes were unable to restore transcriptive function or infectivity to VS-Indiana nucleocapsid template. These experiments again emphasize the relatedness of the Indiana and Cocal serotypes and their unrelatedness or distant relatedness to VS-New Jersey or the antigenically distinct Chandipura viruses.

Having narrowed the candidates for transcriptase activity down to the nucleocapsid proteins L and NS or, of course, a hitherto unidentified protein, experiments were designed to isolate and identify the transcriptase protein or proteins by glycerol gradient centrifugation and phosphocellulose chromatography (Emerson and Wagner, 1973). Only the L protein is capable of restoring transcriptive function to the denuded nucleocapsid template. Soluble L protein rebinds to the ribonucleocapsid when the transcription complex is reconstituted; the RNA synthesized *in vitro* by the L-protein–nucleocapsid complex hybridizes to virion RNA. From these studies it was concluded that the L protein functions as the transcriptase. Recent, more definitive studies prove that the NS protein is also required in conjunction with the L protein to restore full transcriptive activity to the denuded nucleocapsid of VS virus (S.U. Emerson, in press). A hypothesis that the NS protein could also be the replicase is purely speculative and almost entirely based on the negative evidence that none of the other four viral proteins is a likely candidate, except possibly if the L protein turns out to have a dual function. Of some possible functional significance is the fact that the NS protein is the principal VS viral protein phosphorylated *in vitro* and *in vivo* (Sokol and Clark, 1973; Moyer and Summers, 1974*a*; Imblum and Wagner, 1974).

RNA-dependent RNA polymerase activity has been found associated with virions of rhabdoviruses other than VS-Indiana virus. The New Jersey serotype of VS virus also contains a transcriptase in infectious B virions but not in defective T particles (Perrault and Holland, 1972*b*). The antigenically unrelated Kern Canyon rhabdovirus possesses a transcriptase which exhibits all the requirements for *in vitro* activity of the VS-Indiana virus transcriptase, but the specific activity is only 4% that of the VS viral transcriptase (Aaslestad *et al.*, 1971). A transcriptase in the plant rhabdovirus LNYV also appears to have properties similar to those of the VS virus enzyme despite its much lower activity (Francki and Randles, 1972). The LNYV *in vitro* transcription products are all small (3–12 S), single-stranded RNA species homologous to the RNA of the LNYV genome, which is conserved intact during transcription (Francki and Randles, 1973). The nucleocapsid of LNYV is also infectious (Randles and Francki, 1972). These data on rhabdoviruses of widely different sources indicate the likelihood that all rhabdoviruses contain an RNA-dependent RNA polymerase as part of the nucleocapsid. Low specific activity would seem to be responsible for failure to demonstrate transcriptase activity in otherwise fairly classical rhabdoviruses, such as rabies virus.

Chang *et al.* (1974) compared the specific activities of the virion polymerases of five rhabdoviruses. They found that the transcriptase of VS-Indiana virions is 92% more active than the transcriptases of VS-New Jersey and Piry viruses, 87% more active than Chandipura virus and 66% more active than VS-Cocal virus. The polymerases of all five rhabdoviruses efficiently transcribe almost the entire genome as judged by hybridization to homologous virion template RNA. Bukrinskaya (1973) has recently provided an interesting comparative review of the nucleocapsids and transcriptases of rhabdovirus, reovirus, myxovirus, paramyxovirus, and RNA tumor virus.

2.2.1c.   The Transcription Template

It seems quite clear that the transcriptase of VS virus specifically recognizes its own nucleocapsid. In their original studies, Baltimore *et al.* (1970) were unable to detect RNA synthesized on various naked RNA templates added to the VS viral transcription system. Moreover, naked VS viral RNA cannot act as a transcription template. The minimal requirement for template activity is the presence of N protein as the major constituent of an intact nucleocapsid (Emerson and Wagner, 1972, 1973). Although the N protein alone possesses no capacity to serve as transcriptase, it does presumably act as a cofactor for transcription catalyzed by the L protein.

However, Emerson and Wagner (1972) have shown that not all RNA–N-protein complexes can serve as a functional template for the transcriptase. A number of laboratories have reported that the short T particles of VS virus exhibit no capacity to transcribe *in vitro* (Bishop and Roy, 1971a; Perrault and Holland, 1972; Emerson and Wagner, 1972) or *in vivo* (Huang and Manders, 1972) despite seemingly contradictory evidence of Mori and Howatson (1973) that short T and medium T as well as long T defective VS virions derived from the HR strain all synthesize RNA *in vitro*. Bishop and Roy (1971b) have found that long T particles contain about 30% of the transcriptase activity of the infective B virion. This transcriptional defectiveness of noninfectious T particles is evident despite the fact that T particles contain exactly the same proteins as homologous, infectious B particles (Wagner *et al.*, 1969a). A partial solution of this dilemma came from the experiments of Emerson and Wagner (1972), who found that short T particles contain a perfectly good, solubilizable transcriptase which functions when it is recombined with the denuded nucleocapsid template of B virions but not with that of T virions. Conversely, active B-virion transcriptase is completely ineffective when recombined with the nucleocapsid of T virions. It seems clear, therefore, that the transcriptional defect of short T virions derived from standard VS virus resides in its incomplete nucleocapsid template. Since the T nucleocapsid contains RNA (a one-third piece) and N protein, the most cogent alternative hypothesis to explain the transcriptional defectiveness of the T nucleocapsid is absence of appropriate nucleotide signals for initiation of transcription. By extension of this hypothesis, it can be intimated that the RNA of defective long T virions is derived from the opposite segment of the VS viral genome, which contains initiation signals for transcription (Prevec and Kang, 1970; Bishop and Roy, 1971b).

It is a rather remarkable fact that the RNA wrapped up by N protein in the VS nucleocapsid can be transcribed and at the same time is ribonuclease resistant (Cartwright *et al.*, 1970a). Bishop and Roy (1972) tried to resolve this paradox in an interesting series of experiments. First, they found that none of the N protein was dissociated from the nucleocapsid complex during active transcription. If the N protein was partially displaced and replaced, they reasoned, the template RNA should become at least partially ribonuclease sensitive. The template RNA did not become sensitive to RNase A and T_1; in fact, even after deproteinization with phenol, much of the template RNA remained RNase resistant before annealing and all of it after annealing. These data suggest a significant degree of base-paired, template-product, double-stranded RNA during the process of transcription despite the presence of N protein tightly bound to the RNA template. No N protein is found associated with released product RNA. A rolling model of N-protein displacement and replacement as the polymerase moves down the nucleocapsid template during transcription has been entertained by Bishop (personal communication). This model seems logical but the hypothesis may be difficult to test. The origin and role of the recently described homotypic inhibitors of polymerase activity in VS-Indiana and VS-New Jersey virions (Perrault and Kingsbury, 1974) are difficult to fathom.

2.2.1d.   Transcription Mutants

There are two definite genetic complementation groups of VS-Indiana virus mutants (group I and group IV) which exhibit reduced capacity to synthesize viral RNA *in vivo* at the restrictive temperature of 39°C (Pringle and Duncan, 1971; Printz-Ané *et al.*, 1972). The difficulty with exploiting these *ts* mutants is the intrinsic problem that *in vitro* transcription of VS virions is so heat labile that much less RNA is synthesized by wild-type (*wt*) virus at 39°C than at 28–31°C. Despite the fact that the reduction in yield of *wt* RNA transcribed at 39°C is as much as 90%, Szilágyi and Pringle (1972) have shown quite conclusively that six *ts* mutants belonging to VS viral complementation group I synthesize less RNA at 39°C than does the *wt* virus. Three of these group I mutants (*ts* G13, *ts* G16 and *ts* G114) show greater restriction and have a much more heat-labile polymerase activity than three other group I mutants (*ts* G11, *ts* G12, and *ts* G15). Similar studies done with the Winnepeg *ts* mutants derived from the HR variant of VS virus revealed some degree of temperature-sensitive transcription among mutants subsequently designated as belonging to complementation groups I and IV (Cormack *et al.*, 1971; Cairns *et al.*, 1972). These studies, in which kinetics are not always linear, differ from those of Szilágyi and Pringle (1972), who failed to confirm the temperature sensitivity of the *in vitro* transcription of their mutants in group IV. In addition, Cairns *et al.* (1972) have provided some evidence for *in vitro* phenotypic complementation of transcription activity among *in vivo* genetically complementing pairs of their RNA mutants. Similar *in vitro* complementation among *ts* mutants has been found by Bishop (personal communication); these experiments showed cross-complementation at both 31°C and 39°C of *ts* virions fractionated in the two-phase system of dextran–polyethylene glycol.

The most conclusive evidence for the location of the restrictive lesion in group I *ts* mutants was provided by Hunt and Wagner (1974). Our studies confirmed the observation of Szilágyi and Pringle (1972) that different group I mutants varied in their temperature sensitivity to *in vitro* transcription at 39°C, but in each case the transcriptase enzyme and the nucleocapsid template could be fractionated and reconstituted by the method of Emerson and Wagner (1972). Homologous reconstitution of enzyme and template resulted in restored capacity to transcribe at 31°C and 39°C, similar to the unfractionated mutant virion. Recombination of *wt* nucleocapsid template and *ts* group I transcriptase enzyme resulted in no significant restoration of capacity to synthesize RNA at restrictive temperature. In contrast, transcriptive function at 39°C was reconstituted by recombining the *wt* enzyme with the template component of group I *ts* mutants. These data indicate that the transcriptase enzyme, rather than the template, is the temperature-sensitive component of group I VS virus mutants. Very recent data indicate that L protein, not NS protein, is the temperature-sensitive component of group I VS virus mutants *ts* G13 and *ts* G16 (data of D. M. Hunt). Moreover, Ngan *et al.* (1974) have very recently found that at least one group IV mutant, *ts* W16B, is restricted in transcription because of a temperature-sensitive nucleocapsid template.

2.2.1e.   Polyadenylate Synthetase

Infection of cells with VS virus gives rise to cytoplasmic mRNA species which contain tracts of polyadenylic acid (poly A) despite the absence of significant stretches of polyuridylate in VS virion RNA (Ehrenfeld and Summers, 1972; Galet and Prevec, 1973; Soria and Huang, 1973). This finding prompted Villareal and Holland (1973) and Banerjee and Rhodes (1973) to search for and to find an enzyme in VS virions that sequentially adds adenylate sequences, presumably at the 3′ end, to complementary RNA synthesized *in vitro*. Adenylation could be carried out by isolated nucleocapsid cores of VS virus and the functional enzyme was, therefore, presumed to be one of the three nucleocapsid proteins. Further evidence that the poly A synthetase is a viral protein, possibly the transcriptase, was provided by finding that poly A synthesis requires the presence of all four nucleoside triphosphates. Galet and Prevec (1973) found similar evidence for poly A synthesis coupled to *in vitro* transcription by cytoplasmic fractions of cells infected with VS virus. These experiments were confirmed by Banerjee and Rhodes (1973) and by Ehrenfeld (1974) who found poly A tracts in complementary RNA transcribed by VS virions *in vitro*. These poly A sequences range in length from 50 to 200 nucleotides and are demonstrated by resistance to RNase A and T_1, as well as by binding to poly U. The poly A sequences are covalently linked to mRNA but are not added to endogenous RNA in the presence of ATP alone. Virion RNA does not appear to contain any significant regions of poly U as determined by hybridization with poly A or poly dT (Marshall and Gillespie, 1972) or by digestion with RNase U_2 under conditions specific for purines (Ehrenfeld, 1974). Also, cordecypin (3-deoxyadenosine) does not inhibit polyadenylation of VS viral RNA *in vivo* (Ehrenfeld, 1974). Definitive evidence for a role in transcription of the polyadenylate synthetase must await genetic analysis and identification of the enzyme as a specific protein component of the VS virion nucleocapsid.

2.2.2.   Envelope Constituents and Functions

2.2.2a.   Composition

The envelope of VS virus and probably other rhabdoviruses is a bilayered membrane 7–10 nm in thickness which appears to be derived from external or internal membranes of the host cell (Howatson, 1970; Zee *et al.*, 1970). Viral proteins G (the glycoprotein spikes) and M (membrane matrix protein) are inserted into the cell membrane, which is converted into the viral envelope; no cellular protein can be detected in the virion envelope, at least by polyacrylamide gel electrophoresis (Wagner *et al.*, 1969*a*).

The envelope of rhabdoviruses can be stripped off the nucleocapsid by a variety of procedures, most of which result in dissolution of the envelope components. However, the spikes can be removed intact without greatly disturbing the basic structure of the envelope (see Sect. 2.3.3). Only limited success has been achieved in removing the envelope intact. Brown *et al.*, 1967*a*) used Tween 80 and ether to dissect the envelope and spikes, with concomitant loss in infectivity of VS virus. The anionic detergent deoxycholate is also capable of completely dissociating the envelope and spikes, along with proteins G and M, from the nucleocapsid (Kang and Prevec, 1969; Wagner *et al.*, 1969*b*). Disruption of the VS virion by the sterol glycoside digitonin results in release of an envelope component which contains most of the M protein and half of the G protein (Wagner *et al.*, 1969*b*; Wagner and Schnaitman, 1970). Mudd (1973) has reported that treatment with HCl at *p*H 1.5 separated from VS virions a 250 S envelope fraction which contains 57% protein G, 30% protein M, and only 10% and 2% nucleocapsid proteins N and NS, respectively. However, under these conditions of acid dissolution, 66% of protein M appears as a nonsedimentable fraction. In our experience a reliable method for removing the M protein in a relatively pure form is by step-wise degradation, first with Triton X-100 at very low ionic concentration to selectively solubilize the G protein followed by ex-posure of the spikeless virions to Triton X-100 in 0.3 M NaCl, which splits off the M protein with the remainder of the envelope (Emerson and Wagner, 1972). McSharry (personal communication) has been able to isolate and purify the M protein after detergent–salt extraction by gradient centrifugation and column chromatography.

The envelope of rabies virus may be more fragile than the VS virion envelope; Sokol *et al.* (1972) reported that half of rabies strain ERA virions lost their envelope during purification. Neurath *et al.* (1972) found that 0.1% tri(n-butyl)phosphate in the presence of Tween 80 removed all labeled lipids and most of proteins G_1, G_2, and M_1 from rabies virions, but no uridine label or nucleocapsid proteins.

2.2.2b. Structure

A hexagonal lattice structure has been observed by electron mi-croscopy of three negatively stained rhabdoviruses: rabies virus (Hum-meler *et al.*, 1967), broccoli necrotic yellows virus (Hills and Campbell, 1968), and sowthistle yellow vein virus (Peters and Kitajima, 1970). Cartwright *et al.* (1972) have proposed two structural models for the envelope of the VS virion based on their estimate that there are about 1600 copies of the M protein and about 500 copies of the G protein, roughly a ratio of 3:1. One model is visualized as each surface pro-jection (spike) being surrounded by three matrix (M)-protein subunits arranged to fit a tubular structure in which the distribution of M-pro-tein subunits is based on a 92-member icosahedron cut across its inter-lattice axis. In their second model, Cartwright *et al.* (1972) postulate that the matrix-protein units are linked directly to the RNC. Addi-tional chemical data are required to test the validity of these ingenious models.

2.2.2c. The M-Protein Matrix Function

It has been tacitly assumed that the rhabdovirus M protein is the major, or only, structural protein component of the envelope, where it forms a lipoprotein complex with the pre-existing cell lipids. Similar nonglycosylated proteins of about the same molecular weight are found as the sole matrix proteins in the envelopes of myxoviruses (see Chapt. 3 in this volume) and paramyxoviruses (see Chapt. 2 in this volume). In these groups of viruses there is some electron microscopic evidence that the M protein lines the inner surface of the virion envelope, where this additional layer complexes with the nucleocapsid. No such evidence is available for rhabdovirus assembly of nucleocapsid and envelope. In fact, the location of the rhabdovirus M protein within the envelope is poorly understood. The evidence presented by Walter and Mudd (1973) that both the G and M proteins of supposedly intact VS virions are iodinated in the lactoperoxidase reaction may not necessarily signify that the M protein is partly located exterior to the envelope. Evidence that the M protein is closely associated with lipid of the VS viral envelope, possibly as a lipoprotein, is provided by the experiment of Cartwright *et al.* (1969) in which they demonstrated that phospholipase C selectively removes M protein without significantly disturbing the visible spikes, G protein, or infectivity of the virion. These data, along with electron microscopic evidence, have been interpreted as evidence that the spike protein penetrates through the interior of the envelope and is associated with the nucleocapsid (Cartwright *et al.,* 1969; Brown *et al.,* 1974). However, it is well to remember that no proof has been provided that the virion envelope is completely removed by the procedures which do not remove spikes.

2.2.2d.   Cellular Constituents in the Virion Envelope

Cellular constituents have been found associated with VS virions, presumably as part of or tightly adherent to the envelope. An example of an incorporated cellular constituent is the specific ganglioside, hematoside, of BHK cells present in VS virions grown in these cells (Klenk and Choppin, 1971). Cartwright and Pearce (1968) had previously shown that VS virus grown in BHK cells reacts by complement fixation with BHK-cell antibody but not with pig kidney-cell antibody, whereas VS virus grown in pig kidney cells did react with homologous cell antibody. Cartwright and Brown (1972a) extended these observations to show that the glycolipid fraction of VS virions labeled with ^{14}C-choline and ^{3}H-amino acids could be solubilized with SDS and fractionated by filtration through Sephadex G-25 or by polyacrylamide gel electrophoresis (McSharry and Wagner, 1971b). This purified glycolypid fraction reacts specifically by complement fixation with BHK-cell antibody but not with VS viral antibody (Cartwright and Brown, 1972a). These data indicate that at least one of the cellular antigens in the envelope of VS virus is a glycolipid derived from the host cell rather than cellular proteins.

Despite the inability to detect cellular proteins in VS virions by incorporation of labeled amino acid precursors (Wagner *et al.,* 1969*a*; Kang and Prevec, 1969), there is evidence that certain cellular proteins can be detected in VS virions by more sensitive biological or biochemical means. Hecht and Summers (1972) showed that purified VS virions released from infected L cells contained the specific mouse histocompatability (H2) antigen, a plasma membrane glycoprotein. Moreover, infected L cells lost more than 70% of their H2 antigen during the course of VS viral infection.

VS virions also contain enzymes that appear to be derived from the host cell in which the virus is grown. A protein kinase has been demonstrated in association with VS virions (Strand and August, 1971) as well as rabies and Kern Canyon viruses (Sokol and Clark, 1973). Imblum and Wagner (1974) have provided evidence that the protein kinase of VS virus is solubilized, at least to a large extent, by detergent and ionic conditions which disrupt the virion envelope and liberate G and M proteins. However, protein kinase activity is not associated with G or M protein as determined by fractionation on a phosphocellulose column. Although residual protein kinase activity is present in VS nucleocapsids (Imblum and Wagner, 1974; Moyer and Summers, 1974*a*), it is likely to be due to residual contamination of nucleocapsids with virion envelope. Sokol and Clark (1973) did not find protein kinase activity associated with intracellular nucleocapsids of VS virus or Kern Canyon virus, but they did find protein kinase in free nucleocapsids derived from rabies virus-infected cells. Evidence for the cellular origin of the protein kinase in VS virions was indicated by finding different kinetics of enzyme action in virions grown in different cells (Imblum and Wagner, 1974). However, no direct evidence could be obtained for a protein kinase in cellular membrane being incorporated into the envelope of VS virions (Imblum and Wagner, 1974; Moyer and Summers, 1974*a*). The phosphate acceptors of the various rhabdovirus proteins phosphorylated *in vitro* or *in vivo* are serine, predominantly, and also threonine presumably by linkage with a hydroxyl group (Sokol *et al.,* 1974).

Roy and Bishop (1971) have described a nucleoside triphosphate phosphotransferase present in VS virions as well as in influenza and Rauscher leukemia viruses, evidence for the cell-membrane origin of the enzyme. Triton N-101 stimulates the exchange of $\gamma^{32}PO_4$ from all nucleoside triphosphates but purines are the preferred receptors. Also present in VS virions are ATPase, GTPase, UTPase, and CTPase, the

activities of which are somewhat inhibited rather than activated by
Triton N-101.

A proteinase, presumably derived from host cells, is also found in
VS virions activated by nonionic detergent or heat shock (Holland *et
al.,* 1972).

2.2.3.   The Glycoprotein Spikes

2.2.3a.   Polysaccharide Chains

Only preliminary data are available about glycosylation of the VS
viral G protein. Burge and Huang (1970) demonstrated that extensive
pronase digestion results in a residual glycopeptide of approximately
4000 molecular weight as determined by Biogel P-10 filtration. McS-
harry and Wagner (1971*b*) confirmed this observation and by analysis
of the L-cell-grown VS virion glycopeptide by gas–liquid
chromatography found the following sugars: neuraminic acid $\simeq$37.3%,
glucosamine $\simeq$31.1%, glucose $\simeq$21.3%, galactose $\simeq$5.4%, and mannose $\simeq$4.6% (galactosamine $\lessgtr$0.1%, and fucose $\lessgtr$0.1%). Of some
interest is the fact that the VS virion, which has no neuraminidase,
contains considerable neuraminic acid, whereas the glycoproteins
and glycolipids of neuraminidase-containing myxoviruses and
paramyxoviruses are devoid of neuraminic acid (see Chapts. 2 and 3 in
this volume). Only VS virions, but not SV5 or influenza virus, could be
stained with colloidal iron hydroxide, which is specific for neuraminic
acid (Klenk *et al.,* 1970).

However, chemical analysis of the VS viral glycoprotein structure
has hardly begun. Very recent data reveal that ^{3}H-glucosamine is found
in 3 of 5 cyanogen bromide peptides of the VS viral glycoprotein
(Kelley and Emerson, unpublished data). This latter finding indicates
the existence of at least 3 polysaccharide chains and, in all likelihood,
there are more. None of the carbohydrate is dissociated from the intact
glycoprotein by strong alkali, which indicates absence of galactose or
other sugars phosphoester-linked to serine or threonine and presumably means the predominance of histidine– or asparagine–sugar
linkages (Kelley and Emerson, unpublished data).

2.2.3b.   Role in Initiation of Infection

Electron microscopy of VS virus or other rhabdoviruses clearly
shows that the spikes protrude at least 10 nm from the virion envelope

(Howatson, 1970). The spikes of intact virions are readily iodinated in the lactoperoxidase reaction (Walter and Mudd, 1973) and react with glycoprotein antibody (Wagner *et al.*, 1971). Spike protein G can be almost completely removed from intact VS virions without affecting the M protein by exposure to proteolytic enzymes such as trypsin (Cartwright *et al.*, 1969) and pronase (McSharry *et al.*, 1971). These results indicate that by far the greatest portion of the G protein is exterior to the virion envelope. Schloemer and Wagner (unpublished data) were finally able to recover from the virion envelope after thermolysin treatment a hydrophobic peptide fragment with about 50 amino acids comprising the unglycosylated, lipophilic end of the G protein.

Removal of the VS viral spikes by digestion with trypsin results in marked loss in infectivity, whereas considerable solubilization of M protein with phospholipase C does not (Cartwright *et al.*, 1969). It is presumed that the G protein is required for attachment of the VS virion to the cytoplasmic membrane of the susceptible cell. D. F. Summers (personal communication) has found that a pneumococcal endoglycosidase markedly reduces the infectivity of VS virus. Schloemer and Wagner (1974) have found that neuraminidase reduces the infectivity of VS virus by at least 90% merely by cleaving off the terminal neuraminic acid from the glycoprotein. Infectivity is restored by resialylation of the glycoprotein catalyzed by sialyl transferase.

2.2.3c. Hemagglutinin

The rather finicky hemagglutination activity of rhabdoviruses provides another method for studying the virion component responsible for adsorption to cells. Goose erythrocytes under very restricted conditions of *p*H, ionic strength, and temperature can be agglutinated by rather massive concentrations of rabies virus, VS virus, and other rhabdoviruses (Kuwert *et al.*, 1968; Halonen *et al.*, 1968; Arstila *et al.*, 1969). Schneider *et al.* (1971) were able to remove the hemagglutination activity of rabies virus with saponin, which simultaneously also lowered infectivity by 99% and solubilized complement-fixing antigen and immunizing activity. The hemagglutination activity of VS virus was shown by Arstila (1972, 1973) to be due to the spike glycoprotein. These results were confirmed and extended by McSharry and Choppin (personal communication), who found that G protein removed from VS virions by Triton X-100 was capable of hemagglutinating goose erythrocytes, whereas the glycoprotein-denuded virions were not. VS virus antibody blocks hemagglutination by isolated glycoprotein or

whole virions. It is also of interest that the hemagglutination activity of
whole VS virions or solubilized G protein is greater per infective virion
for virus grown in hamster cells (HAK and BHK) than for that grown
in MDBK (Madin-Darby bovine kidney) cells, suggesting that a cell
component, presumably carbohydrate, contributes to hemagglutination
activity. Varying patterns of glycosylation of the G protein are likely to
be the basis for cell modification of the hemagglutination capacity of

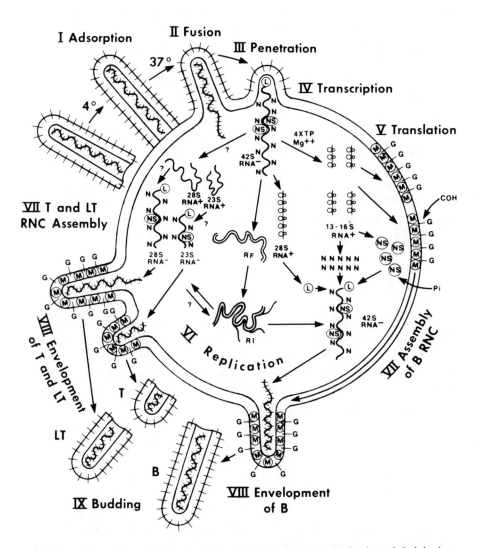

Fig. 8.   Schematic representation of the stages in the cycle of infection of rhabdovirus
prototype VS virus from adsorption to a host cell until progeny infective (B) and defective [T, LT (long T)] virions are released.

VS virions. In this regard it is of interest that neuraminidase can inactivate the hemagglutination activity of VS virions (Schloemer and Wagner, unpublished data) in a manner similar to its reduction of VS viral infectivity reported above.

2.2.3d. Antigenicity

The spike glycoprotein can also be removed almost quantitatively and quite specifically by treatment with nonionic detergents of VS virus (Cartwright *et al.*, 1970*b*; Kelley *et al.*, 1972) and rabies virus (Gyorgy *et al.*, 1971). The specificity of selective solubilization of the G protein is a function of concentration of the detergent and the ionic strength of the reaction mixture. The solubilized G protein forms a single precipitin line after double diffusion in agar with VS viral antiserum (Cartwright *et al.*, 1970*a*). Kelley *et al.* (1972) were able to raise monospecific antiserum by injecting rabbits with purified G protein. This antiglycoprotein is the specific antibody that neutralizes the infectivity of VS-Indiana virus but does not affect the infectivity of VS-New Jersey virus (Kelley and Emerson, unpublished results). Moreover, the partially purified G protein of VS-Indiana virus blocks the antiviral neutralizing activity of the specific antiserum. These data prove conclusively that the spike glycoprotein is the antigen which gives rise to and reacts with neutralizing antibody. Similar antigenic properties are exhibited by the glycoprotein spikes of rabies virus (Wiktor *et al.*, 1973). It seems likely that the protein rather than the carbohydrate moiety provides the principal antigenic determinants of the glycoproteins of rhabdoviruses (Kelley and Emerson, unpublished data).

3. REPLICATION

3.1. Physiology

3.1.1. Composite Model of Infection

Figure 8 illustrates a proposed model for a schematic representation of the entire cycle of infection from the time that VS virus, or presumably any other rhabdovirus, encounters a host cell until the time that progeny virions emerge from the cell. The process of infection is patently an integrated series of overlapping events, some of which occur simultaneously. However, a rational analysis of the entire life cycle of VS virus demands subdivision into separate events in order to scrutinize each of them individually before the overall process can be integrated into a coherent whole. The reader is reminded of the fact that the artificially separated events in replication of a rhabdovirus, or any other virus for that matter, cannot be appreciated when considered in splendid isolation. It is also wise for the reader to remember that certain aspects of the schema presented here are not universally considered to be final truth by all investigators. This section represents a rather superficial overview of the whole process of VS viral replication to serve as a background and framework on which to project the detailed analyses of each step, which will then be suitably documented and annotated. Also to be kept in mind is the point that infection with VS virus can result in two different outcomes: (1) a productive infection, in which the vast majority of progeny virions are infective, and (2) an abortive infection, due to the presence of defective interfering virions or nonpermissive conditions, in which the majority of progeny virions are defective. As noted in Fig. 8, both infective and defective progeny can be and are produced simultaneously.

The initial event in the infectious cycle is random collision of an infective B virion with the host cell. The virus attaches to the surface of the cell (step I), an event which is not energy dependent and can occur at 4°C. The next event (step II) is energy dependent and in our model the virion envelope fuses with the plasma membrane of the host cell. As discussed below, a certain proportion of virions, under perhaps special conditions, can enter the cell by phagocytosis. Those virions that enter the cytoplasm intact would, of course, have to be uncoated (de-enveloped) inside phagocytic vacuoles. On the other hand, when fusion occurs, the virion envelope is stripped off at the plasma membrane with consequent entry of only the nucleocapsid into the cytoplasm (step III).

After entry of the nucleocapsid, the first intracellular event is clearly and incontrovertibly transcription (step IV). Since the template for *in vitro* transcription has been shown to require N protein complexed with virion RNA (Emerson and Wagner, 1972), it follows that no further uncoating of the RNA, beyond removal of the envelope, is required for transcription. In other words, the parental RNA is probably never naked and is presumably not conserved. The transcription products are found on polyribosomes and fall into two size classes, 28 S and a more heterogeneous 12–16 S mRNA, each of which is complementary to virion RNA. The viral messengers are then translated (step V) into five identifiable viral polypeptides which are identical by disk electrophoresis to the five structural polypeptides of the VS virion and are also designated L, G, N, NS, and M. As shown in our schematic representation, the newly synthesized G protein is simultaneously glycosylated, probably in the cell membrane, and the NS protein is specifically phosphorylated. The translation model also presupposes two distinct compartments for synthesis of viral proteins, the cytoplasm for the N, L, and NS nucleocapsid proteins and the plasma membrane for the envelope proteins G and M.

Much more complex and less well understood is the process of replication of the progeny virion RNA (step VI). My schematic model hedges by presenting two alternative pathways, both of them designed to reconcile the requirement for synthesis of progeny RNA of the same nucleotide polarity as parental RNA. Another obstacle to a clear concept of RNA replication is the technical difficulty in identifying the positive-strand RNA template for replication of the progeny negative strand. One scheme, the simplest conceptually, presupposes that the 42 S parental RNA serves as template for 42 S positive-strand RNA which, in turn, serves as template for 42 S progeny RNA. Such a model presupposes formation of a replicative form (RF) and a replicative intermediate (RI). The other possible pathway of viral RNA replication is tied to the common occurrence of defective interfering T particles during the course of rhabdovirus reproduction. This alternative model visualizes as the first stage regular transcription from parental RNA of messengerlike, complementary, positive-stranded RNA species of 28 S and 23 S; in the next stage, the same polymerase or a second, separate enzyme serves to replicate the two or more messengerlike strands to make less-than-virion-sized progeny negative-strand RNA, each of which is encapsidated with N, L, and NS proteins to make defective virions containing 23 S (short T) or 28 S (long T) RNA.

Assembly of progeny RNA and proteins N, L, and NS into nucleocapsids is depicted in Fig. 8 as a separate event (step VII), but in all likelihood this maturation process is a reaction coupled with replication and translation. Coupled replication–translation proceeding to assembly of nucleocapsids would seem to require a reproduction complex containing RNA replicative intermediates, a replicase enzyme, and ribosomes, similar to the replication–translation factories found in poliovirus-infected cells (Baltimore, 1971). None of these components has yet been positively identified in cells infected with rhabdoviruses.

The separate formation of virion envelope probably occurs quite independently of nucleocapsid synthesis by conversion of cellular membrane (surface or intracytoplasmic) by insertion of newly synthesized viral G and M proteins, which replace normal cellular membrane proteins. In this process, the cellular membrane lipids are probably rearranged to conform with the new structural membrane protein.

Given the condition that the viral nucleocapsid and envelope are synthesized and assembled separately, the next stage in the process of VS viral reproduction is for the two components to find each other and assemble. This process of envelopment by viral-converted membrane of standard length (3.5 μm) or shorter (1.1–1.6 μm) nucleocapsids to form B or T virions is probably a unique mechanism (step VIII). Little is known about what controls or promotes envelopment and budding (step IX) of rhabdoviruses, which have been technically more difficult to study by electron microscopy than envelopment and budding of paramyxoviruses or myxoviruses. However, from these and other studies it is assumed that a protein in the rhabdovirus nucleocapsid recognizes and binds to a viral protein in the converted cellular membrane. Envelopment of the nucleocapsid is followed by budding off of a fully infective or defective progeny virion.

The individual steps in replication of VS virus and, where known, of other rhabdoviruses are presented and annotated below.

3.1.2. Growth Cycle

3.1.2a. Production of Infective Virions

The kinetics of VS viral growth was first studied by Franklin (1958), who found that the virus multiplies rapidly and with approximately equal efficiency in primary cultures of chick embryo cells or monkey kidney cells. The rate at which infective virions were produced was about the same for each cell type. In addition, extracellular virus always exceeded cell-associated virus, indicating that the release of mature, infective virions occurs in minutes after maturation and progressively throughout the cycle of infection. Wagner *et al.* (1963) made a detailed analysis of the growth of two variants of VS virus in two cell types. Figure 9 shows the comparative single-cycle growth curves in chick embryo cells infected at an adsorption multiplicity of 10 PFU/cell to ensure infection of every susceptible cell. As noted, a wild-

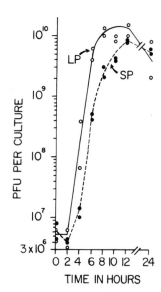

Fig. 9.   Growth curves of VS virus in chick embryo cells infected at a multiplicity of 10 plaque-forming units (PFU) of large-plaque (*LP*) and small-plaque (*SP*) variants. Reprinted with permission from Wagner *et al.* (1963).

type *LP* virus began to produce infectious virions 2 hours after adsorption and reached a maximum yield of approximately 1000 PFU/cell by 6–8 hours. An *SP* mutant of VS virus grew somewhat slower and to slightly lower titer under the same conditions. However, the less-virulent *SP* mutant grew poorly in L cells after a longer lag period and titers reached peak levels of <1 PFU/cell at 12–24 hours. L cells and HeLa cells infected at high multiplicity with VS-New Jersey virus showed maximal titers at 12 hours but antigen was detected by fluorescent-antibody staining in 4–6 hours (Paucker *et al.*, 1970). A small-plaque mutant of VS-New Jersey virus appeared to show retarded intracellular development (Streckfuss and Shechmeister, 1971). The efficiency with which VS virus multiplies is dependent on yet to be determined factors of cellular permissiveness and restriction as well as virus virulence.

   In marked contrast to VS virus, the rabies rhabdovirus grows rather poorly in almost all cultured cells but comparatively better in such cell lines as BHK21, rabbit endothelium (RE), and rabbit kidney (RK$_{13}$), particularly when these cells are infected in the presence of polycations such as DEAE-dextran. A one-step growth curve of rabies virus in BHK cells under optimal conditions reveals the initial presence of virus antigen, as determined by fluorescent-antibody staining, at 8–9 hours after infection; cell-associated rabies virus was detected at 12 hours, released virus was present in the medium at 15 hours, and peak titers were attained by 48 hours after infection (Kaplan *et al.*, 1967; Kuwert *et al.*, 1968).

3.1.2b.   Autointerference

Defective interfering (DI) components of rhabdoviruses and other viruses have recently been extensively reviewed by Huang (1973). Research on VS virus and probably other rhabdoviruses has always been plagued by considerable variation in yields of infective virions, depending on multiplicity of infection, passage level of the viral stocks, and cell type being used as host. We now know that production of high-titered virus requires infection of susceptible cells at low multiplicity with plaque-purified clones of virus (Stampfer *et al.*, 1969). Cooper and Bellett (1959) first described autointerference of VS virus during serial undiluted passage in chick embryo cells and attributed the low yields of infective virus to a transmissible interfering component (T). Reczko (1960) identified by electron microscopy small virus particles in VS virus preparations, and Hackett (1964) correctly assumed that these small virus particles might represent the transmissible component of Cooper and Bellett. Huang *et al.* (1966) conclusively demonstrated that defective T particles purified by rate zonal centrifugation are the interfering component in VS virus stocks. These observations were soon confirmed by other investigators (Crick *et al.*, 1966, 1969; Hackett *et al.*, 1967). These defective T particles were found to be antigenically indistnguishable and identical in other respects to the infectious B virions except that they were about one-third the length and contained about one-third of a piece of RNA (Huang and Wagner, 1966*b*; Brown *et al.*, 1967*c*).

Huang and Wagner (1966*a*) clearly demonstrated that the presence of VS-Indiana T particles markedly inhibited growth of homologous B virions. The degree of interference is a function of the concentration of T particles as well as of the time of superinfection with the T particles. VS-Indiana T virions only partially interfere with growth of VS-New Jersey B virions and are completely without effect on replication of the unrelated encephalomyocarditis virus (Huang and Wagner, 1966*a*). The degree of T-particle autointerference among rhabdoviruses appears to be correlated, at least to some extent, with antigenic relatedness to the infectious B virions (Crick and Brown, 1973). In addition, the interfering action of T particles is quite sensitive to UV irradiation, suggesting a requirement for a function of the T genome despite the inability to detect viral RNA synthesis in cells infected with T particles alone. The demonstration by Sreevalsan (1970) that naked T RNA could induce homologous interference is almost too good to be true.

The long T defective virion derived from the HR strain of VS-Indiana virus shows a much greater capacity to interfere with the growth of heterotypic VS-New Jersey B virions than does short T defective virions of standard VS virus (Prevec and Kang, 1970). Based on the fact that VS-Indiana and VS-New Jersey viruses are related antigenically only by their group-specific N protein, Prevec and Kang have postulated a deletion of the N-protein cistron (as well as of the polymerase cistron) from the short T genome, whereas the long T genome conceivably contains cistrons for N, G, and M proteins and is defective only because of a polymerase cistron deletion. A reasonable map for the complete B-virion genome, therefore, would read, sequentially: cistrons coding for L, N, G, and M proteins.

The origin of the T particle has been debated since it was first described. Presumably, it could arise either from fragmentation of viral RNA at some stage of the replication cycle, or the T RNA could be replicated with B virions as helpers. Probably both hypotheses are partially correct. Stampfer et al. (1969) were able to produce T particles by serial undiluted passage of a T-free clone of B virions, but lower concentrations of T virions in the presence of B virions promoted greater production of progeny T virions. Also worthy of note is the demonstration that the T interfering component of the VS-Brazil serotype could replicate in the presence of the antigenically distinct VS-Indiana B virions; the progeny T particles emerging from this mixed infection were thought to be of the Brazil genotype, based on a somewhat tenuous difference in sedimentation of RNA, but of the Indiana phenotype, as evidenced by their antigenic composition (Wild, 1972). This finding lends additional weight to the hypothesis that all the functional components except the RNA are supplied by the infectious helper virion in this mixed infection. Perrault and Holland (1972a) have emphasized the importance of the host cell in determining the degree of autointerference by T particles of VS-New Jersey virus. In addition, highly purified T virions provide excellent protection against intracerebral infection of mice with homologous B virions (Doyle and Holland, 1973). Cells mixedly infected with infective B virions and defective interfering T virions can become chronically infected due to cyclic production of T nucleocapsids and T virions (Palma and Huang, 1974), similar to the persistent VS viral infection previously described (Wagner et al., 1963). These persistently infected cells resist challenge infection with infective VS virus.

3.1.3. Host Range and Susceptibility to Infection

VS viruses can be propagated in an extraordinarily broad spectrum of vertebrate cells and some invertebrate cells. In our experience, as in that of other investigators, the most satisfactory host cells for bulk production of virus are baby hamster kidney (BHK21/13) cells and primary (or secondary) chick embryo fibroblasts. Mouse L cells and human HeLa cells are quite adequate but the yields are usually lower. Of considerable interest is the finding by Huang and Baltimore (1970) that VS viral infection of the Madin-Darby bovine kidney (MDBK) cell line results in virus progeny devoid of defective T particles. Similar absence of autointerference was found after serial undiluted passage of VS virus in Madin-Darby canine kidney (MDCK) cells (Coward et al., 1971). VS virus also multiplies in a moth cell line (Yang et al., 1969) as well as lines of Aedes albopictus and A. aegypti cells, but the yields of infectious virus are relatively low (Buckley, 1969; Wagner, unpublished data). The remarkable versatility of rhabdoviruses is demonstrated by the finding that fish rhabdoviruses grow as well in mammalian cells as they do in poikilothermic vertebrate cells provided that optimal temperatures under 23°C are maintained (Clark and Soriano, 1974).

The host-dependent functions that determine the rate and extent of replication of VS virus have not been elucidated. Only peripheral data are available, e.g., the finding that actinomycin D causes slight inhibition of VS virus yield (Yamazaki and Wagner, 1970). However, Follett et al. (1974) have shown that VS virus grows perfectly normally in cells enucleated with cytochalasin B, but mature rabies virus was not produced in these enucleated cells despite adequate synthesis of rabies RNA and antigens (Wiktor and Koprowski, 1974).

The beginning of a model system to study intrinsic cellular permissiveness to viral replication has been devised by a number of investigators. Edelman and Wheelock (1968) observed that VS virus grew differently in various kinds of human leukocytes and growth was greatly enhanced in phytohemagglutinin-treated lymphocytes. These results were corroborated by Nowakowski et al. (1973a) who also observed that antigen-induced mutagenesis increased the susceptibility of lymphocytes to VS virus. Interesting comparative model systems to study host factors that control synthesis of VS virus have been reported by Nowakowski et al. (1973b). In this latter study it was found that VS virus was restricted in the Raji cell line of Burkitt lymphoma but grew well in a similar human lymphoblastoid cell line. Restriction in the Raji cells turned out not to be at the transcriptional level but was related to the factors that control production of 42 S virion RNA.

Relatively few studies have been made on the pathogenesis of infection of the intact animal host with VS virus. Mice are extremely susceptible to infection by the intracerebral route but very much less so by the intraperitoneal route. The striking development of encephalitis after intranasal infection suggests a degree of neurotropism (Miyoshi *et al.*, 1971). In contrast, temperature-sensitive mutants of VS virus are not pathogenic but are highly immunogenic (Wagner, 1974).

3.1.4. Initiation of Infection

3.1.4a. Adsorption

Little more can be said about attachment of rhabdoviruses to membranes of their host cells other than to emphasize the key role of the glycoprotein spikes (see Sect. 2.2.3). Experiments performed by Wagner *et al.* (1963) reveal that VS virus adsorbs to susceptible host cells rather slowly and inefficiently. The rate of VS virus attachment was found to be no greater than 60% per hour. Flamand and Bishop (1973) have provided some evidence that VS virus grown in BHK cells adsorbs better on BHK cells than on chick embryo cells and *vice versa*, but these data require confirmation by quantitative techniques other than RNase resistance acquired by the ^{3}H-labeled input RNA strand.

3.1.4b. Penetration and Removal of the Envelope

The controversy between Morgan and Dales over the mode of penetration of animal viruses into host cells extends to VS virus. Simpson, Hauser, and Dales (1969) showed quite conclusively by electron microscopy that whole enveloped VS virus *can* penetrate into L cells by phagocytosis at 37°C within 5 minutes after adsorption at 4°C, while no virions could be found fused with cell membrane. In sharp contrast, Heine and Schnaitman (1969) in our laboratory found equally convincing evidence of fusion of VS virion envelope with the plasma membrane of L cells within minutes after warming the cultures to 37°C after adsorption of virus at 4°C. The only significant difference in technique between these two sets of contradictory experiments is that Simpson *et al.* incubated their virus–cell mixtures in medium containing 20% chicken serum, which should greatly stimulate phagocytosis, whereas Heine and Schnaitman reacted the virus with cells suspended in medium completely devoid of serum. These conflicting reports indicate the danger of studying dynamic events by the inherently static technique of electron microscopy, particularly when the microscopist can hardly be sampling more than a minute fraction of the virus population.

In all likelihood both phagocytosis and fusion of VS virions can occur under varying conditions and possibly both events can lead to productive infection. To determine the more likely process under physiological conditions, Heine and Schnaitman (1971) followed up their electron microscopy studies by the use of biochemical and serological techniques. First, they found that residual VS viral antigen could be detected on the surface of infected cells reacted with antiviral–antiferritin hybrid antibody and ferritin during the several-minute time interval when the penetrated virus could not itself be detected. An even more convincing experiment was performed by fractionating cells recently penetrated by VS virus prelabeled with ^{3}H-amino acids into plasma membrane and cytoplasmic components, each of which was then analyzed by disk gel electrophoresis for the presence of viral envelope and nucleocapsid ^{3}H-proteins. These studies revealed that the plasma membrane of the penetrated L cell contained predominantly viral ^{3}H-proteins G and M, whereas the nucleocapsid N protein was found predominantly in the cytoplasm, not associated with membrane. From these experiments the conclusion can be drawn that VS virions *can* infect cells by fusion of the virion envelope with plasma membrane of the target cell. Only the nucleocapsid, under these conditions, penetrates into the cytoplasm. This hypothesis is consistent with the finding of Cohen *et al.* (1971) that envelope proteins of VS virus, particularly the M protein, have a strong affinity for association with cytoplasmic membrane.

These data do not exclude the possiblity of an alternative pathway of infection by means of phagocytosis of the rhabdovirion. Conceivably, penetration of rabies virus could be slower than that of the VS virus because rabies antibody was found to neutralize the infectivity of the virus up to 15 minutes after interaction with BHK cells (Kaplan *et al.*, 1967).

3.2. RNA Synthesis

3.2.1. Transcription: *In Vitro* Activity of the VS Virion Polymerase

3.2.1a. Kinetics

In their original studies Baltimore *et al.* (1970) delineated the basic requirements for function of the VS virion polymerase. They found that nucleoside triphosphate incorporation was stimulated by Triton N-101, the presence of which was presumably necessary to disrupt the virion envelope. Other nonionic detergents, such as Nonidet P_{40} and Triton X-100, function equally well (Bishop and Roy, 1971a; Emerson and Wagner, 1972). Unenveloped nucleocapsids obtained from the cytoplasm of infected cells transcribe perfectly well without detergents (Galet et al., 1973). Baltimore et al. (1970) found an absolute requirement for Mg^{2+}, the optimal concentration of which is 4–6 mM; Mn^{2+} not only does not substitute for Mg^{2+} but actually inhibits polymerization of RNA in the presence of Mg^{2+}. Bishop et al. (1971) confirmed this observation and compared the VS viral enzyme with the manganese-dependent influenza virion RNA polymerase. NaCl or KCl was also necessary for the polymerase reaction, which is also partially dependent on the presence of 2-mercaptoethanol or dithiothreitol. Ribonuclease destroyed the reaction product but actinomycin D or rifamycin had no effect on transcription. Many of these results were confirmed by Bishop and Roy (1971a).

Baltimore and his colleagues (1970) found linear kinetics of RNA synthesis for 20 minutes in their in vitro polymerase system, but periods up to 10 hours were described by later investigators who achieved more stable conditions (Villareal and Holland, 1973). In their analysis of the polymerase reaction Bishop and Roy (1971a) found that the enzyme would accept no template other than encapsidated virion RNA; the failures included naked VS viral RNA, ribosomal RNA, and a large series of single-stranded and double-stranded polyribo- and polydeoxyribonucleotides. In fact, all extraneous nucleic acids tended to depress the reaction. In addition, the VS virion enzyme would not polymerize deoxyribonucleotides, emphasizing its distinctiveness from the reverse transcriptase.

Transcription in vitro of B virions is rapid and repetitive (Bishop and Roy, 1971b) as well as complete (Bishop, 1971). However, the rate and extent of transcription are greatly dependent on temperature as well as other factors. All investigators have found that in vitro transcription of VS virions is far more efficient at 28–31°C than it is at 37–39°C. Szilágyi and Pringle (1972) were able to solve this problem to some degree by removing the detergent used to activate the reaction. It is of interest in this respect that Galet et al. (1973) found far less temperature sensitivity of wild-type, unenveloped nucleocapsids obtained from infected cells when the reaction was performed without detergent, a finding readily confirmed by Imblum and Wagner (unpublished data). In addition, certain wild-type strains of VS virus are less sensitive to temperature effects during in vitro transcription (Cairns et al., 1972; Bishop and Flamand, 1974).

3.2.1b. *In Vitro* Transcription Products

Only complementary RNA is transcribed *in vitro*, as determined by complete hybridization to excess B-virion RNA (Bishop and Roy, 1971*b*). The RNA transcripts soon become sensitive to ribonuclease, demonstrating that they are rapidly released from the template. The RNA product synthesized *in vitro* is quite heterogeneous (Bishop and Roy, 1971*a*). Roy and Bishop (1972) also presented evidence that *in vitro* transcription is sequential. After transcription at 28°C for periods as short as 30–60 minutes, the product RNA annealed only to B-virion RNA and not to T-virion RNA. Only later in transcription, after several hours, did RNA transcripts hybridize to T RNA as well as B RNA. These data indicate that the defective T genome represents one segment of the fully infective B genome, presumably that part distal to the 3′ end. Under the conditions of these experiments, 3 hours were required to transcribe 90% of the B-RNA template. The very recent, elegant experiments of A. Banerjee (personal communication) solved the problem of heterogeneity of the *in vitro* transcribed mRNA. Removal of all nuclease activity results in transcription *in vitro* of all five VS viral messengers which can translate each respective viral protein.

TABLE 4

Classification of RNA Species Synthesized in Cells Infected with VS Virus
under Conditions Productive of B Virions (Group I) or Autointerference
with T Virions (Group II)[a]

RNA species, $s_{20, w}$	Strandedness	Complementarity[b]	Poly A	Function[c]
Group I				
12–16 S	SS	+	+	mRNA
28 S	SS	+	+	mRNA
42 S	SS	+	+	Template
42 S	SS	−	−	B RNA
25–35 S	DS	±	?	RI, TI
Group II				
6 S	SS	?	?	?
13 S	DS	±	?	RF
23 S	SS	−	?	T RNA
13–19 S	DS	±	?	RI

[a] Adapted from Huang (1974). Her sedimentation coefficients are somewhat modified for purposes of uniformity with text.
[b] + = complementary to virion RNA; − = polarity of virion RNA.
[c] RI = replicative intermediate, TI = transcriptive intermediate, RF = replicative form.

3.2.1c.   Initiation and Direction of Transcription

Roy and Bishop (1973) have opened up an important avenue of research that could lead to a definition of the initiation signals for transcription of VS virion RNA. By using γ^{32}P-nucleoside triphosphates to label the RNA products made during *in vitro* transcription, they found that all complementary RNA species began with pppA or pppG and never pppU or pppC. The ^{32}P-RNA transcripts were digested with alkali, RNase A, or RNase T_1 and chromatographed on a DEAE column along with marker oligonucleotides. By this technique it was possible to determine that the γ^{32}P label was at the 5′ end of the VS viral transcription product. Multiple initiation sequences were observed, two of which were characterized as pppApCpGp . . . and pppGpCp . . . , suggesting different sites for initiation of transcription along the virion genome. Sequential labeling techniques and digestion with exonucleases revealed a 5′ to 3′ direction of synthesis of the RNA polymerase product.

3.2.2.   *In Vivo* Transcription

3.2.2a.   Intracellular VS Viral RNA Species

Early investigations revealed a bewildering array of at least 9 species of VS viral RNA in infected cells (Schaffer *et al.*, 1968; Newman and Brown, 1969; Stampfer *et al.*, 1969; Schincariol and Howatson, 1970; Wild, 1971; Kiley and Wagner, 1972). Some 5 of these species appeared to be single-stranded RNAs that were RNase sensitive, whereas perhaps 2 or 3 were associated with proteins and were RNase resistant. In addition, at least two classes of partially or completely double-stranded RNA can be recovered from infected cells.

Table 4 represents a modified version of the system devised by Huang (1974) for identifying the RNA species synthesized in cells infected with VS virus. According to her classification, group I RNA designates those species made in cells infected by pure clones of infective B virions at relatively low multiplicity. Group II RNA species are those synthesized under conditions of interference with infective B by defective T virions (Stampfer *et al.*, 1969).

3.2.2b.   Messenger RNA Species

Principal credit for identification and categorization of VS viral mRNA belongs to Huang *et al.* (1970) and Mudd and Summers

(1970b). Viral RNA released from polysomes treated with EDTA contained 2 distinguishable size classes of RNA, roughly 28 S and 12–16 S. The larger RNA species was recovered from the more rapidly sedimenting polysomes. Both species of polysome RNA hybridize completely to VS virion RNA, *prima facie* evidence for synthesis of these mRNA species on the VS virion genome. On polyacrylamide gels Wild (1971) found 5–6 species, ranging in molecular weight from 0.24 $\times$ 10^6 to 1.0 $\times$ 10^6 daltons. Perhaps better resolution of the mRNA was obtained by Schincariol and Howatson (1972), who were able by polyacrylamide gel electrophoresis to identify three classes estimated to have molecular weights of 0.75, 0.59, and 0.35 $\times$ 10^6 daltons. Each of the mRNA species hybridized to the RNA of B and long T virions, but the mRNA of molecular weight 0.59 $\times$ 10^6 failed to hybridize with short T-virion RNA. Perhaps the most reliable estimates for molecular weights of complementary mRNA in cells infected with VS-Indiana virus are for three resolvable species, of 2.4 $\times$ 10^6, 0.66 $\times$ 10^6, and 0.31 $\times$ 10^6 daltons, reported by Schaffer and Soergel (1972).

The authenticity of the mRNA species made in cells infected with VS virus has been demonstrated by their capacity to translate VS viral proteins. Grubman and Summers (1973) were able to take crude cytoplasmic extracts of HeLa cells infected with VS virus and synthesize 4 polypeptides that comigrated on polyacrylamide gels with 4 of the 5 VS virion proteins. Morrison *et al.* (1974) were able to go one step further by extracting VS viral mRNA from infected-cell polysomes and get them to translate VS viral proteins in a cell-free system containing ribosomes and other factors derived from various cell types. Of particular interest was the fact that the 28 S mRNA was translated only into a protein similar to the virion L protein, whereas the 12–16 S mRNA made polypeptides that migrated with N, NS, and M proteins but not the L protein. These data point up the distinctiveness of the individual messengers that are presumably derived from separate regions of the VS viral genome.

T particles of VS virus are not capable of undergoing transcription inside an infected cell (Stampfer *et al.*, 1969). Although T particles inhibit RNA synthesis of coinfecting homologous B virions, the defective T virions do not inhibit primary mRNA transcription by B virions (Huang and Manders, 1972). The other effects of T particles on replication of B virions will be discussed in Sect. 3.2.3).

3.2.2c.   Primary Transcription

In vivo synthesis of VS viral mRNA occurs independently of protein synthesis, a process that has been dubbed primary transcription because the template is presumably parental input nucleocapsid with its associated polymerase. Secondary transcription refers to mRNA synthesized by progeny nucleocapsids, the appearance of which later in the course of infection depends on protein synthesis. When protein synthesis is blocked with cycloheximide or puromycin soon after virus penetration, early mRNA synthesis proceeds quite normally and may even exceed transcription in the absence of protein inhibitors (Marcus *et al.*, 1971; Huang and Manders, 1972; Perrault and Holland, 1972*b*). Flamand and Bishop (1973) have examined the kinetics of primary transcription by analyzing the development of RNase resistance of highly labeled input parental strands of RNA. They found that the optimal temperature for primary *in vivo* transcription, unlike that for *in vitro* transcription, was between 36°C and 39.5°C, quite consonant with the earlier report of Huang and Manders (1972). Flamand and Bishop (1973) also found that it takes only 4 minutes to develop complete transcripts of the input genome and the reaction was not affected by actinomycin, cycloheximide, or puromycin. Actually, the mRNA species obtained by primary transcription and secondary transcription are virtually identical 28 S and 12–16 S classes, indicating the absence of significant regulatory mechanisms at the level of transcription in the two stages of infection.

3.2.2d. Adenylation

In their original analysis of the mRNA recovered from polyribosomes of HeLa cells infected with VS virus Mudd and Summers (1970*b*) found a much higher content of adenylic acid than could be accounted for by the uridylic acid content of VS virion RNA. This finding led Ehrenfeld and Summers (1972) to examine the VS viral messengers more carefully and to compare them with adenylate-rich mRNA of uninfected HeLa cells. VS viral 13 S (12–16 S) mRNA from HeLa cell polysomes was found to have segments resistant to digestion by RNase A and T_1; this enzyme-resistant piece contained 93% adenylic acid. The adenylate-rich sequences were more heterogeneous in length than HeLa cell or hemoglobin mRNA and were apparently 70–250 nucleotides in length. Soria and Huang (1973) found that the 28 S mRNA is also adenylated, as are smaller messengers, even in the presence of cordycepin. No function can be attributed to the adenylate-rich region any more than function can be attributed to nuclear adenylation of nonviral cell messengers. The evidence cited in Sect. 2.2.1e that VS virions contain polyadenylate synthetase activity coupled to polymerase (Villareal and Holland,

1973) and that cytoplasmic extracts of VS virus-infected L cells can synthesize polyadenylate (Galet and Prevec, 1973) suggests a potentially important role for adenylation of VS viral mRNA.

3.2.2e.   Temperature-Sensitive Mutants

Rather disappointing results have been obtained in experiments in which *ts* mutants of VS viruses were used to probe the nature of *in vivo* VS viral transcription. Successful localization of the *in vitro* transcription lesion (Szilágyi and Pringle, 1972; Hunt and Wagner, 1974) of group I *ts* mutants can not be easily exploited for studying *in vivo* transcription. Classification of complementation group I and group IV mutants as RNA⁻ was based entirely on reduced synthesis of total viral RNA at restrictive temperature (Pringle and Duncan, 1971; Martinet and Printz-Ané, 1970). By this method, no distinctions could be made of defects at the level of primary transcription, replication, or secondary transcription. Perlman and Huang (1973) used cyclohexi-mide at various stages as well as temperature-shift to pinpoint the lesions in the Glasgow group I mutant *ts* 114. By a rather complicated series of experiments, they concluded that *ts* G114 is temperature-sensitive at 37°C in both primary and secondary transcription but not in replication of virion 42 S RNA. In a follow-up series of experiments Perlman and Huang (1974) found the same behavior of *ts* G114, but the group I mutant *ts* G12 and the group IV mutant *ts* G41 made as much mRNA or more at 37°C than at 31°C. Other effects on 42 S RNA will be discussed in Sect. 3.2.3.

Flamand and Bishop (1973) and Bishop and Flamand (1974) used the very different technique of developing ribonuclease resistance of the input parental RNA strand to study *in vivo* transcription of Orsay *ts* mutants representing each of the five complementation groups. By this technique, no significant difference was noted in primary *in vivo* transcription at the restrictive temperature of 39.5°C compared with permissive conditions of 31°C and 34°C. Even the presumed group I transcriptase mutant *ts* O5 showed no significant *in vivo* decline in RNA synthesis at 39.5°C. However, in our experience (Hunt and Wagner, 1974) the Orsay mutant *ts* O5 may well be leaky by virtue of incomplete switch off of *in vitro* transcription at 39°C.

Contrasting results were obtained by Printz-Ané *et al.* (1972), who reported considerable reduction in synthesis of all RNA species, including 13–15 S (12–16 S) mRNA, by the group I Orsay mutant *ts* O5, even when shifted from permissive to restrictive temperature. They also reported some reduction in mRNA synthesis *in vivo* by a group IV mutant, *ts* O100. Results obtained by Unger and Reichmann (1973) by polyacrylamide gel electrophoretic analyses of the RNA species made at permissive and restrictive temperatures in BHK cells infected with Glasgow *ts* mutants support the data reported by the French workers. The group I mutant *ts* G11 did not synthesize any viral RNA at 39°C and was assumed to be defective in transcription. Among other mutants that had been classified as RNA⁻ by reduced levels of total RNA synthesis at restrictive temperature, group II *ts* G22 and group IV *ts* G41 were found to be capable of synthesizing both classes of mRNA species but not virion RNA, whereas the RNA⁺ group III mutant *ts* G31 made all species of RNA under restrictive conditions.

Many more data, perhaps by even more refined techniques, must be obtained before *ts* mutants can be used successfully to probe *in vivo* transcription mechanisms. Other aspects of the use of mutants for studying viral RNA synthesis will be discussed in Sect. 3.2.3 on replication, including the coupled reactions of transcription and replication.

3.2.3.   Replication of Viral RNA

3.2.3a.   Statement of the Problem

The major hiatus in our understanding of rhabdovirus reproduction is RNA replication, the mechanism by which virion RNA is synthesized. There are three missing links. First, convincing evidence has not been readily available for the existence in cells infected with VS virus of an RNA template on which progeny virion RNA can be replicated. Perlman and Huang (1973) cite the as yet unpublished finding of M. Stampfer of 40 S (42 S) RNA complementary to virion RNA which presumably could serve as such a template. Yet to be published data by Morrison, Stampfer, Lodish, and Baltimore appear to reveal that 80% of 40 S intracellular RNA contains nucleotide sequences identical to virion RNA but 20% of the 40 S RNA is complementary to virion RNA. Second, no one has yet demonstrated conclusively the existence of a replicative intermediate with progeny RNA precursors that can be chased into virions. Many investigators have described partially and completely double-stranded RNA in VS virus-infected cells but it is not possible to say whether these are transcriptive or replicative intermediates (Huang *et al.*, 1970; Mudd and Summers, 1970*b*; Schincariol and Howatson, 1970; Wild, 1971). The third elusive problem is complete failure to identify a replicase, an enzyme capable of catalyzing synthesis of progeny RNA of the same polarity as parental virion RNA. The only polymerase yet found in VS virus-infected cells is a transcriptase which makes only RNA complementary to virion RNA (Galet *et al.*, 1973; Imblum and Wagner, unpublished data). No easily reproducible method has yet been described to switch off transcription in order to study isolated replicative events, although the use of cycloheximide with *ts* mutants may help this approach (Perlman and Huang, 1973).

These difficulties, which also confront those investigators who are studying replication of the related negative-strand myxoviruses and paramyxoviruses, have necessitated indirect approaches to the problem. Quite understandably, these approaches have often led to conflicting and confusing data.

3.2.3b. Intracellular Polymerase

Wilson and Bader (1965) first described an RNA polymerase detectable in cells some hours after infection with VS virus and this observation has been confirmed and extended by Galet *et al.* (1973). The intracellular polymerase appears in cytoplasm about 2 hours after infection and is associated with particulate components which sediment at 140 S and 100 S. It seems likely that these components represent B and long T nucleocapsids which provide the template and enzyme for nucleotide polymerization. No polymerase activity was found in other cytoplasmic components. The *in vivo* polymerase appears to have the same properties as the virion *in vitro* polymerase: it is Mg^{2+} dependent, is blocked by Mn^{2+} and requires all 4 nucleoside triphosphates. However, the enzyme is neither activated nor inhibited by nonionic detergent and appears to be more temperature resistant than the Triton-activated virion polymerase. The only product of the *in vivo* polymerase that could be identified was 6–18 S RNA complementary to virion RNA; however, about 16% of the product seemed to be ribonuclease resistant before hybridization, which might obscure an RNA species of opposite polarity. However, no evidence could be found for the existence of a replicase either in association with the nucleocapsid or as part of another component. Unpublished data of Imblum and Wagner confirm these observations. Very recent studies by Villareal and Holland (1974) also demonstrate 175 S and 110 S nucleocapsids with transcriptase activity in cells infected with VS B virions; under interfering conditions of infection with B + T virions the resulting 110 S nucleocapsid transcribed poorly and only 4 S RNA was made. Of some interest, also, was evidence for a 260 S nucleocapsid with low transcriptase activity in cells infected with rabies virus, whereas rabies virions showed no transcriptase activity.

3.2.3c. RNA Associated with Intracellular Nucleocapsids

Among the numerous species of viral RNA found in VS virus-infected cells, three have been identified as virion RNA. Stampfer *et al.* (1969) were able to identify at least two kinds of virion RNA, depending on whether cells were infected with cloned B virions alone or with B + T virions. The principal virion RNA species which appeared in cells infected with defective T virions were estimated at 19 S (23 S). Petric and Prevec (1970) described a larger RNA species, about 30 S, in cells infected with the HR variant of VS virus, which gives rise to long T defective VS virions. Cells infected with the HR VS virus revealed two kinds of nucleocapsids, one of which sedimented at 140 S and contained 43 S RNA and the other which sedimented at 100 S and contained 30 S RNA. A rather confusing aspect of the problem is the finding that defective virions of the HR strain contain as much as 21% RNA complementary to virion RNA (Roy *et al.*, 1973). Schincariol and Howatson (1970) found identical nucleocapsids in cells infected with 85% B virions and 15% T virions of the HR strain. Similar experiments were performed by Kiley and Wagner (1972) with a standard strain of VS virus which apparently can give rise to short T primarily but also produces long T particles; these latter experiments were performed under conditions in which T particles interfered with normal B development. Kiley and Wagner (1972) were able to identify two distinct nucleocapsids in VS virus-infected cells, one of which sedimented at 100 S and contained 28 S RNA and the other which sedimented at 80 S and contained 23 S RNA. These infected cells released three classes of virions, one of which (long T) contained 28 S RNA, another (short T) contained 23 S RNA, and a third (B virion) which contained 42 S RNA and was infectious. These findings led Kiley and Wagner (1972) to propose the hypothesis that B-virion RNA might be replicated from short pieces of complementary RNA to make progeny RNA that is encapsidated as 100 S nucleocapsids with 28 S RNA (two-thirds piece) and 80 S nucleocapsids with 23 S RNA (one-third piece). This hypothesis requires the existence of a ligase to join the two RNA strands to form infectious virions under permissive conditions and failure of ligation under restrictive interfering conditions resulting in defective short T and long T virions. This hypothesis has never been refuted but has been superseded by a much more likely alternative pathway for producing infectious virions from intact parental RNA by way of a 42 S complementary RNA template (Huang, 1974).

3.2.3d. Evidence for Replicative Forms

The existence of double-stranded RNA in cells infected with VS virus was first described by Schaffer *et al.* (1968) and then confirmed by many investigators. The two heterogeneous classes of double-stranded RNA, 23–35 S and 15–20 S (Stampfer *et al.,* 1969), could just as easily be, and probably are to a considerable extent, transcriptive as well as replicative intermediates. Wild (1971) also described a 13 S double-stranded RNA in VS virus-infected BHK cells and a larger complex which melted out to 38 S and 19 S as well as 10–16 S, the latter presumably mRNA. Schincariol and Howatson (1972) helped to clarify the nature of the double-stranded RNA species by infecting cells with B virions alone or with both B and T virions of the VS virus HR strain followed by fractionation with LiCl. In this way they identified an RF for B virions of 20–21 S with an equivalent molecular weight of 7.0–7.8×10^6 and an RF for long T virions of 15–16 S with an equivalent molecular weight of 3.2–3.8×10^6. Also present in the infected cell was LiCl-precipitable material which was partially ribonuclease digestible; it was not possible to determine whether this heterogeneous viral RNA represents replicative or transcriptive intermediates, or both. Similar types of RNA found after *in vitro* transcription of VS virions have been identified as transcriptive intermediates (Huang *et al.,* 1971). The evidence for a T-virion RI is somewhat more definite because it can be identified under conditions in which B-virion replication and transcription are minimized. These data lead to the observation that during T-particle interference the infected cell contains 13 S RF and 13–19 S RI which give rise to 19 S (23 S) encapsidated T-virion RNA (Huang, 1974).

3.2.3e. RNA Replication by *ts* Mutants

At least four laboratories have been striving by the use of *ts* mutants to uncover the mechanisms by which VS virion RNA is replicated (Perlman and Huang, 1973; Unger and Reichmann, 1973; Combard *et al.,* 1974; Bishop and Flamand, 1974). These experiments are dependent on the ability to inhibit synthesis of 42 S virion RNA at the restrictive temperature without altering transcription of VS viral mRNA. RNA⁻ mutants of complementation group IV are the most likely candidates for a lesion in replication which would permit isolation of this function independent of transcription. Analysis by Unger and Reichmann (1973) of RNA species by polyacrylamide gel electrophoresis revealed that the group IV mutant *ts* G41 makes no 42 S virion RNA at 39°C, but does make mRNA even in the presence of cycloheximide. Similar results were obtained with the group II mutant *ts* G22, but the large amount of 28 S RNA made at 39°C by this mutant could be long T virion RNA rather than the mRNA it is interpreted to be by the authors.

Partial confirmation of these results were obtained by Combard *et al.* (1974), who studied by sucrose gradient centrifugation the RNA species of two Orsay mutants of complementation group IV. These investigators found that these mutants made only 13–15 S RNA at the restrictive temperature of 39.2°C; unlike Unger and Reichmann (1973), they were unable to detect 28 S mRNA at restrictive temperature. Of considerable interest, also, was the marked depression of synthesis of protein N at 39.2°C, suggesting concurrent restriction of RNA and nucleoprotein. We have noted a similar pleiotropic effect in restriction of nucleocapsid propagation by the group IV Glasgow mutants *ts* 41 and *ts* 44 (Wagner, unpublished data). Combard *et al.* (1974) speculated about the possibility that transcription and replication are coupled reactions mediated by a protein other than the transcriptase and presumably defective in group IV mutants. However, these speculations cannot be substantiated without detailed analysis of the origin and polarity of the RNA species made under these complicated conditions.

Interesting experiments with the group I mutant *ts* G114 led Perlman and Huang (1973) to hypothesize interdependence between transcription and replication. This mutant is defective in both primary and secondary transcription at 37°C but will replicate 40 S virion RNA at 37°C, provided preceding transcription is permitted at 31°C. Quite strikingly, when cycloheximide is added to infected cultures at the time of shift up to 37°C, 13–15 S and 28 S mRNA synthesis is enhanced rather than depressed, as it is when transcription is blocked by cycloheximide added at the start of infection. However, cycloheximide causes cessation of replication, as evidenced by inhibition of 40 S RNA synthesis at the same time the mRNA synthesis is enhanced. This effect of cycloheximide can be reversed by a more prolonged period of incubation at 37°C before addition of cycloheximide, in which case 40 S virion RNA synthesis is quite normal at the restrictive temperature. Perlman and Huang (1973) concluded that "replication and transcription appear to be tightly coupled in VSV-infected cells." Apparently, this association of transcription and replication can also be accomplished with wild-type VS virus as well as in 3 other group I mutants and the *ts* G41 group IV mutant (Perlman and Huang, unpublished data). These authors also favor the concept of one enzyme that functions for both transcription and replication, presumably mediated by another, unknown factor.

In a series of rather complicated experiments Perlman and Huang (1974) have provided some additional support for the "hypothesis that transcription and genome replication are distinguishable but interdependent processes." Among *ts* mutants of both groups I and IV that were first incubated at permissive temperature for several hours, a shift to the restrictive temperature (37°C) resulted in inhibition of all species of RNA. Some mutants, however, appeared less able to synthesize 40 S RNA, but other mutants of both groups I and IV replicated 40 S RNA relatively normally but were deficient in mRNA synthesis. These data emphasize the phenotypic variation among different mutants in the same complementation group.

These observations were extended by Palma *et al.* (1974), who tested the combined effects of various restriction procedures on *ts* mutants, primarily coinfection with interfering T particles and cycloheximide, in order to isolate and dissect the events. As previously noted (Huang and Manders, 1972), T particles do not affect transcription of wild-type or mutant VS virus but do inhibit replication of 40 S virion RNA at restrictive temperatures. However, under these conditions 19 S (23 S) T RNA was synthesized, indicating unimpaired replication promoted by the group I mutant *ts* G114 at 37°C. These data can also be interpreted as evidence that the replicative enzyme(s) for synthesis of B virion 40 S RNA provides the helper function as well for synthesis of T-virion 19 S RNA. If this be the case, then a mutant restricted in replication should not serve as helper for synthesis of 19 S RNA of coinfecting T virions. The data reveal 20% reduction in 19 S RNA synthesis at 37°C in cells doubly infected with wild-type T virions and the presumed replication mutant *ts* G41. More convincing than this minor reduction in presumed replicase function is the evidence that ribonuclease-resistant 13 S RNA accumulates in cells doubly infected with *ts* G114 and T virions (Palma *et al.*, 1974). Presumably, this double-stranded RNA represents the replicative form of two hydrogen-bonded 19 S RNA strands that gives rise to T-virion RNA (Schaffer *et al.*, 1968; Stampfer *et al.*, 1969; Wild, 1971).

3.2.3f. The Wagner–Emerson Model for VS Viral RNA Synthesis

This hypothesis is proposed as an experimentally testable working model of integrated transcription and replication. The sequence of events is visualized as follows:

1. Virion RNA is transcribed by the L-protein polymerase to make complementary RNA with NS protein as co-factor.
2. Complementary RNA is synthesized as messenger-sized pieces and released from the template by polyadenylation at the 3′ end. The NS protein is the likely candidate for the polyadenylate synthetase in addition to its polymerase function.
3. When polyadenylation is switched off by alteration of the NS protein, a complete 42 S complementary RNA strand is made by reading through the 42 S parental genome which has lost its termination signals, resulting in a double-stranded replicative form.
4. The 42 S complementary RNA strand of the RF serves as template for replication of progeny RNA catalyzed by the L-protein polymerase which can function as a replicase as well as a transcriptase.
5. The 42 S progeny RNA is displaced from the replicative intermediate as it is encapsidated by N protein in a coupled replication–translation reaction.

3.3. Protein Synthesis and Maturation

3.3.1. Translation

3.3.1a. Cell-Free Systems

Conclusive evidence for the messenger function of the mRNA on polyribosomes of VS virus-infected cells has been provided by Morrison *et al.* (1974). When 13–15 S mRNA was incubated in extracts of rabbit reticulocytes or wheat germ, the polypeptides that were synthesized had the electrophoretic mobility corresponding to authentic VS virion proteins N, NS, M, and possibly G, but not L protein. However, 28 S mRNA translated what is probably a single polypeptide resembling the L protein. These *in vitro*-synthesized polypeptides also cochromatographed on hydroxylapatite columns with virion proteins M, NS, N, and G. The *in vitro*-synthesized NS protein was slightly larger, suggesting cleavage to make the nucleocapsid NS protein. No data have been published on peptide maps to compare virion and *in vitro*-synthesized polypeptides. However, ^{35}S-formyl methionine tryptic peptides derived from the 13–15 S mRNA translation products revealed initiation sites for four distinct polypeptides. The translation product of the 28 S mRNA, on the other hand, contained only one initiator ^{35}S-formyl methionine tryptic peptide, a finding which provides excellent confirmatory evidence for a single 28 S mRNA for the unique L protein (Stampfer and Baltimore, 1973; Emerson and Wagner, 1973). Banerjee (personal communication) has now translated each *in vitro* transcribed mRNA into its viral protein.

The identification by Morrison *et al.* (1974) of a minor component that could correspond to the G protein raises the question of how this complex polypeptide could be synthesized in a cell-free system in the absence of glycosylation. Grubman and Summers (1973) did identify a G protein-like product that was synthesized *in vitro* on polyribosomes isolated from VS virus-infected cells. Similar results of *in vitro* synthesis of all 5 VS viral proteins were obtained with a post-nuclear extract of L cells, but the capacity to synthesize the G protein was lost when membrane-bound polysomes were removed (Ghosh *et al.* 1973). Grubman *et al.* (1974) report that membrane-bound polysomes synthesized primarily unglycosylated G protein and lesser amounts of N, NS, and M proteins but only in the presence of crude L or HeLa cell extracts. Also worthy of note is the failure of Kingsbury (1973) to detect *in vitro* synthesis of a paramyxovirus G protein. Possible differences in the intracellular location of viral messengers could explain some of the data discussed below.

3.3.1b.   Intracellular Synthesis of VS Viral Proteins

The first detailed analyses of the VS viral proteins synthesized in cells infected with VS viruses were made by Wagner *et al.* (1970), Petric and Prevec (1970), and Mudd and Summers (1970*a*). These studies revealed that relatively high-multiplicity infection rapidly switches off cellular protein synthesis, thus allowing detection of virus-specific proteins by the first hour after infection. Thereafter, all five VS viral proteins can be identified by comigration on polyacrylamide gels of cytoplasmic extracts with differentially labeled VS virion proteins (see Fig. 6). Minor intracellular viral protein peaks seen by Wagner *et al.* (1970) and by Mudd and Summers (1970*a*), as well as by many other investigators, are probably artifacts or are of cellular origin. Most investigators now agree that there are no intracellular virus-specific non-structural proteins; each of the five identifiable proteins synthesized in infected cells is incorporated to a greater or lesser extent into virions. Potentially significant is the finding by Kang and Prevec (1971) that the intracellular G protein migrates slightly faster on polyacrylamide gels than does coelectrophoresed virion G protein. This finding has been confirmed in several laboratories, leading to speculation that the faster mobility of the intracellular glycoprotein is a reflection of incomplete glycosylation (Printz and Wagner, 1971). The postulate has also been advanced unofficially for the existence of two virion glycoproteins derived by cleavage of a large intracellular glycoprotein precursor coded by the viral genome. These hypotheses await verification.

All five proteins of VS virus are synthesized throughout the cycle of infection but the amounts of each and their rates of synthesis differ for each protein (Wagner *et al.*, 1970). This lack of evidence for early and late functions suggested the absence of controls at the transcriptional level in contrast to DNA viruses. Differential rates at which each protein is synthesized may imply regulation at the translational level. No evidence could be obtained, however, for synthesis of large precursor polypeptides later cleaved into virion proteins as is the case for picornaviruses (Wagner *et al.*, 1970; Mudd and Summers, 1970).

Kang and Prevec (1971) have provided a detailed analysis of the kinetics of VS viral protein synthesis in L cells; their more extensive data support in most respects the earlier studies of Wagner *et al.* (1970). Total VS viral protein synthesis was found to reach a peak at 4 hours after high-multiplicity infection and to decline somewhat thereafter. The N protein is made earliest and continuously in the greatest amount, representing a relatively constant 40% of the total VS viral proteins synthesized throughout a 7-hour cycle of infection. On the other hand, more NS protein is synthesized early, to the extent of 30% of total proteins during the first hours, but declining to 10% later in infection. The levels of protein L are consistently quite low, but those of G and M protein were found to increase gradually throughout the cycle of infection to reach levels of 25% and 30%, respectively. However, as mentioned below, other investigators using different host cells have found much lower levels of M protein inside the infected cell.

Attempts to inhibit selectively the synthesis of specific viral proteins have thus far been unsuccessful. The sugar analogue 2-deoxy-D-glucose has been shown by Klenk *et al.* (1972) to inhibit glycosylation and biosynthesis of influenza virus glycoproteins without materially altering the synthesis of other viral components. Quite the opposite is the case with VS virus [or Newcastle disease virus (NDV)]. Scholtissek *et al.* (1974) found that 2-deoxy-D-glucose inhibits the synthesis of all VS viral proteins and RNA in cells originally grown in the presence of pyruvate, but not when the cells were grown in glucose-containing medium. In our experience 2-deoxy-D-glucose completely turned off all VS viral functions in infected cells (Wagner, unpublished data). These and other unreported studies have been disappointing because of inability to probe the important question of the role played by glycosylation in the regulation of VS viral glycoprotein synthesis. However, Moyer and Summers (1974*b*) have very recently begun an analysis of the patterns of glycosylation of VS viral glycoprotein under control of host cell glycosyl transferases of BHK cells compared with polyoma virus-transformed BHK cells; their data suggest that the sugar sequences of the VS viral glycoprotein are largely host specified.

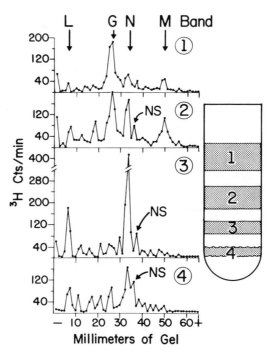

Fig. 10. Electropherograms demonstrating differential association of VS viral proteins with the membranes and other cytoplasmic components of infected L cells fractionated by equilibrium centrifugation in a discontinuous gradient of 0–60% sucrose. Electron microscopy and enzyme markers showed the following predominant composition of the light-scattering bands: 1, smooth (? plasma) membrane; 2, rough membrane; 3, viral nucleocapsids; and 4, ribosomes. Reprinted with permission from Wagner *et al.* (1972).

3.3.2. Morphogenesis

The bulk of available evidence to date strongly indicates that the two major components of the VS virion, the nucleocapsid and the envelope, are synthesized in separate cytoplasmic compartments. One experimental model for this system proposed by Wagner *et al.* (1972, 1974) is illustrated in Fig. 10, which shows that the nucleocapsid with its higher buoyant density is synthesized and assembled in the cytoplasm, whereas the viral envelope is constructed by insertion of viral proteins into pre-existing cell membranes. Assembly of the two components to make the completed VS virion presumably proceeds *pari passu* (Cohen *et al.*, 1971).

3.3.2a. Nucleocapsid

Wagner *et al.* (1970) demonstrated the presence of a sedimentable component in the cytoplasm of L cells from 2 hours after infection with VS virus. This sedimentable component contained N, L, and, although not recognized at the time, NS protein. Petric and Prevec (1970) described a similar cytoplasmic structure with sedimentation coefficients of 140 S and 100 S in cells infected with the HR strain of VS virus; these S values are identical to those of B and long T nucleocapsids, and, in addition, N was the principal protein in each. Fractionation of the cytoplasm by equilibrium centrifugation in sucrose gradients (Fig. 10) revealed by electron microscopy typical nucleocapsid coils in band 3. Pulse labeling with ^{3}H-uridine 2.5 hours post-infection demonstrated 28 S RNA as the principal species in the nucleocapsids of band 3, as would be expected for the RNA in long T nucleocapsids (Wagner *et al.*, 1972).

Morphogenesis of VS viral nucleocapsids has also been followed by electron microscopy. Zajac and Hummeler (1970) found early filamentous material which later accumulated into large nucleocapsid masses to form intracytoplasmic inclusion bodies in BHK21 cells and in 2 of 4 human cell lines. These filamentous strands were found in close proximity to budding virions; they incorporated ^{3}H-uridine and had a buoyant density in CsCl of 1.32 gm/ml. These cytoplasmic filaments in infected BHK21 cells could be specifically labeled with ferritin-conjugated VS viral antiserum and were also identified by autoradiography of incorporated ^{3}H-uridine (Zajac and Hummeler, 1971). Similar studies with Madin-Darby canine kidney cells revealed cytoplasmic filaments stained with ferritin-conjugated VS antibody within

4 hours after infection; later in infection these filaments could be seen in proximity to budding virions (Coward *et al.*, 1971). We await additional studies with ferritin-conjugated antibody directed specifically to VS viral N protein or other nucleocapsid proteins.

The process by which the newly synthesized progeny RNA and proteins are assembled into nucleocapsids is poorly understood. The existence in cytoplasm of only minute amounts of free virion RNA unassociated with nucleocapsids implies rapid protein coating of new progeny RNA strands (Kiley and Wagner, 1972; Huang, 1974). Much of the N protein can be found in a soluble form early in infection but most of it seems to be sedimentable with nucleocapsids at all later times (Wagner *et al.*, 1970; Wagner, unpublished data). No attempts have been made to follow the synthesis of L protein and its incorporation into nucleocapsids, but intracellular nucleocapsids do possess considerable transcriptase activity (Galet *et al.*, 1973) which is probably the function of the L protein (Emerson and Wagner, 1973). Both the L and NS proteins can be stripped off the nucleocapsid with high salt (Kiley and Wagner, 1972; Emerson and Wagner, 1972), indicating a much looser association with RNA than the N protein. The intracellular NS protein is always present in far greater amount as a soluble cytoplasmic component than it is as a nucleocapsid constituent (Mudd and Summers, 1970*b*; Wagner *et al.*, 1970; Cartwright, 1973).

A number of attempts have been made to determine the relationship of the soluble cytoplasmic NS protein to the nucleocapsid NS protein. One rather striking property of the VS virion NS protein is its specific phosphorylation, in contrast to rabies virus in which the N protein is preferentially phosphorylated (Sokol and Clark, 1973). Imblum and Wagner (1974) and Moyer and Summers (1974*a*) found that both the soluble and nucleocapsid-associated NS proteins of VS virus were phosphorylated in infected cells. In addition, VS virions grown in L cells, chick embryo cells, and BHK21 cells also contained an NS phosphoprotein (Imblum and Wagner, 1974). Attempts by pulse-chase experiments to establish a precursor–product relationship between the soluble and nucleocapsid NS phosphoproteins were not successful, but clearly the phosphorylation event occurs very soon after nucleocapsid maturation. No significant differences could be detected in the degree to which the soluble and nucleocapsid NS proteins are phosphorylated. Therefore, despite the great excess of cytoplasmic NS phosphoprotein, it seems likely that it assembles with the nucleocapsid very soon after it is synthesized and phosphorylated. The nature and origin of the protein kinase that phosphorylates the NS protein *in vivo* have not been ascertained, nor are data available to elucidate the role, if any, of the NS phosphoprotein in maturation of the nucleocapsid and its recognition of and assembly with the virion envelope (Imblum and Wagner, 1974; Moyer and Summers, 1974a; Wagner et al., 1974).

An intriguing experimental method for arresting morphogenesis of VS nucleocapsids has been reported by Fiszman et al. (1974). These investigators found that infected L cells produced 90% lower yields of infectious VS virions at pH 6.9 and none at all at pH 6.6 in comparison to yields at physiological pH 7.4. Relatively normal amounts of viral RNA and protein were synthesized in the lower-pH environments. The primary defect noted at pH 6.6 was failure of incorporation of N protein into nucleocapsids despite relatively normal synthesis of 42 S virion RNA in infected cells. Incubation of infected cells at pH 6.9, however, resulted in relatively normal yields of virions and nucleocapsids but in each case the infectivity of these virions and nucleocapsids was only 10% that of virions and nucleocapsids produced by infected cells at pH 7.4. The defect in these virions and nucleocapsids turned out to be in their transcriptive function, which was considerably reduced both *in vivo* and *in vitro*. These experiments, if confirmed, would appear to provide an important probe for investigating the assembly and function of VS viral nucleocapsids.

3.3.2b. Envelope

Several laboratories have obtained conclusive evidence that the G and M proteins synthesized in cells infected with VS virus are rapidly inserted into cytoplasmic membranes. In fact, very little glycoprotein G or matrix protein M is found in a nonsedimentable fraction of infected cells, but both proteins are almost completely pelleted by centrifugation at 130,000g at each stage of infection. Exposure of infected cells to the membrane-dissolving agent, digitonin, results in complete solubilization of protein M and most of protein G (Wagner et al., 1970; Wagner and Schnaitman, 1970). More conclusive evidence that newly synthesized viral proteins G and M are rapidly inserted into smooth membrane, probably plasma membrane, was obtained by Cohen et al. (1971). These investigators found both envelope proteins associated with plasma membrane after a 5-minute pulse of ^{14}C-amino acids. The plasma membrane content of G and M proteins did not increase greatly with successive chases up to 60 minutes but the N protein did. Later experiments on affinity *in vitro* of M protein for eryth-

rocyte and infected HeLa-cell membranes are not convincing because the M protein was probably complexed with lipid (Cohen and
Summers, 1974).

The kinetics of envelope protein incorporation into the plasma
membrane of HeLa cells was studied by David (1973). He found G and
M proteins associated with a putative plasma-membrane fraction after
a 30-second pulse, and their insertion was essentially maximal in 2
minutes. Neither puromycin nor amino acid analogues added at the
end of a 30-second pulse affected membrane incorporation of G and M
proteins during subsequent chases. From these data David (1973) concluded that completed G and M polypeptide chains form small cytoplasmic pools from which they are rapidly inserted into the plasma
membrane. These pools have never been demonstrated *per se,* which
suggests the alternative hypothesis that G and M proteins are
synthesized at and inserted directly into the plasma membrane.

Wagner *et al.* (1972) also found G and M protein in smooth
membrane fractions of cells infected with VS virus (Fig. 10). Based on
electron microscopy and distribution of enzyme markers, the G protein
was determined to be the major viral component of a cell fraction
designated plasma membrane. Another criterion for insertion of newly
synthesized G protein into plasma membrane was membrane antigenic
conversion as determined by specific ferritin labeling with anti-G
serum (Wagner *et al.,* 1971). Much less M protein than G protein
could be found in smooth membranes of infected L cells, a finding
consistent with the total absence of M protein in infected BHK21 cells
(Cartwright, 1973). The hypothesis proposed by Cartwright that
insertion of the M protein is the rate-limiting step, particularly in the
highly permissive BHK cell, is supported by the data of Cohen *et al.*
(1971) and David (1973) which reveal no significant increase in M (or
G) protein on further incubation. Moreover, Kang and Prevec (1971)
showed a marked turnover of protein M during the cycle of infection,
compared with the steady intracellular accumulation of all other viral
proteins. These data indicate the likelihood of greater efficiency of incorporation of protein M into the budding virion, whereas most of the
other viral proteins are made in excess and are wasted by not being incorporated into completed virions.

The rate at which newly synthesized viral proteins are incorporated into virions was also measured by Wagner *et al.* (1970) and by
Kang and Prevec (1971). L cells infected for 2.5 or 3 hours with VS
virus were pulse labeled with ^{3}H- or ^{14}C-amino acids for 30 minutes
and released virions collected after chasing for 1, 2, and 3 hours. The

results showed a roughly linear increase of N protein incorporated into released virions. Intracellular G protein was also incorporated into released virions almost linearly. In sharp contrast, the M protein represented about 50% of the total amino acid label incorporated into released virions during a 30-minute pulse, but this level declined approximately linearly to a level of 18% at the 3-hour chase. This evidence supports our contention and that of Cartwright (1973) that synthesis of M protein may be the final step in virus maturation, and the rate-limiting event in virion assembly and budding. Lazarowitz *et al.* (1971) had advanced a similar proposal for the function of the M protein of influenza virus.

3.3.3. Maturation

3.3.3a. Envelopment of Nucleocapsids

A gap in our knowledge concerning reproduction of rhabdoviruses is how the two newly synthesized subviral components are assembled and released from the infected cell. Envelopment of the nucleocapsid by the converted cell membrane probably takes more time than separate morphogenesis of nucleocapsid and envelope. Cohen *et al.* (1971) have demonstrated almost instantaneous association of M protein with plasma membrane of HeLa cells. However, they also found that no N protein is present in infected-cell plasma membrane after a 5-minute pulse and, in fact, the N protein is barely detectable after a 20-minute chase and increases slowly thereafter. Wagner *et al.* (1972) could find no virion RNA associated with infected-cell plasma membranes after a 10-minute pulse of ^{3}H-uridine, and they found only a comparatively small amount after 90 minutes of labeling. Presumably, therefore, the progeny RNA and nucleocapsid proteins are not directly inserted into virus-converted plasma membrane, and only completed nucleocapsids attach to viral envelope.

No data are available on how the newly assembled nucleocapsid recognizes the inner surface of the plasma membrane that has been converted to viral envelope by insertion of G and M proteins. McSharry *et al.* (1971) and Cartwright *et al.* (1972) have proposed that the M protein provides the recognition site for nucleocapsid attachment to the inner surface of the plasma membrane. Wagner *et al.* (1974) entertained the possibility that the NS protein could be the component that serves to bind the nucleocapsid to the viral membrane.

3.3.3b.   Sites of Envelopment

The tacit assumption that the rhabdoviral nucleocapsid is always enveloped at and buds from the outer cytoplasmic membrane has been challenged by a number of electron microscopists. Hackett *et al.* (1968) found predominant maturation of VS-New Jersey virus at intracytoplasmic vacuoles of chick embryo cells or of the PK(H13) line of pig kidney cells. David-West and Labzoffsky (1968) found maturation and budding of VS virus both from the outer plasma membrane and into cytoplasmic vacuoles of chick embryo cells. Some of the controversy was settled by Zee *et al.* (1970), who examined 100 cells each of 5 different types and found that VS-New Jersey virus was assembled principally in intracytoplasmic membrane vacuoles of PK(H13) cells but almost entirely at the outer plasma membrane of L and Vero cells; assembly and budding at both intracytoplasmic and external membranes were found in infected HeLa and BHK21 cells. It seems quite obvious, therefore, that the sites of maturation of VS virus are cell dependent to a considerable extent. The virus type is obviously also important in determining the site of maturation. The three rhabdoviruses, Navarro, Kwatta, and Mossuril, appear to prefer budding from intracytoplasmic membrane of Vero cells and mouse brain (Karabatsos *et al.*, 1973). Rabies virus matures and accumulates in cytoplasm of BHK21 cells but also buds to some extent from the outer plasma membrane (Hummeler *et al.*, 1967). Three salmonid rhabdoviruses, all identical in morphology and size to VS virus, specifically mature at and bud from the outer plasma membrane of fathead minnow cells (Darlington *et al.*, 1972).

Infection by plant rhabdoviruses has been studied primarily by electron microscopy of host plants and insect vectors. The cycle of development of sowthistle yellow vein virus in aphids has been reported in detail by Sylvester and Richardson (1970). Of some interest is their observation that this rhabdovirus is assembled in the nucleus and passes by stages into perinuclear cisternae, which disintegrate to release virions into the cytoplasm. The presence of rabies virus in perinuclear space should also be noted in this regard (Hummeler, *et al.*, 1967).

All these studies must be considered only as preliminary information on cellular localization of rhabdoviral maturation because of the limitations and vagaries of electron microscopy. Genetic and biochemical studies may help to resolve the question of preferred sites for morphogenesis and budding.

3.3.3c. Translation and Assembly Mutants

Studies of RNA$^+$ *ts* mutants have met with even less success than those of RNA$^-$ *ts* mutants restricted in transcription and replication. In principle, only group I mutants defective in transcription at nonpermissive temperature should be incapable of synthesizing viral proteins because of failure to transcribe messengers. This was the experience of Printz and Wagner (1971), who reported marked deficiency in protein synthesis only with group I mutant *ts* O5 and not to the same extent with mutants representing groups II, III, and V. Wunner and Pringle (1972*b*) also found that Glasgow *ts* mutants in complementation group I were restricted in protein synthesis in BHK21 cells, as were RNA$^-$ mutants of group IV as well as one of two group II mutants. Similar results were obtained with VS-New Jersey mutants (Wunner and Pringle, 1972*c*). In contrast, Perlman and Huang (1974) failed to detect any significant differences in protein components synthesized by group I mutant *ts* G114 or group IV mutant *ts* G41 at 31°C and 37°C. However, Combard *et al.* (1974) found significant reduction in synthesis of N protein at 39°C by RNA$^-$ group IV mutants, a result confirmed by Wagner (unpublished data). The discrepancies in these results cannot be explained. The recently published data of Obijeski and Simpson (1974) on host-restricted mutants are not readily amenable to comparative analysis.

RNA$^+$ mutants should exhibit no restriction in synthesis of viral proteins because they presumably are not defective in either primary or secondary transcription. However, certain observations have been made with RNA$^+$ mutants which, if confirmed, might indicate faulty function of a specific protein or deficiency in its incorporation into subviral components, leading, in either case, to arrested assembly or a defectively assembled virion. Printz and Wagner (1971) reported that the group II mutant *ts* O52 appeared to synthesize a glycoprotein precursor which failed to be glycosylated at restrictive temperature, and could not, therefore, be inserted into cell membrane. No viral antigen was detected on the cell surface and no mature virions could be visualized. These experiments have not been repeated successfully nor have other mutants been found to be arrested in maturation because of a defective glycoprotein. Moreover, Flamand and Lafay (1973) have described partial defectiveness in RNA synthesis of *ts* mutants O52 and O63 which, of course, may not be the primary lesion. Of potential interest, however, is the report that VS-New Jersey virus mutant *ts* D1 at restrictive temperature synthesizes G and N proteins that migrate faster on polyacrylamide gels than do G and N proteins of ts^+ VS-New Jersey virus (Pringle and Wunner, 1974).

An RNA^+ group III mutant, ts O23 also merits some attention because of low levels of protein synthesis at nonpermissive temperature and complete failure to detect intracellular M protein (Printz and Wagner, 1971). This observation could, of course, be fortuitous because of inherent difficulties in detecting M protein even in productively infected cells (Cartwright, 1973). However, some confirmation of this observation comes from the experiments of Lafay (1971), who reported reduced incorporation of M protein into ts O23 virions released after infected cells labeled at restrictive temperature were shifted down to the permissive temperature. These findings, if confirmed, would be evidence of maturation arrest of mutants blocked at the level of translation due to inability to insert M protein into membrane. However, Wunner and Pringle (1972b) did not detect restriction of M protein in 2 Glasgow group III mutants.

A faulty envelope may be responsible for low infectivity of mutant ts O45 of complementation group V. Deutsch and Berkaloff (1971) have shown that the virion envelope of this thermolabile mutant breaks down at 40°C, thus releasing morphologically intact nucleocapsids. F. Lafay (*J. Virol.*, in press) has recently found that group V ts mutants show restricted insertion of G protein into cell membrane, resulting in maturation arrest.

None of these experiments has gone far enough to pinpoint specific lesions responsible for defective assembly. Much more sophisticated techniques are required before the mutants of rhabdoviruses can be exploited to probe important physiological questions of virus assembly.

3.3.3d.   Mixed Phenotypes and Pseudotypes

An important clue to the role of the envelope in maturation of VS virions was provided by an intriguing discovery of Choppin and Compans (1970). When cells persistently infected with the paramyxovirus simian virus 5 (SV5) are superinfected with VS virus, they give rise to three kinds of progeny: SV5, VS virus, and a phenotypic mixture of VS virus and SV5. Of the total yield of virions released by these doubly infected cells, 10–45% were hybrid particles, most of which were bullet-shaped but adsorbed to chicken erythrocytes in the manner of SV5. About 2% of these virions were neutralized only by SV5 antiserum (pseudotypes), but the infectivity of most was neutralized by both SV5 and VS viral antiserum. Specific labeling of bullet-shaped VS virions could be demonstrated with ferritin-labeled SV5 antiserum. McSharry *et al.* (1971) were then able to demonstrate that these phenotypically mixed VS virions contained both SV5 glycoproteins as well as the VS viral glycoprotein, but no SV5 M or nucleocapsid proteins could be detected in the VS viral mixed phenotypes. These phenotypic mixtures of SV5–VS virus hybrids or VSV(SV5) pseudotypes gave rise only to VS virus on passage in the absence of SV5, providing proof for retention of a VS viral genotype. These data indicate that other viral glycoproteins can substitute for VS viral G protein to make a functional envelope with spikes.

These observations have been extended by finding other VS viral mixed phenotypes and pseudotypes. Závada and Rosenbergová (1972) were able to produce mixed populations of VS virus and influenza fowl plague virus (FPV) in which approximately 20% of virions were neutralized only by anti-FPV serum. Mixed VSV(FPV) phenotypes could also be produced *in vitro* by combining disrupted fowl plague virions with intact VS virions. Mixed phenotypes produced *in vivo* or *in vitro* exhibited the thermal stability of FPV more closely than that of VS virus.

Závada (1972*a,b*) has also produced an extremely interesting group of pseudotypes of VS virion with the envelope of murine leukemia virus (MLV) or of avian myeloblastosis virus (AMV). A considerable proportion of these virions of pseudotype VSV(MLV) and VSV(AMV) were resistant to neutralization by VS viral antiserum and exhibited the host range specificity and interference properties of the leukosis virus which donated the envelope. Cells infected with these viruses gave rise only to progeny VS virions, indicating that the genetic characteristic is purely rhabdoviral.

Another interesting finding was the capacity of avian myeloblastosis virus to complement the group V VS virus mutant *ts* O45, but not *ts* mutants of groups I and III. Cells previously infected with AMV were able to support the production at restrictive temperature of *ts* O45 virions (Závada, 1972*a,b*). The leukosis virus not only serves as helper for growth of *ts* O45 VS virus but also gives rise to a pseudotype virion at permissive temperature that exhibits the thermostability of wild-type VS virus rather than that of the thermolabile mutant *ts* O45 (Deutsch and Berkaloff, 1971). The thermostable pseudotype is neutralized by AMV antiserum but not by VS virus antiserum. Závada (1972*b*) also isolated thermolabile mutants by selection of VS virus grown in the presence of specific VS virus antiserum. These mutants were rapidly heat inactivated but could form VSV(AMV) pseudotypes which were heat stable and were neutralized by AMV antiserum. Závada *et al.* (1972) also produced a pseudotype of VS virus by growth in a human mammary carcinoma cell line (MaTu). A small fraction of these VSV(MaTu) pseudotype virions resisted neutralization by anti-VSV-serum; these human tumor VSV pseudotypes also exhibited strict host specificity for growth in human diploid cells and would not infect hamster, chick, or mouse cells.

Huang *et al.* (1973) confirmed the results of Závada and his colleagues by constructing a VSV(M-MuLV) pseudotype by growing VS virus in a BALB/c murine cell line which is a producer of Moloney murine leukemia virus. The ability of this pseudotype with N-tropic MuLV coat to grow in cells resistant to N-tropic and B-tropic viruses is an intracellular, not a surface, function under genetic control of the host cell. More recent exploitation of this technique has been accomplished by Love and Weiss (1974) with avian RNA tumor virus and by Huang *et al.* (personal communication) with herpes virus membrane glycoproteins.

3.4. Cellular Reactions to Infection

3.4.1. Cytotoxicity

Virulent animal viruses cause cytopathic effects that are often preceded by inhibition of cellular macromolecular synthesis. Two types of viral cytopathology have been identified: (1) a rapid cellular response which may not require active virus replication and has been likened to a toxic reaction, and (2) a much later reaction of the infected cell in response to active replication of the virus, usually accompanied by production of progeny virions. Both of these cytopathic effects can be produced by infection with VS virus.

Probably the first observation of the cytotoxic activity of VS virus was made by Cantell *et al.* (1962), who showed that large doses of UV-irradiated VS virus could kill L cells even if interference had been previously induced by Newcastle disease virus. This observation was extended by Huang and Wagner (1965), who demonstrated that infection with nonreplicating VS virus at high multiplicity rapidly switched off RNA synthesis of Krebs-2 ascites cells. This 80–90% inhibition of cellular RNA synthesis occurred under conditions in which viral functions were suppressed and no progeny virions were being produced. This cytotoxic effect was evident with heavily UV-irradiated virus, under conditions in which viral protein synthesis was blocked with puromycin (Huang and Wagner, 1965), and when cells were infected with defective T virions (Huang *et al.*, 1966). This inhibition of cellular RNA synthesis by VS virus also results in failure of the cells to synthesize interferon (Wagner and Huang, 1966). It was tempting to speculate that this cytotoxic effect of VS virus is caused by marked perturbation of membrane function.

These experiments were repeated by Yaoi *et al.* (1970), who found that at multiplicities of approximately 500 PFU/cell both infective and UV-inactivated VS-New Jersey virus rapidly switched off RNA synthesis in chick embryo cells. DNA and protein synthesis were also inhibited, though to a lesser extent, and no increased degradation of cellular nucleic acids was noted. A subsequent series of papers (Yaoi and Amano, 1970; Yaoi and Ogata, 1972) purport to show that DNA synthesis and cell division were inhibited by UV-inactivated VS-New Jersey virus infection of partially synchronized chick embryo cells in the G phase, but not when they entered the S phase of the growth cycle. A high proportion of mitotic figures in late telophase was taken as evidence for selective inhibition of G1 functions in Vero cells infected with VS virus (Osunkoya and David-West, 1972). Doyle and Holland (1973) were able to show similar but less striking effects of highly purified T virions on RNA and protein synthesis of BHK cells. Marcus and Sekellick (1974) have recently reported single-cell killing by non-plaque-forming as well as by plaque-forming B virions but not T virions of VS virus; they postulate that the virion *per se* is not toxic but that cytopathogenicity may require virion-associated transcription. The validity of this hypothesis may be implicit in recent findings by McAllister and Wagner (ms. in preparation) that transcription-restricted group I *ts* mutants of VS virus fail to switch off L-cell protein synthesis at nonpermissive temperature.

Wertz and Youngner (1970) tested wild-type VS virus (L_1) and a small-plague variant (S_2) for their effect on macromolecular synthesis and interferon production in different cells. Shutoff of macromolecular synthesis was found to be the critical factor in induction of interferon synthesis. Little difference could be detected in the capacity of L_1 VS and S_2 VS viruses to switch off L-cell protein synthesis which was, in any case, highly multiplicity dependent. Farmilo and Stanners (1972) also found that the HR strain of VS-Indiana virus at an input multiplicity of approximately 20 PFU/cell could switch off DNA synthesis in serum-stimulated primary hamster embryo cell cultures. Cellular proliferation was impeded by wild-type virus and mutant *ts* 54 but not by *ts* 1026.

VS virus also shuts off cellular protein synthesis, as well as cellular RNA synthesis, in primary rabbit kidney cells (Yamazaki and Wagner, 1970). These effects are also rapid and multiplicity dependent.

This inhibition by VS virus of cellular protein synthesis is completely unaffected by potent interferon, which is capable of blocking all detectable synthesis of VS viral proteins in the same cells. These results clearly demonstrate that VS viral protein synthesis, possibly including VS viral transcription which should also be blocked by interferon (Marcus *et al.,* 1971; Manders *et al.,* 1972), is not required for the cytotoxic action of the virus on cellular macromolecular synthesis.

McSharry and Choppin (personal communication) have examined macromolecular synthesis of BHK21 cells exposed to VS viral G protein isolated and purified by extraction with Triton X-100 and precipitation with butanol. The G protein alone causes moderate reduction in cellular RNA and DNA synthesis, more slowly than is the case with whole virions. Cellular protein synthesis is less well inhibited, if at all, by G protein. Specific anti-G serum reverses the inhibition of cellular RNA and DNA synthesis, and virions rendered spikeless by proteolytic enzyme have no detectable effect on cell functions. Although more data are required, these results of McSharry and Choppin strongly suggest that the G-protein spikes are responsible for the cytotoxic effect of VS virions on cellular macromolecular synthesis.

3.4.2. Late Effects of VS Viral Infection

Wertz and Youngner (1972) have provided evidence that host cell protein synthesis can be shut off late in infection as well as by "initial" inhibition soon after high-multiplicity infection. Experiments by reversal of cycloheximide inhibition and with UV-irradiated virus seem to indicate that VS viral protein synthesis is required for later, progressive inhibition of cellular protein synthesis. This effect was presumed not to be due to primary transcription of input virions, which was also blocked by pretreatment of host cells with cycloheximide. Late functions of the virus presumably explain the failure of mouse L cells infected with VS virus to regenerate H2 histocompatability antigen (Hecht and Summers, 1972). More experiments are required to implicate specific viral functions that inhibit macromolecular synthesis of the host cell, but the available data implicate two mechanisms, the cytotoxic action of input virions and the later expression of viral functions in the infected cell.

3.5. Inhibition of Growth

VS virus has been a favorite target for studies of viral chemotherapy for many reasons, among them: rapid growth of the virus, distinctive morphology, wide spectrum of cellular susceptibility, and reliable quantitative assays. Therefore, the literature on antiviral agents for this virus is voluminous; future volumes will deal with physical and chemical agents that inactivate the virus or inhibit its growth in cells. Only a few examples with very limited documentation can be cited here.

Growth of VS virus is quite susceptible to interferon, and this system has served as a model for many studies of interferon action. VS viral protein synthesis is effectively blocked in interferon-treated cells (Yamazaki and Wagner, 1970), but this inhibition is likely to be a secondary effect. Marcus *et al.* (1971) and Manders *et al.* (1972) showed that primary transcription of VS virus is inhibited in interferon-treated cells even when protein synthesis is blocked with cycloheximide. This effect of interferon on transcription, the primary event in VS viral infection, is not easy to reconcile with the observations that translation of viral mRNA *in vitro* is effectively inhibited on ribosomes from interferon-treated cells (Kerr *et al.*, 1974; Samuel and Joklik, 1974). In fact, very recent data by Repik *et al.* (1974) support an interpretation that interferon does not act at the level of primary transcription but at a step intermediate between primary and secondary transcription, possibly translation.

Three other putative inhibitors of VS viral growth may provide interesting probes for dissecting the stages of replication. One is poliovirus, which effectively shuts off VS viral protein synthesis in HeLa cells without affecting viral RNA synthesis (Doyle and Holland, 1972). This effect of poliovirus late in the cycle of VS viral replication is almost undoubtedly due to disruption of polyribosomes. Another compound that may turn out to be of some importance is chloroquine, which inhibits VS viral growth in chick embryo cells, probably by affecting viral RNA synthesis (Shimizu *et al.*, 1970). It has also been reported that rifampicin reversibly inhibits multiplication of VS virus in L cells (Moreau, 1972).

ACKNOWLEDGMENTS

I am grateful to Suzanne U. Emerson and Purnell W. Choppin for their thoughtful and critical review of the manuscript. Preprints and other materials have been graciously contributed by many colleagues, among them: Alice S. Huang, David H. L. Bishop, Ludwik Prevec, Frederick A. Murphy, Robert E. Shope, John F. Obijeski, Donald F. Summers, and James J. McSharry.

4. REFERENCES

Aaslestad, H. G., and Urbano, C., 1971, Nucleotide composition of the RNA of rabies virus, *J. Virol.* **8**, 922.

Aaslestad, H. G., Clark, H. F., Bishop, D. H. L., and Koprowski, H., 1971, Comparison of the ribonucleic acid polymerase of two rhabdoviruses, Kern Canyon virus and vesicular stomatitis virus, *J. Virol.* **7**, 726.

Ahmed, M. E., Block, L. M., Perkins, E. G., Walker, B. L., and Kummerviv, F. A., 1964, Lipids in potato yellow dwarf virus, *Biochem. Biophys. Res. Commun.* **17**, 103.

Almeida, J. D., Waterson, A. P., and Simpson, D. I. H., 1971, Morphology and morphogenesis of the Marburg agent, *in* "Marburg Virus Disease" (G. A. Martini and R. Siegert, eds.), pp. 84–97, Springer-Verlag, Berlin.

Amend, D. F., and Chambers, V. C., 1970, Morphology of certain viruses of salmonid fishes. I. *In vitro* studies of some viruses causing hematopoietic necrosis, *J. Fish. Res. Bd. Can.* **27**, 1285.

Arstila, P., 1972, Two hemagglutinating components of vesicular stomatitis virus, *Acta Pathol. Microbiol. Scand. (B)* **80**, 33.

Arstila, P., 1973, Small-sized hemagglutinin of vesicular stomatitis virus released spontaneously and with Nonidet P_{40}, *Acta Pathol. Microbiol. Scand. (B)* **81**, 27.

Arstila, P., Halonen, P. E., and Salmi, A., 1969, Hemagglutinin of vesicular stomatitis virus, *Arch. Ges. Virusforsch.* **27**, 198.

Baer, G. M., ed., 1973, "The Natural History of Rabies," Academic Press, New York.

Baltimore, D., 1971, Expression of animal virus genomes, *Bacteriol. Rev.* **35**, 235.

Baltimore, D., Huang, A. S., and Stampfer, M., 1970, Ribonucleic acid synthesis of vesicular stomatitis virus. II. An RNA polymerase in the virion, *Proc. Natl. Acad. Sci. USA* **66**, 572.

Banerjee, A. K., and Rhodes, D. P., 1973, *In vitro* synthesis of RNA that contains polyadenylate by virion-associated RNA polymerase of vesicular stomatitis virus, *Proc. Natl. Acad. Sci. USA* **70**, 3566.

Bates, S. R., and Rothblat, G. H., 1972, Incorporation of L cell sterols into vesicular stomatitis virus, *J. Virol.* **9**, 883.

Bergold, G. H., and Munz, K., 1970, Characterization of Piry virus, *Arch. Ges. Virusforsch.* **31**, 152.

Berkaloff, A., Bregliano, J. C., and Ohanessian, A., 1965, Mise en évidence de virions dans des drosophiles infectées par le héréditaire sigma, *C. R. Acad. Sci. Hebd. Seances Ser. D Sci. Nat.* **260**, 5956.

Bishop, D. H. L., 1971, Complete transcription by the transcriptase of vesicular stomatitis virus, *J. Virol.* **7**, 486.

Bishop, D. H. L., and Flamand, A., 1974, The transcription of VSV and its mutants *in vivo* and *in vitro in* "Negative Strand Viruses" (R. D. Barry and B. W. J. Mahy, eds.), Academic Press, London.

Bishop, D. H. L., and Roy, P., 1971*a*, Kinetics of RNA synthesis by vesicular stomatitis virus particles, *J. Mol. Biol.* **57**, 513.

Bishop, D. H. L., and Roy, P., 1971*b*, Properties of the product synthesized by vesicular stomatitis virus particles, *J. Mol. Biol.* **58**, 799.

Bishop, D. H. L., and Roy, P., 1972, Dissociation of vesicular stomatitis virus and relation of the virion proteins to the viral transcriptase, *J. Virol.* **10**, 234.

Bishop, D. H. L., Obijeski, J. F., and Simpson, R. W., 1971, Transcription of the influenza ribonucleic acid genome by a virion polymerase, *J. Virol.* **8**, 66.

Bishop, D. H. L., Repik, P., Roy, P., Flamand, A., and Obijeski, J. F., 1974*a*, Evidence for sequence homology and genome size of rhabdovirus RNAs, *in* "Negative Strand Viruses" (R. D. Barry and B. W. J. Mahy, eds.), Academic Press, London.

Bishop, D. H. L., Emerson, S. V., and Flamand, A., 1974*b*, Reconstitution of infectivity and transcriptase activity of homologous and heterologous viruses: Vesicular stomatitis (Indiana serotype), and Chandipura, vesicular stomatitis (New Jersey serotype) and Cocal viruses, *J. Virol.* **14**, 139.

Blough, H. A., and Tiffany, J. M., 1973, Lipids in viruses, *Adv. Lipid Res.* **11**, 267.

Bradish, C. J., and Kirkham, J. B., 1966, The morphology of vesicular stomatitis virus (Indiana C) derived from chick embryos or cultures of BHK 21/13 cells, *J. Gen. Microbiol.* **44**, 359.

Bradish, C. J., Brookbsy, J. B., and Dillon, J. F., 1956, Biophysical studies of the virus system of vesicular stomatitis, *J. Gen. Microbiol.* **14**, 290.

Brown, F., and Cartwright, B., 1966, The antigens of vesicular stomatitis virus. II. The presence of two low-molecular-weight immunogens in virus suspensions, *J. Immunol.* **97**, 612.

Brown, F., Cartwright, B., and Almeida, J. D., 1966, The antigens of vesicular stomatitis virus. I. Separation of immunogenicity for three complement-fixing components, *J. Immunol.* **96**, 537.

Brown, F., Cartwright, B., and Smale, C. J., 1967*a*, The antigens of vesicular stomatitis virus. III. Structure and immunogenicity of antigens derived from the virion with Tween and ether, *J. Immunol.* **99**, 171.

Brown, F., Cartwright, B., Crick, J., and Smale, C. J., 1967*b*, Infective virus substructure from vesicular stomatitis virus, *J. Virol.* **1**, 368.

Brown, F., Martin, S., Cartwright, B., and Crick, J., 1967*c*, The ribonucleic acids of the infective and interfering components of vesicular stomatitis virus, *J. Gen. Virol.* **1**, 479.

Brown, F., Smale, C. J., and Horzinek, M. C., 1974, Lipid and protein organization in vesicular stomatitis and Sindbis viruses, *J. Gen. Virol.* **22**, 455.

Buckley, S. M., 1969, Susceptibility of the *Aedes albopictus* and *A. aegypti* cell lines to infection with arboviruses, *Proc. Soc. Exp. Biol. Med.* **131**, 625.

Bukrinskaya, A. G., 1973, Nucleocapsids of large RNA viruses as functionally active units in transcription, *Adv. Virus Res.* **18**, 195.

Burge, B. W., and Huang, A. S., 1970, Comparison of membrane protein glycopeptides of Sindbis virus and vesicular stomatitis virus, *J. Virol.* **6**, 176.

Cairns, J. E., Holloway, A. F., and Cormack, D. V., 1972, Temperature-sensitive mutants of vesicular stomatitis virus: *In vitro* studies of virion-associated polymerase, *J. Virol.* **10**, 1130.

Cantell, K., Skurska, Z., Paucker, K., and Henle, W., 1962, Quantitative studies on viral interference in suspended L cells. II. Factors affecting interference by UV-irradiated Newcastle disease virus against vesicular stomatitis virus, *Virology* **17**, 312.

Cartwright, B., 1973, The distribution of virus proteins in BHK 21 cells infected with vesicular stomatitis virus, *J. Gen. Virol.* **21**, 407.

Cartwright, B., and Brown, F., 1972*a*, Glycolipid nature of the complement-fixing host cell antigen of vesicular stomatitis virus, *J. Gen. Virol.* **15**, 243.

Cartwright, B., and Brown, F., 1972*b*, Serological relationship between different strains of vesicular stomatitis virus, *J. Gen. Virol.* **16**, 391.

Cartwright, B., and Pearce, C. A., 1968, Evidence for a host cell component in vesicular stomatitis virus, *J. Gen. Virol.* **2**, 207.

Cartwright, B., Smale, C. J., and Brown, F., 1969, Surface structure of vesicular stomatitis virus, *J. Gen. Virol.* **5**, 1.

Cartwright, B., Smale, C. J., and Brown, F., 1970*a*, Dissection of vesicular stomatitis virus into infective ribonucleoprotein and immunizing components, *J. Gen. Virol.* **7**, 19.

Cartwright, B., Talbot, P., and Brown, F., 1970*b*, The proteins of biologically active subunits of vesicular stomatitis virus, *J. Gen. Virol.* **7**, 267.

Cartwright, B., Smale, C. J., Brown, F., and Hull, R., 1972, A model for vesicular stomatitis virus, *J. Virol.* **10**, 256.

Chang, S. H., Hefti, E., Obijeski, J. F., and Bishop, D. H. L., 1974, RNA transcription by the virion polymerase of five rhabdoviruses, *J. Virol.* **13**, 652.

Choppin, P. W., and Compans, R. W., 1970, Phenotypic mixing of envelope proteins of the parainfluenza virus SV5 and vesicular stomatitis virus, *J. Virol.* **5**, 609.

Chow, T. L., Chow, F. H., and Hanson, R. P., 1954, Morphology of vesicular stomatitis virus, *J. Bacteriol.* **68**, 724.

Clark, H. F., and Koprowski, H., 1971, Isolation of temperature-sensitive conditional lethal mutants of "fixed" rabies virus, *J. Virol.* **7**, 295.

Clark, H. R., and Soriano, E. Z., 1974, Fish rhabdovirus replication in cell culture: new system for the study of rhabdovirus-cell interaction in which the virus and cell have different temperature optima, *Infect. Immunity* **10**, 180.

Cohen, G. H., and Summers, D. F., 1974, *In vitro* association of vesicular stomatitis virus proteins with purified HeLa and erythrocyte plasma membranes, *Virology* **57**, 566.

Cohen, G. H., Atkinson, P. H., and Summers, D. F., 1971, Interactions of vesicular stomatitis virus structural proteins with HeLa plasma membrane, *Nat. New Biol.* **231**, 121.

Combard, A., Martinet, C., Printz-Ané, C., Friedman, A., and Printz, P., 1974, Transcription and replication of vesicular stomatitis virus: Effects of temperature-sensitive mutations in complementation group IV, *J. Virol.* **13**:922.

Cooper, P. D., and Bellett, A. J. D., 1959, A transmissible interfering component of vesicular stomatitis virus preparations, *J. Gen. Microbiol.* **21**, 485.

Cormack, D. V., Holloway, A. F., Wong, P. K. Y., and Cairns, J. D., 1971, Temperature-sensitive mutants of vesicular stomatitis virus. II. Evidence of defective polymerase, *Virology* **45**, 824.

Cormack, D. V., Holloway, A. F., and Pringle, C. R., 1973, Temperature-sensitive mutants of vesicular stomatitis virus: Homology and nomenclature, *J. Gen. Virol.* **19**, 295.

Coward, J. E., Harter, D. H., Hsu, K. C., and Morgan, C., 1971, Electron microscopic study of development of vesicular stomatitis virus using ferritin-labeled antibodies, *J. Gen. Virol.* **13**, 27.

Crick, J., and Brown, F., 1973, Interference as a measure of cross-relationship in the vesicular stomatitis group of rhabdoviruses, *J. Gen. Virol.* **18**, 79.

Crick, J., and Brown, F., 1974, An interfering component of rabies virus which contains RNA, *J. Gen. Virol.* **22**, 147.

Crick, J., Cartwright, B., and Brown, F., 1966, Interfering component of vesicular stomatitis virus, *Nature (Lond.)* **211**, 1204.

Crick, J., Cartwright, B., and Brown, F., 1969, A study of the interference phenomenon in vesicular stomatitis replication, *Arch. Ges. Virusforsch.* **27**, 221.

Danglot, C., Vilagines, R., de Teinmerum, N., and Pascu, A., 1973, Etude de l'activité protein-kinase associée au virus de la stomatite vésiculaire (VSV), *C. R. Acad. Sci. Hebd. Seances Ser. D Sci. Nat.* **276**, 2749.

Darlington, R. W., Trafford, R., and Wolk, K., 1972, Fish rhabdoviruses: Morphology and ultrastructure of North American salmonid isolates, *Arch. Ges. Virusforsch.* **39**, 257.

David, A. E., 1973, Assembly of the vesicular stomatitis virus envelope: Incorporation of viral polypeptides into the host plasma membrane, *J. Mol. Biol.* **76**, 135.

David-West, T. S., and Labzoffsky, N. A., 1968, Electron microscopic studies in the development of vesicular stomatitis virus, *Arch. Ges. Virusforsch.* **23**, 105.

Deutsch, V., and Berkaloff, A., 1971, Analyse d'un mutant thermolabile du virus de la stomatite vésiculaire (VSV), *Ann. Inst. Pasteur (Paris)* **121**, 101.

Dietzschold, B., Schneider, L. G., and Cox, J. H., 1974, Serological characterization of the three major proteins of vesicular stomatitis virus, *J. Virol.* **14**, 1.

Doyle, M., and Holland, J. J., 1972, Virus-induced interference in heterologously infected HeLa cells, *J. Virol.* **9**, 22.

Doyle, M., and Holland, J. J., 1973, Prophylaxis and immunization in mice by virus-free defective T particles to protect against intracerebral infection by vesicular stomatitis virus, *Proc. Natl. Acad. Sci. USA* **70**, 2105.

Edelman, R., and Wheelock, E. F., 1968, Specific role for each human leukocyte type in viral infection. II. Phytohemagglutinin-treated lymphocytes as host cells for vesicular stomatitis virus, *J. Virol.* **2**, 440.

Ehrenfeld, E., 1974, Polyadenylation of vesicular stomatitis virus messenger RNA, *J. Virol.* **13**:1055.

Ehrenfeld, E., and Summers, D. F., 1972, Adenylate-rich sequences in vesicular stomatitis virus messenger ribonucleic acid, *J. Virol.* **10**, 683.

Emerson, S. U., and Wagner, R. R., 1972, Dissociation and reconstitution of the transcriptase and template activities of vesicular stomatitis B and T virions, *J. Virol.* **10**, 297.

Emerson, S. U., and Wagner, R. R., 1973, L protein requirement for *in vitro* RNA synthesis by vesicular stomatitis virus, *J. Virol.* **12**, 1325.

Farmilo, A. V., and Stanners, C. P., 1972, Mutant of vesicular stomatitis virus which allows DNA synthesis and division of cells synthesizing viral RNA, *J. Virol.* **10**, 605.

Federer, K. B., Burrows, R., and Brooksby, J. B., 1967, Vesicular stomatitis virus—The relationship between some strains of the Indiana serotype, *Res. Vet. Sci.* **8**, 103.

Fiszman, M., Leauté, J.-B., Chany, C., and Girard, M., 1974, Mode of action of acid pH on the development of vesicular stomatitis virus, *J. Virol.* **13**, 801.

Flamand, A., 1969, Etude des mutants thermosensibles du virus de la stomatite vésiculaire. Mise au point d'un test de complementation, *C. R. Acad. Sci. Hebd. Seances Ser. D Sci. Nat.* **268**, 2305.

Flamand, A., 1970, Etude génétique du virus de la stomatite vésiculaire: Classement de mutants thermosensible spontanés en group de complementation, *J. Gen. Virol.* **8**, 187.

Flamand, A., and Bishop, D. H. L., 1973, Primary *in vivo* transcription of vesicular stomatitis virus and temperature-sensitive mutants of five vesicular stomatitis virus complementation groups, *J. Virol.* **12**, 1238.

Flamand, A., and Lafay, A., 1973, Etude des mutants thermosensibles du virus de la stomatite vésiculaire appartenant au groupe de complementation II, *Ann. Inst. Pasteur (Paris)* **124**, 261.

Flamand, A., and Pringle, C. R., 1971, The homologies of spontaneous and induced temperature-sensitive mutants of vesicular stomatitis virus isolated in chick embryos and and BHK-21 cells, *J. Gen. Virol.* **11,** 81.

Follett, E. A. C., Pringle, C. R., Wunner, W. H., and Skehel, J. J., 1974, Virus replication in enucleate cells: Vesicular stomatitis virus and influenza virus, *J. Virol.* **13,** 394.

Francki, R. I. B., 1973, Plant rhabdoviruses, *Adv. Virus Res.* **18,** 257.

Francki, R. I. B., and Randles, J. W., 1972, RNA-dependent RNA polymerase associated with particles of lettuce necrotic yellows virus, *Virology* **47,** 270.

Francki, R. I. B., and Randles, J. W., 1973, Some properties of lettuce necrotic yellows virus RNA and its *in vitro* transcription by virion-associated transcriptase, *Virology* **54,** 359.

Francki, R. I. B., and Randles, J. W., 1974, Composition of the plant rhabdovirus lettuce yellows necrotic virus in relation to its biological properties, *in* "Negative Strand Viruses" (R. D. Barry and B. W. J. Mahy, eds.), Academic Press, London.

Franklin, R. M., 1958, Studies on the growth of vesicular stomatitis virus in tissue culture, *Virology* **5,** 408.

Galasso, G. J., 1967, Enumeration of VSV particles and a demonstration of their growth kinetics by electron microscopy, *Proc. Soc. Exp. Biol. Med.* **124,** 43.

Galet, H., and Prevec, L., 1973, Polyadenylate synthesis by extracts from L cells infected with vesicular stomatitis virus, *Nat. New Biol.* **243,** 200.

Galet, H., Shedlarski, J. G., Jr., and Prevec, L., 1973, Ribonucleic acid polymerase induced in L cells infected with vesicular stomatitis virus, *Can. J. Biochem.* **51,** 721.

Ghosh, H. P., Toneguzzo, F., and Wells, S., 1973, Synthesis *in vitro* of vesicular stomatitis virus proteins in cytoplasmic extracts of L cells, *Biochem. Biophys. Res. Comm.* **54,** 228.

Grubman, M. J., and Summers, D. F., 1973, *In vitro* protein synthesizing activity of vesicular stomatitis virus-infected cell extracts, *J. Virol.* **12,** 265.

Grubman, M. J., Ehrenfeld, E., and Summers, D. F., 1974, *In vitro* synthesis of proteins by membrane-bound polysomes from VSV-infected HeLa cells, *J. Virol.* **14,** in press.

Gyorgy, E., Sheehan, M., and Sokol, F., 1971, Release of envelope glycoprotein from rabies virus by a nonionic detergent, *J. Virol.* **8,** 649.

Hackett, A. J., 1964, A possible morphologic basis for the autointerference phenomenon in vesicular stomatitis virus, *Virology* **24,** 51.

Hackett, A. J., Schaffer, F. L., and Martin, S. H., 1967, The separation of infectious and autointerfering particles in vesicular stomatitis virus preparations, *Virology* **31,** 114.

Hackett, A. J., Zee, Y. C., Schaffer, F. L., and Talens, L., 1968, Electron microscopic study of the morphogenesis of vesicular stomatitis virus, *J. Virol.* **2,** 1154.

Halonen, P. E., Murphy, F. A., Fields, B. N., and Reese, D. R., 1968, Hemagglutinin of rabies and some other bullet-shaped viruses, *Proc. Soc. Exp. Biol. Med.* **127,** 1037.

Hanson, R. P., 1952, The natural history of vesicular stomatitis, *Bacteriol. Rev.* **16,** 179.

Hecht, T. T., and Summers, D. F., 1972, Effect of vesicular stomatitis virus infection on the histocompatibility antigen of L cells, *J. Virol.* **10,** 578.

Heine, J. W., and Schnaitman, C. A., 1969, Fusion of vesicular stomatitis virus with cytoplasmic membrane of L cells, *J. Virol.* **3,** 619.

Heine, J. W., and Schnaitman, C. A., 1971, Entry of vesicular stomatitis virus into L cells, *J. Virol.* **8,** 786.

Hills, G. J., and Campbell, R. N., 1968, Morphology of broccoli necrotic yellows virus, *J. Ultrastruct. Res.* **24,** 134.

Holland, J. J., Doyle, M., Perrault, J., Kingsbury, D. T., and Etchison, J., 1972, Proteinase activity in purified animal viruses, *Biochem. Biophys. Res. Commun.* **46,** 634.

Holloway, A. F., Wong, P. K. Y., and Cormack, D. V., 1970, Isolation and characterization of temperature-sensitive mutants of vesicular stomatitis virus, *Virology* **42,** 917.

Howatson, A. F., 1970, Vesicular stomatitis and related viruses, *Adv. Virus Res.* **16,** 195.

Howatson, A. F., and Whitmore, G. F., 1962, The development and structure of vesicular stomatitis virus, *Virology* **16,** 466.

Huang, A. S., 1973, Defective interfering viruses, *Annu. Rev. Microbiol.* **27,** 101.

Huang, A. S., 1974, Ribonucleic acid synthesis of vesicular stomatitis virus, *in* "Negative Strand Viruses" (R. D. Barry and B. W. J. Mahy, eds.), Academic Press, London.

Huang, A. S., and Baltimore, D., 1970, Defective viral particles and viral disease processes, *Nature (Lond.)* **226,** 325.

Huang, A. S., and Manders, E., 1972, Ribonucleic acid synthesis of vesicular stomatitis virus. IV. Transcription by standard virus in the presence of defective interfering particles, *J. Virol.* **9,** 909.

Huang, A. S., and Wagner, R. R., 1965, Inhibition of cellular RNA synthesis by nonreplicating vesicular stomatitis virus, *Proc. Natl. Acad. Sci. USA* **54,** 1579.

Huang, A. S., and Wagner, R. R., 1966a, Defective T particles of vesicular stomatitis virus. II. Biologic role in homologous interference, *Virology* **30,** 173.

Huang, A. S., and Wagner, R. R., 1966b, Comparative sedimentation coefficients of RNA extracted from plaque-forming and defective particles of vesicular stomatitis virus, *J. Mol. Biol.* **22,** 381.

Huang, A. S., Greenawalt, J. W., and Wagner, R. R., 1966, Defective T particles of vesicular stomatitis virus. I. Preparation, morphology and some biologic properties, *Virology* **30,** 161.

Huang, A. S., Baltimore, D., and Stampfer, M., 1970, Ribonucleic acid synthesis of vesicular stomatitis virus. III. Multiple complementary messenger RNA molecules, *Virology* **42,** 946.

Huang, A. S., Baltimore, D., and Bratt, M. A., 1971, Ribonucleic acid polymerase in virions of Newcastle disease virus: Comparison with the vesicular stomatitis virus polymerase, *J. Virol.* **7,** 389.

Huang, A. S., Besmer, P., Chu, L., and Baltimore, D., 1973, Growth of pseudotypes of vesicular stomatitis virus with N-tropic murine leukemia virus coats in cells resistant to N-tropic viruses, *J. Virol.* **12,** 659.

Hummeler, K., 1971, Bullet-shaped viruses, *in* "Comparative Virology" (K. Maramorosch and E. Kurstak, eds.), pp. 361–386, Academic Press, New York.

Hummeler, K., Koprowski, H., and Wiktor, T. J., 1967, Structure and development of rabies virus in tissue culture, *J. Virol.* **1,** 152.

Hunt, D. M., and Wagner, R. R., 1974, Location of the transcriptase defect in group I temperature-sensitive mutants of vesicular stomatitis virus, *J. Virol.* **13,** 28.

Imblum, R. L., and Wagner, R. R., 1974, Protein kinase and phosphoproteins of vesicular stomatitis virus, *J. Virol.* **13,** 113.

Kang, C. Y., and Prevec, L., 1969, Proteins of vesicular stomatitis virus. I. Polyacrylamide gel analysis of viral antigens, *J. Virol.* **3,** 403.

Kang, C. Y., and Prevec, L., 1970, Proteins of vesicular stomatitis virus. II. Immunological comparisons of viral antigens, *J. Virol.* **6**, 20.

Kang, C. Y., and Prevec, L., 1971, Proteins of vesicular stomatitis virus. III. Intracellular synthesis and extracellular appearance of virus specific proteins, *Virology* **46**, 678.

Kaplan, M. M., Wiktor, T. J., Maes, R. F., Campbell, J. B., and Koprowski, H., 1967, Effect of polyanions on the infectivity of rabies virus in tissue culture: Construction of a single-cycle growth curve, *J. Virol.* **1**, 145.

Karabatsos, N., Lipman, M. B., Garrison, M. S., and Mongillo, C. A., 1973, The morphology, morphogenesis, and serological characteristics of the rhabdoviruses Navarro, Kwatta, and Mossuril, *J. Gen. Virol.* **21**, 429.

Kelley, J. M., Emerson, S. U., and Wagner, R. R., 1972, The glycoprotein of vesicular stomatitis virus is the antigen that gives rise to and reacts with neutralizing antibody, *J. Virol.* **10**, 1231.

Kerr, I., Friedman, R. M., Brown, R. E., Ball, L. A., and Brown, J. C., 1974, Inhibition of protein synthesis in cell-free systems from interferon-treated, infected cells: Further characterization and effect of formylmethionyl-tRNA$_F$, *J. Virol.* **13**, 9.

Kiley, M. P., and Wagner, R. R., 1972, Ribonucleic acid species of intracellular nucleocapsids and released virions of vesicular stomatitis virus, *J. Virol.* **10**, 244.

Kingsbury, D. W., 1973, Cell-free translation of paramyxovirus messenger RNA, *J. Virol.* **12**, 1020.

Klenk, H.-D., and Choppin, P. W., 1971, Glycolipid content of vesicular stomatitis virus grown in baby hamster kidney cells, *J. Virol.* **7**, 416.

Klenk, H.-D., Compans, R. W., and Choppin, P. W., 1970, An electron microscopic study of the presence or absence of neuraminic acid in enveloped viruses, *Virology* **42**, 1158.

Klenk, H.-D., Scholtissek, C., and Rott, R., 1972, Inhibition of glycoprotein biosynthesis of influenza virus by D-glucosamine and 2-deoxy-D-glucose, *Virology* **47**, 723.

Knudson, D. L., 1973, Rhabdoviruses, *J. Gen. Virol.* **20**, 105.

Knudson, D. L., and MacLeod, R., 1972, The proteins of potato yellow dwarf virus, *Virology* **47**, 285.

Kuwert, E., Wiktor, T. J., Sokol, F., and Koprowski, H., 1968, Hemagglutination by rabies virus, *J. Virol.* **2**, 1381.

Lafay, F., 1971, Etudes des functions du virus de la stomatite vésiculaire alterées par une mutation thermosensible: Mise en evidence de la protein structural affectée par la mutation *ts* 23, *J. Gen. Virol.* **13**, 449.

Lafay, F., 1974, Envelope proteins of vesicular stomatitis virus: Effect of temperature sensitive mutations in complementation groups III and V, *J. Virol:* in press.

Lazarowitz, S. G., Compans, R. W., and Choppin, P. W., 1971, Influenza virus structural and nonstructural proteins in infected cells and their plasma membranes, *Virology* **46**, 830.

Leamnson, R. N., and Reichmann, M. E., 1974, The RNA of defective vesicular stomatitis virus particles in relation to viral cistrons, *J. Mol. Biol.,* **85**, 551.

Love, D. N., and Weiss, R. A., 1974, Pseudotypes of vesicular stomatitis virus determined by exogenous and endogenous avian RNA tumor virus, *Virology* **57**, 271.

McCombs, R. M., Benyesh-Melnick, M., and Brunschwig, J. P., 1966, Biophysical studies on vesicular stomatitis virus, *J. Bacteriol.* **91**, 803.

McSharry, J. J., and Wagner, R. R., 1971a, Lipid composition of purified vesicular stomatitis virus, *J. Virol.* **7**, 59.

McSharry, J. J., and Wagner, R. R., 1971b, Carbohydrate composition of vesicular stomatitis virus, *J. Virol.* **7**, 412.

McSharry, J. J., Compans, R. W,, and Choppin, P. W., 1971, Proteins of vesicular stomatitis virus and of phenotypically mixed vesicular stomatitis virus–simian virus 5 virions, *J. Virol.* **8**, 722.

Manders, E. K., Tilles, J. G., and Huang, A. S., 1972, Interferon-mediated inhibition of virion-directed transcription, *Virology* **49**, 573.

Marcus, P. I., and Sekellick, M. J., 1974, Cell killing by viruses. I. Comparison of cell-killing, plaque-forming and defective-interfering particles of vesicular stomatitis virus, *Virology* **57**, 321.

Marcus, P. I., Engelhardt, D. L., Hunt, J. M., and Sekellick, M. J., 1971, Interferon action: Inhibition of vesicular stomatitis virus RNA synthesis induced by virion-bound polymerase, *Science (Wash., D.C.)* **174**, 593.

Marshall, S., and Gillespie, D., 1972, Poly U tracts absent from viral RNA, *Nat. New Biol.* **240**, 43.

Martinet, C., and Printz-Ané, C., 1970, Analyse de la synthese de l'ARN viral du virus de la stomatite vésiculaire (VSV). Utilisation des mutants thermosensibles, *Ann. Inst. Pasteur (Paris)* **119**, 411.

Matsumoto, S., 1970, Rabies virus, *Adv. Virus Res.* **16**, 257.

Miyoshi, K., Harter, D. H., and Hsu, K. C., 1971, Neuropathological and immuno-fluorescence studies of experimental vesicular stomatitis virus encephalitis in mice, *J. Neuropathol. Exp. Neurol.* **30**, 266.

Moreau, M.-C., 1972, Action de la rifampicine sur le virus de la stomatite vésiculaire, *C. R. Acad. Sci. Hebd. Seances Ser. D Sci. Nat.* **274**, 611.

Mori, H., and Howatson, A. F., 1973, *In vitro* transcriptase activity of vesicular stomatitis virus B and T particles: Analysis of product, *Intervirology* **1**, 168.

Morrison, T., Stampfer, M., Baltimore, D., and Lodish, H. F., 1974, Translation of vesicular stomatitis messenger RNA by extracts from mammalian and plant cells, *J. Virol.* **13**, 62.

Moyer, S. A., and Summers, D. F., 1974a, Phosphorylation of vesicular stomatitis virus *in vivo* and *in vitro, J. Virol.* **13**, 455.

Moyer, S. A., and Summers, D. F., 1974b, Vesicular stomatitis virus envelope glyco-protein alterations induced by host cell transformation, *Cell* **2**, 63.

Mudd, J. A., 1973, Effects of *p*H on the structure of vesicular stomatitis virus, *Virology* **55**, 546.

Mudd, J. A., and Summers, D. F., 1970a, Protein synthesis in vesicular stomatitis virus-infected HeLa cells, *Virology* **42**, 238.

Mudd, J. A., and Summers, D. F., 1970b, Polysomal ribonucleic acid of vesicular stomatitis virus-infected HeLa cells, *Virology* **42**, 958.

Mudd, J. A., Leavitt, R. W., Kingsbury, D. T., and Holland, J. J., 1973, Natural selection of mutants of vesicular stomatitis virus by cultured cells of *Drosophila melanogastor, J. Gen. Virol.* **20**, 341.

Murphy, F. A., and Fields, B. N., 1967, Kern Canyon virus: Electron microscopic and immunological studies, *Virology* **33**, 625.

Murphy, F. A., Coleman, P. H., and Whitfield, S. G., 1966, Electron microscopic observations of Flanders virus, *Virology* **30**, 314.

Murphy, F. A., Shope, R. E., Metselvar, D., and Simpson, D. I. H., 1970, Characterization of Mount Elgon bat virus, a new member of the rhabdovirus group, *Virology* **40**, 288.

Murphy, F. A., Taylor, W. P., Mims, C. A., and Whitfield, S. G., 1972, Bovine ephemeral fever virus in cell culture and mice, *Arch. Ges. Virusforsch.* **38**, 234.

Murphy, F. A., Bauer, S. P., Harrison, A. K., and Winn, W. C., 1973a, Comparative pathogenesis of rabies and rabies-like viruses: Viral infection and transit from inoculation site to the central nervous system, *Lab. Invest.* **28**, 361.

Murphy, F. A., Harrison, A. K., Winn, W. C., and Bauer, S. P., 1973b, Comparative pathogenesis of rabies and rabies-like viruses: Infection of the central nervous system and centrifugal spread of virus to peripheral tissues, *Lab. Invest.* **29**, 1.

Nakai, T., and Howatson, A. F., 1968, The fine structure of vesicular stomatitis virus, *Virology* **35**, 268.

Neurath, A. R., Vernon, S. K., Dobkin, M. B., and Rubin, B. A., 1972, Characterization of subviral components from treatment of rabies virus with tri(n-butyl)phosphate, *J. Gen. Virol.* **14**, 33.

Newman, J. F. E., and Brown, F., 1969, Induced ribonucleic acids in cells infected with vesicular stomatitis virus, *J. Gen. Virol.* **5**, 305.

Ngan, J. S. C., Holloway, A. F., and Cormack, D. V., 1974, Temperature-sensitive mutants of vesicular stomatitis virus: comparison of the *in vitro* RNA polymerase defects of group I and group IV mutants, *J. Virol.* **14**, in press.

Nowakowski, M., Feldman, J. D., Kano, S., and Bloom, B. R., 1973a, The production of vesicular stomatitis virus by antigen- or mitogen-stimulated lymphocytes and continuous lymphoblastoid lines, *J. Exp. Med.* **137**, 1042.

Nowakowski, M., Bloom, B. R., Ehrenfeld, E., and Summers, D. F., 1973b, Restricted replication of vesicular stomatitis virus (VSV) in human lymphoblastoid cells, *J. Virol.* **12**, 1272.

Obijeski, J. F., and Simpson, R. W., 1974, Conditional lethal mutants of vesicular stomatitis virus. II. Synthesis of virus-specific polypeptides in non-permissive cells infected with "RNA" host-restricted mutants, *Virology* **57**, 369.

Obijeski, J. F., Marchenko, A. T., Bishop, D. H. L., Cann, B. W., and Murphy, F. A., 1974, Comparative electrophoretic analysis of the virus proteins of four rhabdoviruses, *J. Gen. Virol.* **22**, 21.

Osunkoya, B. O., and David-West, T. S., 1972, Telophase arrest of cultured cells by vesicular stomatitis virus, *Arch. Ges. Virusforsch.* **38**, 228.

Palma, E. L., and Huang, A. S., 1974, Cyclic production of vesicular stomatitis virus caused by defective interfering particles, *J. Infect. Dis.* **129**, 402.

Palma, E. L., Perlman, S. M., and Huang, A. S., 1974, Ribonucleic acid synthesis of vesicular stomatitis virus. VI. Correlation of defective particle RNA synthesis with standard RNA replication, *J. Mol. Biol.* **85**, 127.

Paucker, K., Shechmeister, I. L., and Birch-Andersen, A., 1970, Studies on the multiplication of vesicular stomatitis virus with fluorescein and ferritin-conjugated antibodies, *Acta Pathol. Microbiol. Scand. (B)* **78**, 317.

Perlman, S. M., and Huang, A. S., 1973, RNA synthesis of vesicular stomatitis virus. V. Interaction between transcription and replication, *J. Virol.* **12**, 1395.

Perlman, S. M., and Huang, A. S., 1974, Intracellular RNA and proteins specified by temperature-sensitive mutants of vesicular stomatitis virus, *Intervirology* in press.

Perrault, J., and Holland, J. J., 1972a, Variability of vesicular stomatitis autointerference with different host cells and virus serotypes, *Virology* **50**, 148.

Perrault, J., and Holland, J. J., 1972b, Absence of transcriptase activity or transcription-inhibiting ability in defective interfering particles of vesicular stomatitis virus, *Virology* **50**, 159.

Perrault, J., and Kingsbury, D. T., 1974, Inhibitor of vesicular stomatitis virus transcriptase in purified virions, *Nature* (*Lond.*) **248**, 45.

Peters, D., and Kitajima, E. W., 1970, Purification and electron microscopy of sowthistle yellow vein virus, *Virology* **41**, 135.

Petric, M., and Prevec, L., 1970, Vesicular stomatitis virus—A new interfering particle, intracellular structures and specific RNA, *Virology* **41**, 615.

Prevec, L., 1974, Physiological properties of vesicular stomatitis virus and some related rhabdoviruses, *in* "Viruses, Evolution and Cancer" (E. Kurstak and K. Maramorosch, eds.), Academic Press, New York.

Prevec, L., and Kang, C. Y., 1970, Homotypic and heterotypic interference by defective particles of vesicular stomatitis virus, *Nature* (*Lond.*) **228**, 25.

Prevec, L., and Whitmore, G. F., 1963, Purification of vesicular stomatitis virus and the analysis of P^{32}-labeled virus components, *Virology* **20**, 464.

Pringle, C. R., 1970, Genetic characteristics of conditional lethal mutants of vesicular stomatitis virus induced by 5-fluorouracil, 5-azacytidine and ethyl methane sulfonate, *J. Virol.* **5**, 559.

Pringle, C. R., and Duncan, I. B., 1971, Preliminary physiological characterization of temperature-sensitive mutants of vesicular stomatitis virus, *J. Virol.* **8**, 56.

Pringle, C. R., and Wunner, W. H., 1973, Genetic and physiological properties of temperature-sensitive mutants of Cocal virus, *J. Virol.* **12**, 677.

Pringle, C. R., and Wunner, W. H., 1974, A comparative investigation of the structure and function of the VSV genome, *in* "Negative Strand Viruses" (R. D. Barry and B. W. J. Mahy, eds.), Academic Press, London.

Pringle, C. R., Duncan, I. B., and Stevenson, M., 1971, Isolation and characterization of temperature-sensitive mutants of vesicular stomatitis virus, New Jersey serotype, *J. Virol.* **8**, 836.

Printz, P., 1973, Relationship of sigma virus to vesicular stomatitis virus, *Adv. Virus Res.* **18**, 143.

Printz, P., and Wagner, R. R., 1971, Temperature-sensitive mutants of vesicular stomatitis virus: synthesis of virus specific proteins, *J. Virol.* **7**, 651.

Printz-Ané, C., Combard, A., and Martinet, C., 1972, Study of the transcription and the replication of vesicular stomatitis virus by using temperature-sensitive mutants, *J. Virol.* **10**, 889.

Randles, J. W., and Francki, R. I. B., 1972, Infectious nucleocapsid of lettuce necrotic yellows virus with RNA-dependent RNA polymerase activity, *Virology* **50**, 297.

Reczko, E., 1960, Elektronmikroskopische Untersuchungen am Virus der Stomatitis vesicularis, *Arch. Ges. Virusforsch.* **10**, 588.

Reeder, G. S., Knudson, D. L., and MacLeod, R., 1972, The ribonucleic acid of potato yellow dwarf virus, *Virology* **50**, 301.

Reichmann, M. E., Pringle, C. R., and Follett, E. A. C., 1971, Defective particles in BHK cells infected with temperature-sensitive mutants of vesicular stomatitis virus, *J. Virol.* **8**, 154.

Repik, P., and Bishop, D. H. L., 1973, Determination of the molecular weight of animal RNA viral genomes by nuclease digestions, *J. Virol.* **12**, 969.

Repik, P., Flamand, A., Clark, H. F., Obijeski, J. F., Roy, P., and Bishop, D. H. L., 1974a, The detection of homologous RNA sequences among six rhabdovirus genomes, *J. Virol.* **13**, 250.

Repik, P., Flamand, A., and Bishop, D. H. L., 1974b, Effect of interferon upon the primary and secondary transcription of vesicular stomatitis and influenza viruses, *J. Virol.* **14**, in press.

Roy, P., and Bishop, D. H. L., 1971, Nucleoside triphosphate phosphotransferase. A new enzyme activity of oncogenic and non-oncogenic "budding" viruses, *Biochim. Biophys. Acta* **235**, 191.

Roy, P., and Bishop, D. H. L., 1972, The genome homology of vesicular stomatitis virus and defective T particles and evidence for the sequential transcription of the virion RNA, *J. Virol.* **9**, 946.

Roy, P., and Bishop, D. H. L., 1973, Initiation and direction of RNA transcription by vesicular stomatitis virion transcriptase, *J. Virol.* **11**, 487.

Roy, P., Repik, P., Hefti, P., and Bishop, D. H. L., 1973, Complementary RNA species isolated from vesicular stomatitis (HR strain) defective virions, *J. Virol.* **11**, 915.

Samuel, C. E., and Joklik, W. K., 1974, A protein synthesizing system from interferon-treated cells that discriminates between cellular and viral messenger RNAs, *Virology,* **58**, 476.

Schaffer, F. L., and Soergel, M. E., 1972, Molecular weight estimates of vesicular stomatitis virus ribonucleic acids from virions, defective particles, and infected cells, *Arch. Ges. Virusforsch.* **39**, 203.

Schaffer, F. L., Hackett, A. J., and Soergel, M. E., 1968, Vesicular stomatitis virus RNA: Complementarity between infected cell RNA and RNAs from infectious and autointerfering virus fractions, *Biochem. Biophys. Res. Commun.* **31**, 685.

Schaffer, F. L., Soergel, M. E., Tegtmeier, G., and Shechmeister, I. L., 1972, Unusual molecular size of RNA from a long rod mutant of vesicular stomatitis virus, *Virology* **47**, 236.

Schincariol, A. L., and Howatson, A. F., 1970, Replication of vesicular stomatitis virus. I. Viral specific RNA and nucleoprotein in infected cells, *Virology* **42**, 732.

Schincariol, A. L., and Howatson, A. F., 1972, Replication of vesicular stomatitis virus. II. Separation and characterization of virus-specific RNA species, *Virology* **49**, 766.

Schlesinger, H. R., Wells, H. J., and Hummeler, K., 1973, Comparison of the lipids of intracellular and extracellular rabies viruses, *J. Virol.* **12**, 1028.

Schloemer, R. H., and Wagner, R. R., 1974, Sialoglycoprotein of vesicular stomatitis virus: role of the neuraminic acid in infection, *J. Virol.* **14**, 270.

Schneider, L. G., Horzinek, M., and Novicky, R., 1971, Isolation of a hemagglutinating, immunizing and noninfectious subunit of the rabies virion, *Arch. Ges. Virusforsch.* **34**, 360.

Schneider, L. G., Dietzschold, B., Dierks, R. E., Matthaeus, W., Enzmann, P. J., and Strohmaier, K., 1973, Rabies group-specific ribonucleoprotein antigen and a test system for grouping and typing of rhabdoviruses, *J. Virol.* **11**, 748.

Scholtissek, C., Rott, R., Hau, G., and Kalinza, G., 1974, Inhibition of the multiplication of vesicular stomatitis and Newcastle disease virus by 2-deoxy-D-glucose, *J. Virol.* **13**:1186.

Shechmeister, I. L., Streckfuss, J., and St. John, R., 1967, Comparative pathogenicity of vesicular stomatitis virus and its plaque type mutant, *Arch. Ges. Virusforsch.* **21**, 127.

Shimizu, Y., Yamamoto, S., Homma, M., and Ishida, N., 1972, Effect of chloroquine on the growth of animal viruses, *Arch. Ges. Virusforsch.* **36**, 93.

Shope, R. E., 1973, Rabies virus antigenic relationships, *in* "The Natural History of Rabies" (G. M. Baer, ed.), Academic Press, New York.

Shope, R. E., Murphy, F. A., Harrison, A. K., Causey, O. R., Kemp, G. E., Simpson, D. I. H., and Moore, D. L., 1970, Two African viruses serologically and morphologically related to rabies virus, *J. Virol.* **6**, 690.

Simpson, R. W., and Hauser, R. E., 1966, Structural components of vesicular stomatitis virus, *Virology* **29**, 654.

Simpson, R. W., and Obijeski, J. F., 1974, Conditional lethal mutants of vesicular stomatitis virus. I. Phenotypic characterization of single and double mutants exhibiting
host restriction and temperature sensitivity, *Virology* **57**, 357.

Simpson, R. W., Hauser, R. E., and Dales, S., 1969, Viropexis of vesicular stomatisis
virus by L cells, *Virology* **17**, 285.

Sokol, F., and Clark, H. F., 1973, Phosphoproteins, structural components of
rhabdoviruses, *J. Virol.* **52**, 246.

Sokol, F., Kuwert, E., Wiktor, T. J., Hummeler, K., and Koprowski, H., 1968, Purification of rabies virus grown in tissue culture, *J. Virol.* **2**, 836.

Sokol, F., Schlumberger, H. D., Wiktor, T. J., and Koprowski, H., 1969, Biochemical
and biophysical studies on the nucleocapsid and on the RNA of rabies virus,
Virology **38**, 651.

Sokol, F., Stancek, D., and Koprowski, H., 1971, Structural proteins of rabies virus, *J.
Virol.* **7**, 241.

Sokol, F., Clark, H. F., and Gyorgy, E., 1972, Heterogeneity of phospholipid content
of purified rabies virus (ERA strain) particles, *J. Gen. Virol.* **16**, 173.

Sokol, F., Tan, K. B., McFalls, M. L., and Madore, P., 1974, Phosphate acceptor
amino acid residues in structural proteins of rhabdoviruses, *J. Virol.* **14**, 145.

Soria, M., and Huang, A. S., 1973, Association of polyadenylic acid with messenger
RNA of vesicular stomatitis virus, *J. Mol. Biol.* **77**, 449.

Sreevalsan, T., 1970, Homologous viral interference: Induction by RNA from defective particles of vesicular stomatitis virus, *Science (Wash., D.C.)* **169**, 991.

Stampfer, M., and Baltimore, D., 1973, Identification of the vesicular stomatitis virus
large protein as a unique viral protein, *J. Virol.* **11**, 520.

Stampfer, M., Baltimore, D., and Huang, A. S., 1969, Ribonucleic acid synthesis of
vesicular stomatitis virus. I. Species of ribonucleic acid found in Chinese hamster
ovary cells infected with plaque-forming and defective particles, *J. Virol.* **4**, 154.

Strand, M., and August, J. T., 1971, Protein kinase and phosphate acceptor proteins in
Rauscher murine leukemia virus, *Nat. New Biol.* **233**, 137.

Streckfuss, J. L., and Shechmeister, I. L., 1971, The intracellular development of vesicular stomatitis virus and two of its mutants, *Arch. Ges. Virusforsch.* **35**, 208.

Sylvester, E. S., and Richardson, J., 1970, Infection of *Hyperomyzas lactucae* by
sowthistle yellow vein virus, *Virology* **42**, 1023.

Sylvester, E. S., Richardson, J., and Wood, P., 1968, Comparative electron micrographs of sowthistle yellow vein and vesicular stomatitis viruses, *Virology* **36**,
693.

Szilágyi, J. F., and Pringle, C. R., 1972, Effect of temperature-sensitive mutations on
the virion-associated RNA transcriptase of vesicular stomatitis virus, *J. Mol. Biol.*
71, 281.

Szilágyi, J. F., and Uryvayev, L., 1973, Isolation of an infectious ribonucleoprotein
from vesicular stomatitis virus containing an active RNA transcriptase, *J. Virol.* **11**,
279.

Szilágyi, J. F., and Uryvayev, L., 1974, Studies on the virion-associated transcriptase
in VSV, *in* "Negative Strand Viruses" (R. D. Barry and B. W. J. Mahy, eds.),
Academic Press, London.

Unger, J. T., and Reichmann, M. E., 1973, RNA synthesis in temperature-sensitive
mutants of vesicular stomatitis virus, *J. Virol.* **12**, 570.

Villareal, L. P., and Holland, J. J., 1973, Synthesis of poly(A) *in vitro* by purified
virions of vesicular stomatitis virus, *Nat. New Biol.* **245**, 17.

Villareal, L. P., and Holland, J. J., 1974, Transcribing complexes in cells infected by vesicular stomatitis virus and rabies virus, *J. Virol.* **14,** in press.

Wagner, R. R., 1974, Pathogenicity and immunogenicity for mice of temperature-sensitive mutants of vesicular stomatitis virus, *Infect. Immun.,* **10,** 309.

Wagner, R. R., and Huang, A. S., 1966, Inhibition of RNA and interferon synthesis in Krebs-2 cells infected with vesicular stomatitis virus, *Virology* **28,** 1.

Wagner, R. R., and Schnaitman, C. A., 1970, Proteins of vesicular stomatitis virus, *in* "The Biology of Large RNA Viruses" (R. D. Barry and B. W. J. Mahy, eds.), pp. 655–671, Academic Press, London.

Wagner, R. R., Levy, A. H., Snyder, R. M., Ratcliff, G. A., Jr., and Hyatt, D. F., 1963, Biological properties of two plaque variants of vesicular stomatitis virus (Indiana serotype), *J. Immunol.* **91,** 112.

Wagner, R. R., Schnaitman, T. C., and Snyder, R. M., 1969*a*, Structural proteins of vesicular stomatitis viruses, *J. Virol.* **3,** 395.

Wagner, R. R., Schnaitman, T. C., Snyder, R. M., and Schnaitman, C. A., 1969*b*, Protein composition of the structural components of vesicular stomatitis virus, *J. Virol.* **3,** 611.

Wagner, R. R., Snyder, R. M., and Yamazaki, S., 1970, Proteins of vesicular stomatitis virus: Kinetics and cellular sites of synthesis, *J. Virol.* **5,** 548.

Wagner, R. R., Heine, J. W., Goldstein, G., and Schnaitman, C. A., 1971, Use of antiviral–antiferritin hybrid antibody for localization of viral antigen in plasma membrane, *J. Virol.* **7,** 274.

Wagner, R. R., Kiley, M. P., Snyder, R. M., and Schnaitman, C. A., 1972, Cytoplasmic compartmentalization of the proteins and ribonucleic acid species of vesicular stomatitis virus, *J. Virol.* **9,** 672.

Wagner, R. R., Emerson, S. U., Imblum, R. L., and Kelley, J. M., 1974, Structure-function relationships of proteins of vesicular stomatitis virions, *in* "Negative Strand Viruses" (R. D. Barry and B. W. J. Mahy, eds.), Academic Press, London.

Walter, G., and Mudd, J. A., 1973, Iodination of vesicular stomatitis virus with lactoperoxidase, *Virology* **52,** 574.

Ware, B. R., Raj, T., Flygare, W. H., Lesnaw, A., and Reichmann, M. E., 1973, Molecular weights of vesicular stomatitis virus and its defective particles by laser light scattering spectroscopy, *J. Virol.* **11,** 141.

Wertz, G. W., and Levine, M., 1973, RNA synthesis by vesicular stomatitis virus and a small plaque mutant: Effects of cycloheximide, *J. Virol.* **12,** 253.

Wertz, G. W., and Youngner, J. S., 1970, Interferon production and inhibition of host synthesis in cells infected with vesicular stomatitis virus, *J. Virol.* **6,** 476.

Wertz, G. W., and Youngner, J. S., 1972, Inhibition of protein synthesis in L cells infected with vesicular stomatitis virus, *J. Virol.* **9,** 85.

Wiktor, T. J., and Koprowski, H., 1974, Rhabdovirus replication in enucleated host cells. *J. Virol.* **14,** 300.

Wiktor, T. J., Gyorgy, E., Schlumberger, H. D., Sokol, F., and Koprowski, H., 1973, Antigenic properties of rabies virus components, *J. Immunol.* **110,** 269.

Wild, T. F., 1971, Replication of vesicular stomatitis virus: Characterization of the virus-induced RNA, *J. Gen. Virol.* **13,** 295.

Wild, T. F., 1972, Replication of vesicular stomatitis virus: The effect of purified interfering component, *J. Gen. Virol.* **17,** 295.

Wilson, R. G., and Bader, J. P., 1965, Viral ribonucleic acid polymerase: Chick-embryo cells infected with vesicular stomatitis virus or Rous-associated virus, *Biochim. Biophys. Acta* **103,** 549.

Wong, P. K. Y., Holloway, A. F., and Cormack, D. V., 1971, A search for recombination between temperature-sensitive mutants of vesicular stomatitis virus, *J. Gen. Virol.* **13**, 477.

Wong, P. K. Y., Holloway, A. F., and Cormack, D. V., 1972, Characterization of three complementation groups of vesicular stomatitis virus, *Virology* **50**, 829.

Wunner, W. H., and Pringle, C. R., 1972*a*, Comparison of structural polypeptides from vesicular stomatitis virus (Indiana and New Jersey serotypes) and Cocal virus, *J. Gen. Virol.* **16**, 1.

Wunner, W. H., and Pringle, C. R., 1972*b*, Protein synthesis in BHK 21 cells infected with vesicular stomatitis virus. I. *ts* mutants of the Indiana serotype, *Virology* **48**, 104.

Wunner, W. H., and Pringle, C. R., 1972*c*, Protein synthesis in BHK 21 cells infected with vesicular stomatitis virus. II. *ts* mutants of the New Jersey serotype, *Virology* **50**, 250.

Yamazaki, S., and Wagner, R. R., 1970, Action of interferon: Kinetics and differential effects on viral functions, *J. Virol.* **6**, 421.

Yang, Y. J., Stoltz, D. B., and Prevec, L., 1969, Growth of vesicular stomatitis virus in a continuous culture line of *Antheraea eucalypti* moth cells, *J. Gen. Virol.* **5**, 473.

Yaoi, Y., and Amano, M., 1970, Inhibiting effect of ultraviolet-inactivated vesicular stomatitis virus in initiation of DNA synthesis in cultured chick embryo cells, *J. Gen. Virol.* **9**, 69.

Yaoi, Y., and Ogata, M., 1972, The fate of vesicular stomatitis virus in cultured chick embryo cells. *J. Gen. Virol.* **16**, 419.

Yaoi, T., Mitsui, H., and Amano, M., 1970, Effect of UV-irradiated vesicular stomatitis virus on nucleic acid synthesis in chick embryo cells, *J. Gen. Virol.* **8**, 165.

Youngner, J. S., and Wertz, G., 1968, Interferon production in mice by vesicular stomatitis virus, *J. Virol.* **2**, 1360.

Zajac, B. A., and Hummeler, K., 1970, Morphogenesis of the nucleoprotein of vesicular stomatitis virus, *J. Virol.* **6**, 243.

Zajac, B. A., and Hummeler, K., 1971, Identification of vesicular stomatitis virus nucleoprotein *in situ*, *J. Gen. Virol.* **13**, 215.

Závada, J., 1972*a*, Pseudotypes of VSV with the coat of murine leukemia and of avian myeloblastosis virus, *J. Gen. Virol.* **15**, 183.

Závada, J., 1972*b*, VSV pseudotype particles with the coat of avian myeloblastosis virus, *Nat. New Biol.* **240**, 122.

Závada, J., and Rosenbergová, M., 1972, Phenotypic mixing of vesicular stomatitis virus with fowl plague virus, *Acta Virol.* **16**, 103.

Závada, J., Závadova, Z., Malik, A., and Kocent, A., 1972, VSV pseudotypes produced in cell line derived from human mammary carcinoma, *Nat. New Biol.* **240**, 124.

Zee, Y. C., Hackett, A. J., and Talens, L., 1970, Vesicular stomatitis virus maturation sites in six different host cells, *J. Gen. Virol.* **7**, 95.

Zwillenberg, L. O., Jensen, M. H., and Zwillenberg, H. H. L., 1965, Electron microscopy of the virus of viral hemorrhagic septicaemia of rainbow trout (Egtved virus), *Arch. Ges. Virusforsch.* **17**, 1.

CHAPTER 2

Reproduction of Paramyxoviruses

Purnell W. Choppin and Richard W. Compans

The Rockefeller University
New York, New York 10021

1. INTRODUCTION

1.1. Members of the Paramyxovirus Group

The paramyxovirus group is a large one which includes the parain-fluenza viruses types 1–5, Newcastle disease, and mumps viruses. Measles, canine distemper, and rinderpest viruses form a distinct subgroup on the basis of antigenicity, hemagglutinating characteristics, and lack of evidence for a virion-associated neuraminidase or neuraminic acid-containing cellular receptors. However, it is now generally accepted that these viruses should also be included in the paramyxovirus group because of their similar structural properties. Other more recently isolated viruses which have been classified as paramyxoviruses on the basis of morphological and biological properties are Yucaipa (Dinter *et al.,* 1964) and Nariva (Walder, 1971) viruses. Table 1 lists paramyxoviruses and their primary hosts.

On the basis of their properties such as adsorption to mucoprotein receptors on erythrocytes and host cells and neuraminidase activity, mumps and Newcastle disease viruses were originally classified as myxoviruses together with the influenza viruses (Andrewes *et al.,* 1955). It soon became clear that there were significant differences in physical and biological properties among the members of this large group, and that actually two distinct groups existed. It was initially

TABLE 1

Paramyxoviruses

Virus type	Other names or subtypes	Some natural hosts
Newcastle disease	Avian pneumo-encephalitis	Chicken, other birds
Mumps	Epidemic parotitis	Man
Parainfluenza 1	Sendai, hemagglutinating virus of Japan	Mouse
	Hemadsorption type 2	Man
Parainfluenza 2	Croup-associated (CA)	Man
Parainfluenza 3	Hemadsorption type 1	Man
	Shipping fever	Cow, sheep
Parainfluenza 4		Man
Parainfluenza 5	SV5, DA	Dog, monkey
Measles	Rubeola	Man, monkey
Canine distemper		Dog
Rinderpest	Cattle plague	Bovines, sheep, goats
Yucaipa		Chicken
Nariva		Rodents

proposed that the myxoviruses be divided into subgroups I and II (Wa-terson, 1962). Subsequently, the term myxovirus (or orthomyxovirus) group was adopted to include the various influenza viruses, and paramyxovirus group to include the viruses listed in Table 1. The major differences that distinguish these two virus groups are that the paramyxoviruses contain a larger helical nucleocapsid than the myxoviruses and they have a genome which is a single continuous RNA molecule, as opposed to the segmented genome of the myxoviruses, and that paramyxovirus replication is not inhibited by actinomycin D. The properties and reproduction of myxoviruses are described in Chapt. 3 of this volume.

Respiratory syncytial virus and pneumonia virus of mice have shown certain properties in common with the myxoviruses and paramyxoviruses, but they differ significantly in the morphology of their nucleocapsid (Compans et al., 1967; Zakstelskaya et al., 1967; Joncas et al., 1969; Norrby et al., 1970). Thus these viruses appear to represent another distinct group for which the term metamyxoviruses has been proposed (Melnick, 1973) and which will not be discussed further in this chapter.

Much of our knowledge of the structure and replication of paramyxoviruses is derived from studies on three viruses, Newcastle disease virus (NDV), Sendai virus (also designated hemagglutinating virus of Japan, HVJ), and simian virus 5 (SV5), and this chapter will draw largely on work with these viruses, with some discussion of the results obtained with mumps virus and with measles virus, in which there is now an increasing amount of interest. Previous reviews of paramyxoviruses include: Chanock and Parrott (1965), Katz and Enders (1965), Robinson and Duesberg (1968), Blair and Duesberg (1970), Compans and Choppin (1971), Choppin *et al.* (1971), Hsiung (1972), and Kingsbury (1973*a*). The proceedings volume of a recent conference on "Negative Strand Viruses," edited by Barry and Mahy (1974), describes much of the recent work on paramyxoviruses.

1.2. General Biological Properties

The various members of the paramyxovirus group cause a wide spectrum of diseases in man and animals, ranging from mild respiratory diseases, to mumps and measles, to acute and chronic neurological diseases. Although many of the paramyxoviruses replicate in and cause diseases of the respiratory tract of the susceptible hosts, some are capable of infecting a wide variety of tissues. For example, mumps virus may infect many tissues of the body, and several viruses may cause disease of the central nervous system, e.g., measles virus, canine distemper virus, and NDV. The paramyxoviruses are widely distributed in nature and most animal species that have been adequately investigated have been found to be susceptible to infection by one or more paramyxovirus.

One of the important biological properties of members of this group, which was recognized some time ago, is their ability to cause persistent infection of cultured cells [see review by Walker (1968)]. Almost every member of the paramyxovirus group has been shown to produce a persistent, noncytocidal infection in one or more cell types. The biological importance of this property has been recently emphasized by the extensive evidence obtained in many laboratories that a fatal neurological disease of man, subacute sclerosing panencephalitis (SSPE), has been shown to be caused by persistent infection with measles virus. In addition, evidence raising the question of involvement of paramyxoviruses in the etiology of other chronic diseases such as multiple sclerosis has also been obtained, including reports of elevated antibody levels to measles virus in patients with this disease, the findings of structures resembling paramyxovirus nucleocapsids in brain cells, and the isolation of measles and parainfluenza viruses from such cells (Adams and Imagawa, 1962; Prineas, 1972; ter Meulen *et al.*,

1972*a*; Field *et al.,* 1972). A review of the extensive literature on this question is not within the scope of this chapter, but the proven involvement of measles virus in SSPE alone indicates that persistent infection by paramyxoviruses *in vitro* has its counterpart in disease of the whole organism.

Another biological property which the paramyxoviruses possess is the ability to cause cell fusion and lysis of erythrocytes. Giant cell formation in the course of paramyxovirus infection of man was recognized by Virchow (1858) in the 19th century, and in cultured cells by Henle *et al.* (1954), Enders and Peebles (1954), and Okada (1958), and subsequently has been studied extensively in many laboratories. The ability to fuse cells and create hybrids has become an important tool in somatic cell genetics and studies of cellular regulation [reviewed by Harris (1970) and Ruddle (1974)].

2. VIRIONS

2.1. Morphology

2.1.1. Size and Shape

The paramyxovirus virion consists of a membrane-containing envelope, covered with surface projections or spikes, which encloses a helical ribonucleoprotein (RNP) nucleocapsid (Figs. 1–4). Early electron microscopic studies (Elford *et al.,* 1947; Cunha *et al.,* 1947; Bang, 1946, 1948, 1955; Dawson and Elford, 1949; Schäfer *et al.,* 1949) suggested that NDV virions were larger and more pleomorphic than influenza virions. With the advent of negative-contrast electron microscopy, it was found with several different paramyxoviruses that the virions vary considerably in size; most are 150–200 nm in diameter and are roughly spherical in shape; however, larger particles of 500–600 nm are occasionally observed (Horne *et al.,* 1960; Horne and Waterson, 1960; Horne and Wildy, 1961; Rott and Schäfer, 1961; Hosaka *et al.,* 1961; Choppin and Stoeckenius, 1964). Fig. 1 shows a negatively stained SV5 virion. On the basis of negative-contrast studies, it was originally thought that filamentous forms of paramyxovirus were rare or did not occur (Waterson, 1962); however, when fixed thin sections of infected cells were examined, it became apparent that filamentous forms of paramyxoviruses are not infrequent (Compans *et al.,* 1966; Howe *et al.,* 1967) (see Figs. 15–17). Apparently, disruption of the larger filamentous virions frequently occurs

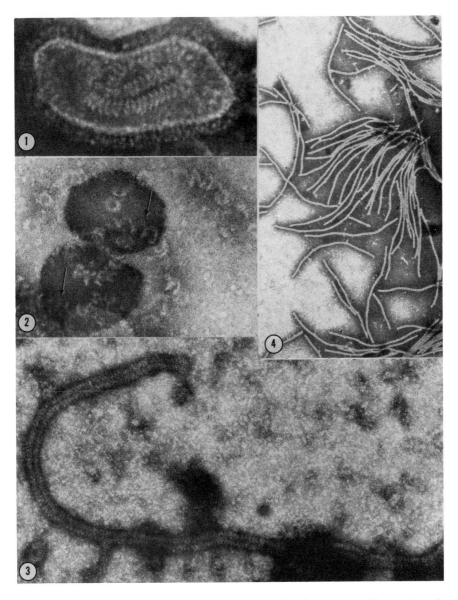

Fig. 1. SV5 virion negatively stained with sodium phosphotungstate. The envelope is covered with a layer of closely spaced projections about 1000 nm in length. The helical nucleocapsid is coiled inside. ×280,000. From Choppin and Stoeckenius (1964).

Fig. 2. Segments of the nucleocapsid released from disrupted SV5 virions. The helical nucleocapsid is extended and the individual turns of the single helix are clearly resolved (arrows). ×304,500. From Choppin and Stoeckenius (1964).

Fig. 3. A tightly coiled nucleocapsid about 0.9 μm in length which was released from an SV5 virion by treatment with phospholipase C. Negative staining with uranyl acetate. ×210,000. From Choppin and Stoeckenius (1964).

Fig. 4. SV5 nucleocapsids purified in a cesium chloride gradient. The nucleocapsids are tightly coiled, and most measure about 1 μm in length. ×26,600. From Compans and Choppin (1973).

under conditions of negative staining, and this accounts for the absence of these particles and the abundance of free nucleocapsids that are frequently seen in such preparations. It is also likely that some of the very large pleomorphic virions that are observed in negatively stained preparations may have been released as filaments and have then become distorted under the conditions of preparation and staining.

2.1.2. Mass

Due to the pleomorphism discussed above, exact measurements of the mass of paramyxoviruses cannot be made. However, since most of the virions are of approximately the same size, some rough estimates can be made. An estimate of the mass of an SV5 virion which contains a single copy of the virus genome can be made (Klenk and Choppin, 1969a) on the basis of an estimated particle weight for the nucleocapsid of approximately 165×10^6 daltons and the nucleocapsid comprising approximately 22% of the dry weight of the virion, or from the 0.91% RNA content of the virus and an estimated weight of genome of approximately 6×10^6. Estimates obtained from such calculations agree quite well and yield values of $6-7 \times 10^8$ daltons for the particle weight and $1.0-1.2 \times 10^{-15}$ g for the weight of a single virion (Klenk and Choppin, 1969a). Sedimentation coefficients of 1000–1100 S have been obtained for several paramyxoviruses; however, in view of the pleomorphism described above, such values can also be viewed only as representing the average or standard-sized particle, which presumably contains a single copy of the genome. This is emphasized by the fact that different populations of virions, presumably containing different numbers of nucleocapsids, can be separated by sedimentation (Dahlberg and Simon, 1969; Kingsbury et al., 1970; Simon, 1972).

2.2. Composition

2.2.1. Overall Chemical Composition

Chemical analyses of highly purified SV5 virions indicated the following composition, expressed as percent of dry weight: 0.91% RNA, 73% protein, 20% lipid, and 6.1% carbohydrate (Klenk and Choppin, 1969a). Roughly similar, though not identical, values were obtained by Nakajima and Obara (1967) for NDV. It is likely that the earlier value of Cunha et al. (1947) of 3.5% RNA for NDV virions purified only by differential centrifugation was falsely high due to contamination with cellular RNA.

2.2.2. RNA

Because of the structural similarities between SV5 nucleocapsids and tobacco mosaic virus, and the finding of intact pieces of SV5 nucleocapsid > 0.9 μm in length, Choppin and Stoeckenius (1964) suggested that the SV5 might contain several times the 2×10^6 daltons of RNA that TMV contains, and this was subsequently found to be the case. The RNA of Newcastle disease was the first genome of the paramyxovirus shown to be of high molecular weight; this was determined on the basis of a sedimentation coefficient in sucrose gradients of 50–57 S in most studies (Adams, 1965; Duesberg and Robinson, 1965; Kingsbury, 1966a; Sokol, et al. 1966; Nakajima and Obara, 1967). Similar values have been obtained for Sendai virus (Iwai et al., 1966; Barry and Bukrinskaya, 1968; Blair and Robinson, 1968), SV5 (Compans and Choppin, 1968), measles virus (Schluederberg, 1971; Hall and Martin, 1973; Winston et al., 1973), mumps virus (East and Kingsbury, 1971), and Yucaipa virus (Kingsbury, 1973). The most frequently used designations for the sedimentation coefficient of paramyxovirus RNAs are "57 S" and "50 S." These differences are in most instances due to differences in the conditions in the various laboratories because when two paramyxovirus RNAs are sedimented in the same gradient they sediment at similar rates (Compans and Choppin, 1968). A small but definite difference on cosedimentation has been reported between the RNAs of measles virus (52.2 S) and SV5 (50 S) (Schluederberg, 1971). However, the general significance of this finding is not yet clear since it has also been reported that the RNAs of measles and Newcastle disease virus cosedimented in the same gradient (Winston et al., 1973). In this chapter the term 50 S will be used for convenience, following the convention of Kingsbury (1973).

The size of the single-stranded RNA genomes have been estimated on the basis of their sedimentation coefficients in sucrose gradients and also by calculation from the percent RNA composition of the nucleocapsid and the estimated particle weight of that structure (Compans and Choppin, 1967a, 1968). The values obtained have been in the range of $5.5–7.5 \times 7.5 \times 10^6$ daltons. Using an empirical equation obtained by Strauss et al. (1968), Duesberg (1968) estimated the molecular weight of NDV RNA to be 6.3×10^6 on the basis of sedimentation under denaturing conditions in dimethyl sulfoxide (DMSO).

Under similar conditions the RNA of Rous sarcoma virus gave a sedimentation coefficient of 36 S, indicating that the paramyxovirus RNA is the largest covalently linked animal virus genome thus far examined. Subsequently, Kolakofsky and Bruschi (1973) estimated a value of 2.3 $\times$ 10^6 for Sendai RNA on the basis of sedimentation in sucrose containing DMSO, using ribosomal RNAs as markers, but confirmed the value of approximately 6 $\times$ 10^6 calculated on the basis of sedimentation under non-denaturing conditions. However, Kolakofsy et al. (1974) found that electron microscopic measurements of Sendai virus and NDV RNAs suggested values of 5.2–5.6 $\times$ 10^6 and concluded that the lower value obtained in their earlier study was due to less denaturation of the paramyxovirus RNA than of the marker RNAs by DMSO. Thus, all the available information now indicates that the paramyxovirus genome is a single, covalently linked, single-stranded RNA molecule of 5–6 $\times$ 10^6 daltons. Small amounts of 4 S RNA obtained from paramyxovirus virions (Duesberg and Robinson, 1965) have been found not to be within the nucleocapsid (Adams, 1966; Kingsbury and Darlington, 1968). As will be discussed in Sect. 4, defective virions are produced under certain conditions and contain RNA smaller than 50 S, i.e., 19–24 S.

Base compositions of the RNAs of NDV (Duesberg and Robinson, 1965; Kingsbury, 1966a), Sendai virus (Iwai et al., 1966; Blair and Robinson, 1968), and SV5 (Compans and Choppin, 1968) have been determined and are in general similar; in particular, they each have a relatively high content of uracil. Annealing studies using virion RNA and complementary RNA obtained from infected cells showed that different strains of NDV were closely related (Kingsbury, 1966b; Blair and Robinson, 1968), but that NDV, Sendai, and mumps viruses were not sufficiently related to be detected by this procedure (Blair and Robinson, 1968; Robinson and Duesberg, 1968; East and Kingsbury, 1971).

An interesting property of the RNAs extracted from some strains of paramyxoviruses is their ability to self-anneal. Robinson (1970) found that as much as 60% of the 50 S RNA from Sendai virions became ribonuclease resistant under conditions permitting self-annealing, and that NDV self-annealed up to 30%. Self-annealing was also found with Sendai virus (Portner and Kingsbury, 1971) and mumps virus (East and Kingsbury, 1971), but no more than about 30% and 20%, respectively, and Portner and Kingsbury (1970) found no self-annealing with the C strain of NDV. These results indicate that the extent of self-hybridization depends on both the strain and the given lot of virus. The available evidence suggests that it is not intramolecular hybridization, but rather the incorporation into virions, in some instances, of RNA which is complementary to the genome RNA. The biological significance of these observations is still obscure.

For previous detailed reviews of paramyxovirus RNAs, the reader is referred to Robinson and Duesberg (1968), Kingsbury (1970, 1973*a*), and Blair and Duesberg (1970).

2.2.3. Proteins

The initial reports on the virion proteins of NDV analyzed by polyacrylamide gel electrophoresis described the presence of three major proteins and a variable number of minor proteins (Evans and Kingsbury, 1969; Haslam *et al.*, 1969; Bikel and Duesberg, 1969). Subsequently, studies with SV5, NDV, and Sendai virus (Caliguiri *et al.*, 1969; Klenk *et al.*, 1970*a*; Mountcastle *et al.*, 1971) indicated that there were 5–7 proteins in the virion, and possibly 1 or 2 additional minor proteins. Comparison of the proteins of these three virions revealed some differences among them, but also that there were features common to the group (Mountcastle *et al.*, 1970, 1971). Each had a nucleocapsid protein with a molecular weight of around 60,000 daltons. Each has at least two glycoproteins; the larger, which is the most abundant, has a molecular weight of 65,000–74,000 daltons, the smaller one has a molecular weight of 53,000–56,000. These molecular weight estimates are based on migration in SDS gels, which are not exact for glycoproteins. Finally, each paramyxovirus has a nonglycosylated protein which appears to be associated with the virion envelope and has a molecular weight of 38,000–41,000 daltons. The differences among these paramyxoviruses lie in the 2–4 other nonglycosylated proteins which differ in number, size, and abundance in the virions. The available evidence suggests that most if not all of these proteins are not exposed on the surface of the virion (Chen *et al.*, 1971; Scheid and Choppin, 1974*b*; Moore *et al.*, 1974). The function of these proteins remains to be determined.

Because of the finding of a protein band near the origin of polyacrylamide gels of NDV and Sendai virus proteins, several groups of investigators have suggested that a high-molecular-weight protein may exist in the virion (Bratt *et al.*, 1974; Lamb and Mahy, 1974; Moore *et al.*, 1974). An alternative explanation is that this material represents an aggregate rather than a primary gene product. This interpretation is based on the fact that the amount of protein in this region of the gel and the amount of carbohydrate label vary greatly in different preparations of the same strain of virus, and that this material is at times almost completely absent (Caliguiri *et al.*, 1969; Klenk *et al.*, 1970a; Mountcastle *et al.*, 1970, 1971; Scheid *et al.*, 1972) (see also Fig. 7B). In addition, in gels of doubly labeled virus, the ratios of two different amino acid labels vary greatly across this peak, in contrast to their uniformity across the virion protein peaks (Caliguiri *et al.*, 1969). These results do not completely exclude the presence of a small amount of a high-molecular-weight protein in paramyxovirus virions, and this question requires further study. It is perhaps pertinent that, in the case of vesicular stomatitis (VS) virus, the large protein, once considered to be an aggregate, is now known to be an authentic protein (see Chapt. 1 in this volume).

Hall and Martin (1973) have analyzed the proteins of measles virions. Although some significant differences were found, the measles virus protein pattern did share most of the features common to the other paramyxoviruses.

The estimated sums of the molecular weights of the known structural proteins of the various paramyxoviruses are between 300,000 and 400,000 daltons, excluding a very large protein; thus, with a genome molecular weight around 6×10^6 daltons, there is potential information for coding for another 200,000 daltons or more of other proteins, such as non-structural proteins and possibly as yet unrecognized minor structural proteins. However, some of this information may not be expressed, or there may be redundant sequences in the genome (Kingsbury and Granoff, 1970).

As in the case of other enveloped RNA viruses, enzymes such as ATPases or protein kinases have been in some instances found associated with paramyxoviruses (Neurath and Sokol, 1963; Neurath, 1965; Roux and Kolakofsky, 1974). It is not yet clear whether these enzymes are merely adsorbed to the virus or are a minor but integral component of the virion. There is no evidence that they are coded by the virus, and in those cases where they are present, they are apparently not present in large enough amounts to be detected by polyacrylamide gel electrophoresis. It is, therefore, not likely that these enzymes are important as structural components of the virion. In the case of rhabdoviruses, which also have been found to have an associated protein kinase, the available evidence suggests that this is a host-coded enzyme (Imblum and Wagner, 1974). Phosphorylation of paramyxovirus proteins *in vivo* and *in vitro* has been reported (Lamb and Mahy, 1974; Roux and Kolakofsky, 1974). However, the significance of such enzymes, if any, in the replication and functions of the virion is unknown.

The details of the structure, location, and functions of the virion proteins of paramyxoviruses are discussed below in Sect. 2.3.

2.2.4. Lipids

The weight of the available evidence suggests that the lipids of the paramyxovirus virion are largely determined by the host cell. Early studies suggested that the lipids of myxoviruses resembled those of the host (Kates *et al.*, 1962) and that prelabeled host lipids were incorporated into the virus particle (Wecker, 1957). Blough and his coworkers examined the lipids of NDV and Sendai virions, as well as of three strains of influenza virions, grown in the chick embryo and found differences among the various strains (Blough and Lawson, 1968; Tiffany and Blough, 1969*a,b*; Blough and Tiffany, 1973). On the basis of these findings, these authors proposed that the viral envelope proteins determine the lipid composition of the virion by selective association with lipids. However, the differences that were observed were largely in the fatty acids of the neutral lipids; the fatty acids of the polar glycolipids were, in general, similar among the various strains. Since the fatty acids of the neutral lipids represent a small portion of the total in the virion, the significance of these differences is not clear. Further, these analyses were done on virus grown under multiple cycle conditions, and analyses which were done on virions grown in the chick embryo at different times were compared.

Klenk and Choppin (1969*b*, 1970*a,b*) and Choppin *et al.* (1971, 1972) examined the lipids of the plasma membranes of four different types of cultured cells and of SV5 virions grown in these cells. The plasma membranes of the various cells differed significantly, both quantitatively and qualitatively, with respect to their lipid composition, and the virions grown in these cells contained lipids which, with few exceptions, resembled closely those of the host cell membrane. For example, concentrations in plasma membranes of certain phospholipids such as phosphatidylethanolamine and phosphatidylserine differed over a threefold range, and there were also qualitative differences in neutral glycolipids; each of these differences was reflected closely in the virion. Major differences were also found in the fatty acid composition of plasma membranes, which in turn reflected the fatty acid composition of the serum in the medium, and these same large differences were found in the virions grown in the respective cells. In addition, by growing SV5 virions in the presence or absence of an essential fatty acid (linoleic acid), the concentration of the fatty acid in the virion could be varied by fourfold (Klenk and Choppin, 1970*b*). The finding of such major variations in the fatty acid composition of the virions of the same strain of paramyxovirus, which therefore contain the same proteins, raises questions concerning the significance of lesser differences in the fatty acid composition of the neutral lipids of different strains of viruses. In one instance in the comparative studies of SV5 virions and plasma membranes, a significant difference was noted between the phospholipid concentration of the plasma membrane and that of virions. Virions grown in the MDBK line of bovine kidney cells had a higher phosphatidylethanolamine content and lower phosphatidylcholine content than the membrane. This was the one finding in the studies of Klenk and Choppin which was compatible with the hypothesis of Blough and co-workers that the viral proteins have an effect on virion lipid composition. Quigley *et al.* (1971) examined the plasma membranes of chick embryo fibroblasts and of NDV and Sendai virions grown in these cells and found that in general the lipid composition of the virions resembled that of the cells, but that the virions had a somewhat higher sphingomyelin content and lower phosphatidylcholine content than the membrane. However, the lipid compositions of the two paramyxoviruses were similar, as were those of Rous sarcoma and Sindbis viruses examined in the same study. Thus, there was no evidence that different viral proteins specified different lipids.

Further evidence that in general the lipids of the plasma membrane are incorporated quantitatively into the virion was derived from studies showing that during continuous production of SV5 virions by MDBK cells the synthesis of sphingolipids is altered so that the sphingomyelin content of the cell decreases and that of the glycosphingolipid globoside increases. These changes in cellular sphingolipid content are reflected in the virions produced, so that SV5 virions produced on the first day after infection contain more sphingomyelin and less globoside than those produced by the same cells four days after infection (Scheid and Choppin, 1971).

One major qualitative exception to the rule that the virion contains the same lipids as the plasma membrane is that the virions of paramyxoviruses and myxoviruses, which contain the enzyme neuraminidase, do not contain the neuraminic acid-containing glycolipids, the gangliosides (Klenk and Choppin, 1970*b*, 1971; Klenk *et al.*, 1970*a,b*), presumably due to the incorporation of the viral neuraminidase into the membrane. However, VS virus, which does not contain neuraminidase, was found to contain the same ganglioside which was present in the plasma membrane (Klenk and Choppin, 1971).

In summary, the bulk of the evidence indicates that the lipid composition of the viral membrane is determined chiefly by the host cell, and that the composition of virions of the same strain can vary widely, depending on the composition of the plasma membrane of the host. However, exceptions have been found which keep open the possibility that, within narrow limits, some selective incorporation of available lipids may occur. Correlation of the lipid composition of various plasma membranes with the yield of SV5 virions from these cells and the susceptibility of these cells to fusion has suggested that there may be a cell membrane lipid pattern which is optimal for virus production, characterized by a relatively high phosphatidylethanolamine content and lower phosphatidylcholine content. There may also be a correlation between susceptibility to cell fusion and a relatively high ganglioside content and low phosphatidylethanolamine content in the membrane (Klenk and Choppin, 1969*b*, 1970*a*; Choppin *et al.*, 1971, 1972). However, the significance of this apparent correlation remains to be established.

2.2.5. Carbohydrates

Paramyxoviruses contain carbohydrate bound to both glycoproteins and glycolipids. Approximately 6% of the dry weight of the virions is carbohydrate, and in SV5 virions grown in MDBK cells, approximately two-thirds of this is found covalently linked to glycoproteins and one-third to glycolipids (Klenk *et al.*, 1970*a*). These proportions may vary, however, depending on the cell; MDBK cells possess a relatively high concentration of neutral glycolipid (Klenk and Choppin, 1970*b*), and therefore relatively more of the total carbohydrate in the virion may be found in glycolipid than in virions grown in cells whose membranes contain less glycolipid. Galactose, mannose, fucose, and glucosamine were found in glycoproteins, and galactose, glucose, and galactosamine in glycolipids (Klenk *et al.*, 1970*a*; Klenk and Choppin, 1970*b*). No major differences were found in the overall carbohydrate content of virions grown in different cells (Klenk *et al.*, 1970*a*). There is little information available on the exact structure of the carbohydrate chains. It is known that the carbohydrate associated with glycolipid in the virion is determined by the host cell (Klenk and Choppin, 1970*b*), and it is thought that this is also the case with the carbohydrate side chains of glycoproteins, as is apparently the case with other enveloped viruses (see Chapts. in this volume, 1 and 3, on rhabdoviruses and myxoviruses, respectively). Unlike the myxoviruses and rhabdoviruses, the paramyxoviruses do have enough genetic information to code for a few glycosyl transferases, but there is no evidence that they do so. Host cell carbohydrate antigens such as blood group or Forssman antigens have been found to be associated with paramyxoviruses (Isacson and Koch, 1965; Rott *et al.*, 1966).

Presumably because of the viral neuraminidase, paramyxoviruses lack neuraminic acid bound to either glycolipids or glycoproteins. This has been shown by chemical analyses and by electron microscopy using colloidal iron as a specific stain for neuraminic acid; these studies revealed the localized loss of these residues only in those areas of membrane where virions were budding (Klenk and Choppin, 1970*b*, 1971; Klenk *et al.*, 1970*a,b*; Choppin *et al.*, 1971). On the other hand, VS virions, which lack neuraminidase, do contain neuraminic acid (Burge and Huang, 1970; McSharry and Wagner, 1971; Klenk and Choppin, 1971; Klenk *et al.*, 1970*b*). The absence of neuraminic acid is apparently due to the presence of the neuraminidase in that area of membrane which becomes the viral envelope. It is possible that the localized loss of these residues may play a role in virus assembly, although this has not been established (Klenk *et al.*, 1970*b*; Choppin *et al.*, 1971).

The role of the carbohydrate moieties in the biological functions of the virion is not yet clear. Because all virion glycoproteins thus far discovered have been external glycoproteins and the external proteins of enveloped RNA viruses have been found to be glycosylated, it appears that glycosylation is important for positioning of the proteins as projections on the viral surface. Whether the carbohydrate is required for the function of the paramyxovirus glycoproteins, such as receptor binding, hemolysis, or cell fusion, has not been established.

Purified paramyxovirus particles as well as other enveloped RNA viruses and cells infected with these viruses have been shown to be agglutinable by lectins such as concanavalin A, which react with carbohydrate receptors (Becht *et al.*, 1972; Klenk *et al.*, 1972). In the case of influenza virus, the lectin has been shown to react with the glycoprotein spikes (Klenk *et al.*, 1972), and it is likely that this is the case with all of the enveloped RNA viruses.

2.3. Fine Structure and Arrangement of Virion Components

2.3.1. Envelope

2.3.1a. Spikes

The paramyxovirus virion is covered with surface projections or spikes 8–12 nm in length (Horne *et al.*, 1960; Horne and Wildy, 1961;

Rott and Schäfer, 1961; Hosaka *et al.*, 1961; Choppin and Stoeckenius, 1964). These spikes can be removed from the virions by treatment with proteolytic enzymes (Calberg-Bacq *et al.*, 1967; Maeno *et al.*, 1970; Chen *et al.*, 1971). Chen and co-workers (1971) showed that the only proteins affected by treatment of SV5 virions with pronase were the glycoproteins of the virion, establishing that these proteins comprised the spikes, and that the other proteins were protected from the enzyme by the lipid layer. In these studies, no detectable portion of the glycoprotein remained associated with the membrane after protease treatment, indicating that the entire glycoprotein was accessible to the enzyme, and thus suggesting that the spikes do not penetrate deeply into the bilayer. Furthermore, removal of the spikes with the proteolytic enzyme did not disrupt the virion, suggesting that the spike glycoproteins do not play a significant structural role in maintaining the integrity of the viral membrane. Finally, when the spikes were removed from the SV5 virions, hemagglutinating and neuraminidase activities were lost, indicating that these activities are associated with virion glycoproteins.

2.3.1b. Isolation and Functions of the Glycoproteins

Hemagglutinin and Neuraminidase. Because of the extensive evidence that the hemagglutinating and neuraminidase activities of myxoviruses reside on separate glycoproteins, it was initially assumed that this would also be the case with paramyxoviruses. The two glycoproteins have been isolated from SV5 virions by extraction with the nonionic detergent Triton X-100, and separated from each other on sucrose gradients containing Triton and 1 M KCl (Scheid *et al.*, 1972). Under these conditions, full neuraminidase and hemagglutinin activities were retained, and both activities were associated with the larger glycoprotein (molecular weight *ca.* 67,000 daltons); neither activity was associated with the smaller glycoproteins (molecular weight approximately 56,000 daltons). Subsequently, the glycoproteins of NDV (Scheid and Choppin, 1973) and Sendai virus were isolated (Scheid and Choppin, 1974*a,b*), and in each case the larger virion glycoprotein possessed both activities, and the smaller, neither activity. Tozawa *et al.* (1973) also found that both activities of Sendai virus were associated with a single protein.

Other recent evidence which is compatible with the existence of both biological activities on the same glycoprotein is the failure to separate these two activities in *ts* mutants (Pierce and Haywood, 1973; Preble and Youngner, 1973*b*; Portner *et al.*, 1974). In this chapter, the large paramyxovirus glycoprotein will be referred to as HN and the smaller as F, as suggested previously by Scheid and Choppin (1974*a,b*).

The previous reports that hemagglutinating and neuraminidase subunits of paramyxoviruses could be separated (Haslam *et al.*, 1969; Iinuma *et al.*, 1971; Brostrom *et al.*, 1971) were not based on isolation of individual purified proteins, and were complicated by factors such as significant inactivation of neuraminidase in some cases and the probable formation of mixed aggregates of different sizes which differed in biological activities. The failure of the neuraminidase released from virions by a proteolytic enzyme (Maeno *et al.*, 1970) to bind to or agglutinate red blood cells can probably now be explained by removal of the hydrophobic base of the large glycoprotein as discussed below, so that it was able to aggregate, was monovalent, and did not bind firmly to the cell surface.

When purified SV5 glycoprotein spikes are removed from a Triton-containing solution, they form rosettelike clusters aggregating by their bases (Scheid *et al.*, 1972). This type of aggregation in aqueous solution suggests that the spikes have hydrophobic bases. This conclusion has been supported by the observation that treatment of the isolated HN glycoprotein with chymotrypsin removed about 6000 daltons of protein, and the remaining glycoprotein was soluble in aqueous solution and retained neuraminidase activity (Scheid and Choppin, unpublished experiments). The aggregates formed by the isolated HN and F proteins are morphologically distinguishable (Scheid *et al.*, 1972); the HN protein forms berrylike clusters, and the F protein forms rosettes with more distinct radiating spikes. This suggests the possibility that two different types of spikes are present on paramyxovirus virions, although they cannot be distinguished on the intact virion by electron microscopy. There is considerable evidence that this is the case with myxoviruses (see Chapt. 3 in this volume). However, the possibility has not yet been completely excluded that both HN and F proteins of paramyxoviruses might be present in a single morphological spike unit on the intact virions, and that when purified and separated from each other by detergents and then allowed to aggregate, homogeneous aggregates form which do not represent the configuration present on the intact virion.

On the basis of the size of the spikes in the electron microscope, the sedimentation constant of spikes in Triton-containing sucrose gradients (8.9 S and 6.7 S for the HN and F proteins of SV5, and 9.3 S and 6.1 S for NDV, respectively), and suggestive evidence that monomers of spike proteins may be linked by disulfide bonds, it appears likely that each morphological spike contains at least two glycoprotein monomers (Scheid *et al.*, 1972; Scheid and Choppin, 1973, and unpublished experiments). The precise fine structure of the spikes remains to be determined.

Isolation by Affinity Chromatography. A recent improvement in the isolation and separation of the glycoproteins of paramyxoviruses has been the use of affinity chromatography on fetuin-Sepharose (Scheid and Choppin, 1974*a,b*). This method is based on the specific adsorption of the HN protein to the neuraminic acid-containing receptor on the fetuin. It yields glycoproteins in preparative quantities, and is therefore very useful for obtaining pure proteins for biochemical studies. Further, it should prove useful for vaccine production since it can be used to produce, in one simple step, large amounts of the pure proteins which are important in inducing immmunity to infection.

The Smaller Virion Glycoprotein. When it was found that the larger glycoprotein of SV5 and NDV possessed both hemagglutinating and neuraminidase activities, it was postulated that the smaller glycoprotein was involved in virus-induced cell fusion and hemolysis (Scheid *et al.*, 1972; Scheid and Choppin, 1973). Evidence to support this concept was subsequently obtained independently by Scheid and Choppin (1974*a,b*) and Homma and Ohuchi (Homma and Ohuchi, 1973; Homma, 1974) with Sendai virus. Sendai virions grown in MDBK cells (Scheid and Choppin, 1974*a,b*) contain, in addition to the large HN glycoprotein, another large glycoprotein (molecular weight *ca.* 65,000 daltons). This protein (designated F_0) has been shown to be a precursor of the smaller virion glycoprotein (F), which is derived from F_0 by proteolytic cleavage. This cleavage does not occur to a significant extent in MDBK cells, but does occur when virus is grown in the chick embryo. The MDBK cell-grown virions, which contain the precursor, do not cause cell fusion or hemolysis and are not infective, whereas the chick embryo-grown virions possess these activities. Cleavage of the precursor on MDBK cell-grown virions can be accomplished *in vitro* with trypsin, and virions so treated induce cell fusion and hemolysis and become infective. Thus, the small paramyxovirus glycoprotein is synthesized as an approximately 65,000-dalton protein which appears to be biologically inactive, but is activated by a host-dependent proteolytic cleavage to yield the biologically active smaller glycoprotein. The significance of this protein in the initiation of infection will be discussed below in Sect. 3.2. Essentially similar results were obtained by Homma and co-workers with Sendai virions grown in L cells, which were biologically inactive, and in the chick embryo, which were fully active (Homma and Ohuchi, 1973; Homma, 1974). Homma had found previously that L cell-grown virions were not infective for L cells and did not cause hemolysis or cell fusion, but did so after trypsin treatment (Homma, 1971, 1972; Homma and Tamagawa, 1973). It was originally suggested in these earlier studies that trypsin treatment removed a host-specific inhibitor from the virions; however, the recent studies on the virion proteins by Homma and Ohuchi (Homma and Ohuchi, 1973; Homma, 1974) and those of Scheid and Choppin (1974a,b) cited above are now in complete agreement. Lamb and Mahy (1974) also found evidence for host-dependent differences in virion glycoproteins. Thus, it appears well established that cleavage of a precursor of the small virion glycoprotein is required for activation of cell fusion, hemolysis, and infectivity of Sendai virions, and that whether such cleavage occurs depends on the host cell. Such a precursor protein has not yet been identified with certainty on mature SV5 or NDV virions, presumably because cleavage had occurred on those virions before maturation. A minor but inconsistent peak was seen in this region of gels of NDV by Mountcastle et al. (1971). Further, a protein has been found in NDV-infected cells which may correspond to this protein (Lomniczi et al., 1971), and evidence has been obtained for a precursor–product relationship (Kaplan and Bratt, 1973; Samson and Fox, 1973; Hightower and Bratt, 1974).

The requirement for cleavage of a presursor glycoprotein for activation of biological activities and the variation in the extent of cleavage, depending on the cell in which the virus is grown, provide a biochemical basis for the host-dependent variation in virus-induced cell fusion, hemolysis, and infectivity of paramyxoviruses that has been previously observed by a number of investigators (Ishida and Homma, 1960; Matsumoto and Maeno, 1962; Young and Ash, 1970; Homma, 1971, 1972; Homma and Tamagawa, 1973). In addition, it now appears likely that strain-dependent variation in hemolysis and cell fusion may be explained ultimately on the basis of differences in the sensitivity to cleavage of the precursor of the smaller glycoprotein.

The mechanism by which the smaller virion glycoprotein is involved in cell fusion and hemolysis is not yet clear. It is pertinent to indicate that protein alone is insufficient to cause fusion. Evidence from many laboratories, using different paramyxoviruses, has indicated that the association of lipid with protein is necessary for fusion, and it has recently been found in reassembly experiments with viral envelope proteins and lipids that both lipids and proteins are required to obtain biologically active aggregates (Hosaka and Shimizu, 1972; Hosaka, 1974).

2.3.1c. Lipid Bilayer and Nonglycosylated Envelope Protein

Spin-label electron spin resonance (ESR) studies have provided evidence that the lipids of the paramyxovirus membrane are present in a bilayer (Landsberger *et al.*, 1973). Stearic acid derivatives with a nitroxide group at different positions on the acyl chain were incorporated into the viral membrane, and a flexibility gradient was obtained which is characteristic of a lipid bilayer (McConnell and McFarland, 1972). By growing SV5 and influenza virions, which have different membrane proteins, in MDBK cells and BHK21 cells, which have significantly different lipid composition (Klenk and Choppin, 1969*b*, 1970*a,b*), it was possible to vary independently the lipid and protein compositions of the viral membrane and to examine the structure of the lipid of these membranes by ESR methods (Landsberger *et al.*, 1973). Growing the two different viruses in the same cell produced membranes with different proteins but similar lipids, and in this case the ESR spectra were indistinguishable. Conversely, growing the same virus in the two different cell types permitted a comparison of membranes with similar proteins but different lipids. In this case, there were significant differences in the ESR spectra. These results indicate that the rigidity of the lipid phase of the viral membrane depends largely on the lipid composition and is not affected by the differences in the membrane protein composition of two viruses. These results are compatible with the previous finding that removal of the spikes from the surface of influenza (Compans *et al.*, 1970) or parainfluenza (Chen, *et al.*, 1971) virions does not result in disruption of the membrane nor change the ESR spectra (Landsberger *et al.*, 1971). In addition, removal of the spikes by proteolytic enzymes left no detectable residual portion of the glycoproteins associated with the membrane, suggesting that the spikes did not penetrate through the bilayer. These results can best be interpreted as indicating that the major portion of the viral membrane is organized as a bilayer, that the structural rigidity of this bilayer depends on the lipid composition and not on differences in membrane-associated proteins, and that the spike glycoproteins neither penetrate deeply into the bilayer nor contribute significantly to the structure of the lipid phase (Landsberger *et al.*, 1973). The precise mechanism of attachment of the spikes to the viral membrane remains to be determined.

Associated with the envelope of paramyxoviruses is a nonglycosylated protein with a molecular weight of 38,000–41,000 daltons. This protein is referred to as the M or membrane protein. It can be solubilized by Triton X-100 in the presence of high salt such as

1 M KCl or 30% CsCl (McSharry *et al.*, 1972; Scheid *et al.*, 1972; Scheid and Choppin, 1973). Both the detergent and high salt are required to keep it in solution. In aqueous solution, this protein forms fibrous aggregates, and an amino acid analysis of this protein from SV5 virions has revealed a moderately hydrophobic pattern (McSharry *et al.*, 1972, and unpublished experiments). Analogous proteins are present in rhabdoviruses and myxoviruses (see Chapts 1 and 3 in this volume). The available evidence suggests that these proteins are located just beneath the lipid bilayer. Such evidence, which is most complete in the case of myxoviruses, includes electron microscopic and preliminary X-ray diffraction studies; it indicates a layer of protein on the underside of the viral envelope, the failure to label this protein with reagents specific for surface proteins, the resistance of this protein to proteolytic enzymes, and the transfer of fluorescence from the aromatic residues of an internal protein to a fluorescent probe incorporated in the lipid bilayer. The reader is referred to the Chapt. 3 in this volume on myxoviruses for discussion of this evidence.

The assignment of functions to this nonglycosylated membrane protein is largely based on circumstantial evidence. However, it appears that interaction between this protein and the lipid of the membrane may play a role in maintaining the structure and integrity of the viral envelope. As pointed out above, the spikes do not appear to play such a role. Further, if migration of host cell proteins in the plane of the membrane occurs, as an increasing body of evidence suggests, then there must be a mechanism for excluding host proteins from those areas of membranes which become the viral membrane, and which therefore represent localized domains within the plasma membrane of the cell (Choppin *et al.*, 1972). The M protein appears to be the best candidate for such a role because of its location in the virion and the apparent exclusion of the spikes as important in this capacity. Finally, this protein may function during virus assembly as the site which is recognized by the viral nucleocapsid when it aligns under those areas of cell membrane which contain viral proteins and are destined to become the viral membrane. This would follow from the location of the proteins on the underside of the membrane. Evidence supporting this concept was obtained in phenotypic mixing experiments between SV5 and VS virus in which it was shown that the spike glycoproteins of the two viruses could be freely intermixed, or even totally exchanged, on virions. In contrast, virions containing the VS virus nucleocapsid contained only the VS virus M protein, suggesting that a specific recognition must occur between these two components during assembly (Choppin and Compans, 1970; McSharry *et al.*, 1971).

A more extensive discussion of the structure and assembly of viral membranes will appear in a subsequent volume in this series (Choppin and Compans, 1975).

2.3.2. The Nucleocapsid

2.3.2a. Structure

Early electron microscopic studies using the negative-contrast method revealed that the nucleocapsids of paramyxoviruses were flexible helical structures 17–18 nm in diameter with a central hole about 5 nm in diameter (Horne et al., 1960; Horne and Waterson, 1960). It was proposed in those studies that the nucleocapsid was a double-helical structure; however, it was subsequently shown to be a single-helical structure (Choppin and Stoeckenius, 1964) (Figs. 2 and 3). Hosaka et al. (1966) estimated the lengths of nucleocapsids within Sendai virions of various sizes and found multiples of 1 μm. Compans and Choppin (1967a,b) isolated the nucelocapsids from SV5- and NDV-infected cells and obtained a unit-length distribution of approximately 1.0 μm (see Fig. 4), and such a value has also been found by several other workers with the isolated nucleocapsids from various paramyxoviruses (Hosaka, 1968; Hosaka and Shimizu, 1968; Kingsbury and Darlington, 1968; Finch and Gibbs, 1970; Nakai et al., 1969; Waters et al., 1972). This length of nucleocapsid is therefore assumed to contain one copy of the viral genome. The paramyxovirus nucleocapsids have been found to contain between 4 and 5% RNA (Compans and Choppin, 1967a; Hosaka, 1968; Kingsbury and Darlington, 1968; Hall and Martin, 1973; Waters et al., 1972). Buoyant densities in CsCl have ranged from 1.27 to 1.31 g/ml (Compans and Choppin, 1967a; Hosaka, 1968; Kingsbury and Darlington, 1968, Blair and Robinson, 1970; Hall and Martin, 1973).

Finch and Gibbs (1970) carried out a thorough study of paramyxovirus nucleocapsids using optical diffraction methods on electron micrographs. They concluded that there are 11–13 structure units per turn of the nucleocapsid helix, which has a pitch of 5 nm. This number of units per turn would give a total of 2200–2600 subunits for a 1-μm nucleocapsid with 200 turns. These authors suggested that the subunits were hour-glass shaped and arranged at an angle of about 60° to the long axis of the helix, which may contribute to the flexibility of the structure which is essential for its being enclosed within the virion. Using a goniometer stage in the electron microscope, Compans *et al.* (1972) examined stretched out segments of SV5 and mumps virus nucleocapsids, and by observing the effects of tilting on the images of the turn of the helix, determined that the sense of the helix of these paramyxoviruses is left-handed.

2.3.2b. Protein Subunit

As discussed above, the protein subunits of the nucleocapsids of paramyxoviruses have molecular weights of about 60,000 daltons (56,000–61,000). In the course of examining the nucleocapsids released from paramyxovirus-infected cells which had been dispersed with trypsin, it was found that nucleocapsids isolated under these conditions were composed of subunits of smaller size, i.e., SV5, about 43,000, Sendai, 46,000, and NDV, 47,000 daltons (Mountcastle *et al.*, 1970). Thus, the addition of trypsin to the cells before disruption results in the cleavage of every subunit of every nucleocapsid to a smaller size, with the loss of about 10,000–18,000 daltons of protein, which has not yet been recovered as an intact piece. Examination of the nucleocapsids composed of the smaller, cleaved subunits indicated that they were more tightly wound and less flexible helices than the nucleocapsids composed of the larger, native protein subunits. Subsequent studies have revealed that the cleavage can be accomplished by other enzymes, such as chymotrypsin and ficin, either by dispersing cells with the enzymes, or by treating the isolated nucleocapsids *in vitro* (Mountcastle *et al.*, 1974). These results suggest that there is a segment of the nucleocapsid polypeptide chain that is extremely susceptible to cleavage by proteolytic enzymes, and the remainder, i.e., the 43,000- to 47,000-dalton cleavage product, is resistant. In addition, this cleavage product apparently contains the necessary configuration to bind to the nucleic acid and to maintain the helical structure. Further, since the helix formed by this cleaved subunit is more stable and rigid than that formed by the native, 60,000-dalton subunit, it appears that the smaller portion of the molecule removed by the enzymes confers flexibility on the helix. It has also been postulated that this portion of the nucleocapsid protein may be exposed on the outer surface of the native subunit where it is accessible to the enzyme, and that it therefore might be involved in the recognition by the nucleocapsid of specific areas of membrane during maturation (Mountcastle *et al.*, 1970, 1974). The evidence supporting an external location of this portion of the protein includes its accessibility to proteases and the observation that the native nucleocapsid behaves as a hydrophobic structure, aggregating in aqueous solution, whereas the nucleocapsid composed of the cleaved 45,000-dalton subunits is more freely dispersed in aqueous solution. This suggests a hydrophobic, externally disposed portion of the molecule, and since the membrane protein (M) discussed above also behaves hydrophobically, the postulated recognition interaction between these two proteins may involve hydrophobic interactions (Mountcastle *et al.*, 1974).

The extreme susceptibility of the nucleocapsid protein subunits to proteolytic cleavage raises the question that under some conditions this cleavage might occur intracellularly. If so, this might result in inability of such nucleocapsid to be incorporated into budding virions because of both the decreased flexibility of the structure and the possible loss of the necessary recognition site discussed above. Such an event could play a role in the intracellular accumulation of paramyxovirus nucleocapsids which frequently occurs, particularly in abortive or persistent infections (Compans *et al.*, 1966; Mountcastle *et al.*, 1970, 1974).

2.3.2c.   Other Proteins Associated with the Nucleocapsid

In addition to the protein subunit of the nucleocapsid, another protein has been found associated with paramyxovirus nucleocapsids in some cases. The largest protein in Sendai virus is a nonglycosylated protein with a molecular weight of about 69,000 daltons (Mountcastle *et al.*, 1971). Stone and co-workers (1972) found that a transcriptive complex isolated from infected cells contaied this protein, which will be designated here as P, in addition to the nucleocapsid protein. Marx and co-workers (1974) subsequently found that the disruption of Sendai virions with Triton released a structure which contained these same two polypeptides and which had RNA transcriptase activity. In the case of SV5, a nonglycosylated protein with a molecular weight of about 50,000 daltons sediments with the nucleocapsid after disruption of the virion with Triton X-100 (McSharry *et al.*, 1972); however, this protein can be largely removed from the nucleocapsid by repeated centrifugation in CsCl (Mountcastle *et al.*, 1970; McSharry *et al.*, 1972, and unpublished experiments). This protein was originally designated protein 5 (Caliguiri *et al.*, 1969). It appears to be analogous to the largest Sendai virion protein in that is is associated with the nucleocapsid, but it is apparently not tightly bound since it can be removed by CsCl. These proteins will be discussed further in Sect. 3.3.1, which deals with RNA transcriptase activity.

TABLE 2

**Summary of Properties of Some Paramyxovirus Proteins
and Suggested Designations for These Proteins**[a]

Mol. wt.,[b] daltons	Presence of carbohydrate	Function	Suggested designation
69,000[c]	−	In virion RNA polymerase complex	P
67,000–74,000	+	Hemagglutinin, neuraminidase	HN
65,000[d]	+	Precursor of F protein	F_0
56,000–61,000	−	Nucleocapsid subunit	NP
53,000–56,000	+	Cell fusion, hemolysis	F
38,000–41,000	−	Membrane protein	M

[a] Modified from Scheid and Choppin (1974a, b). It should be noted that other proteins have been identified in various paramyxoviruses, but sufficient evidence is not available on their function or location to permit designations on this basis.

[b] Based on estimates of Mountcastle et al. (1971) for SV5, Sendai virus, and NDV. Others have reported estimates somewhat different in some cases.

[c] Estimate for Sendai virus protein. An analogous protein has not yet been definitely identified in other paramyxoviruses. An SV5 protein which may have comparable function has a molecular weight of approximately 50,000 daltons.

[d] Estimate for Sendai virus protein. An analogous protein. An analogous protein has not yet been definitely identified with other paramyxoviruses. An NDV protein with a molecular weight of 62,000–66,000 daltons may have this function.

2.3.3. Summary of Properties of Virion Proteins

Table 2 shows a summary of properties of some of the paramyxovirus proteins for which there is persuasive evidence concerning their location and functions. Suggested designations based on these functions are listed. Figures 5, 6, and 7 show polyacrylamide gel electropherograms of the proteins of SV5, NDV, and Sendai virus, respectively.

2.3.4. Diagram of the Structure of a Paramyxovirus

Figure 8 shows a schematic diagram of the arrangement of the components in a paramyxovirus virion. The spikes covering the surface are not drawn with two distinctly different appearances because their existence as such on the virion has not been conclusively established; however, for convenience and because it is at present thought to be the most likely arrangement, the two glycoproteins are indicated on different spikes. The P protein is thought to be associated with the nucleocapsid, but is not depicted there because there is no information available on the arrangement of this protein in the nucleocapsid. There are other proteins present in virions of some types of paramyxoviruses, but these are not indicated because of lack of evidence for their location.

3. REPLICATION

3.1. General Comments

As would be expected with such a diverse group of viruses, the kinetics of replication of paramyxoviruses differ widely, depending on virus type, host cell, and multiplicity of infection. The length of the latent period varies considerably; for example, it can be as short as 2.5 hours with NDV (Wheelock and Tamm, 1961b) and as long as 15 hours with Sendai virus (Darlington *et al.*, 1970). Similarly, depending on the virus–cell system involved, virus production may terminate

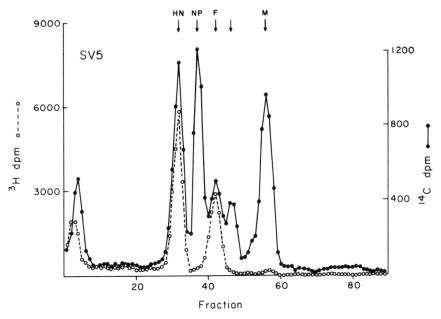

Fig. 5. Polyacrylamide gel electrophoresis of the polypeptides of the parainfluenza virus SV5 labeled with ^{14}C-amino acid mixture(—●——●) and ^{3}H-glucosamine (O----O-). The properties of these proteins and the designations used are described in the text. The designations are those suggested by Scheid and Choppin (1974a,b). The function of the polypeptide indicated by the unlabeled arrow (molecular weight approximately 50,000 daltons) has not yet been definitely established; therefore, a letter designation has not been given, but this protein appears to be associated with the nucleocapsid and may correspond to protein P of Sendai virus (see text). The origin is at the left and anode at the right. Modified from Chen *et al.* (1971).

within 8 hours when cell death occurs, or it may continue for many days, and the yield of infective virus may vary from less than one to over a thousand infective virions per cell. Among the most productive systems yet described is SV5 in primary rhesus monkey kidney cells, in which 1500 PFU/cell may be produced in the first 24 hours after infection, and production continues for many days without cell death (Choppin 1964). On the other hand, infection of the BHK21-F line of baby hamster kidney cells with the same virus yields only about 10 PFU/cell; nucleocapsid accumulates in the cytoplasm due to a block in maturation at the cell membrane; and the cells die following massive cell fusion (Holmes and Choppin, 1966; Compans *et al.*, 1971). Thus, there is no single growth curve, virus yield, or fate of the infected cell which is characteristic of paramyxovirus infection, and events at the

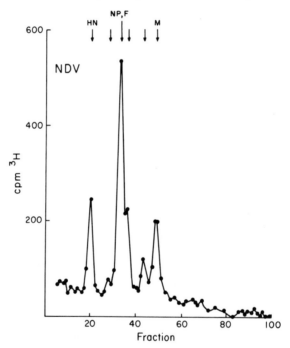

Fig. 6. Polyacrylamide gel electrophoresis of the polypeptides of NDV labeled with ^{3}H-leucine. The nucleocapsid protein (NP) and the smaller virion glycoprotein (F) comigrate. The functions of the proteins indicated by the unlabeled arrows (molecular weights approximately 62,000, 53,000, and 46,000 daltons) have not been established, and thus no letter designations have been given. The largest of these, which is a very small peak, may correspond to the F_0 protein of Sendai virus (see text). Modified from Mountcastle *et al.* (1971).

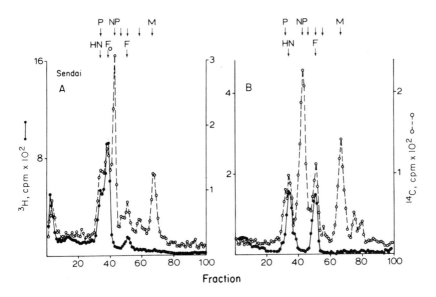

Fig. 7.   Polyacrylamide gel electrophoresis of the polypeptides of Sendai virus labeled with ^{14}C-amino acids (O———O) and ^{3}H-glucosamine (●———●). (A) Virions grown in MDBK cells. (B) Virions grown in the embryonated chicken egg. The properties of these proteins are described in the text. The largest nonglycosylated protein, P, and the glycoprotein HN frequently comigrate (panel A) but are sometimes resolved (panel B). Protein F_0 is present in large amounts in the virions grown in MDBK cells and absent in virions grown in the chick embryo. F is derived from F_0 by proteolytic cleavage, which occurs in the embryonated egg but to only a very limited extent in MDBK cells (see text). The functions of the polypeptides indicated by the unlabeled arrows have not been determined. A nonglycosylated protein also migrates in the region of the smaller glycoprotein. Modified from Scheid and Choppin (1974a,b).

cell membrane which are dependent on both the virus strain and the host cell type are particularly important in determining the outcome of infection.

3.2.   Adsorption

3.2.1.   Adsorption to Glycoprotein Receptors

Soon after the discovery of hemagglutination by influenza virus (Hirst, 1941; McClelland and Hare, 1941), it was found that NDV (Burnet, 1942) and mumps (Levens and Enders, 1945) also hemagglutinated. It was subsequently established that, as with influenza virus, the receptor for paramyxoviruses on the cell surface was a mucoprotein containing neuraminic acid and that the virion possessed the enzyme neuraminidase, which was capable of destroying these receptors.

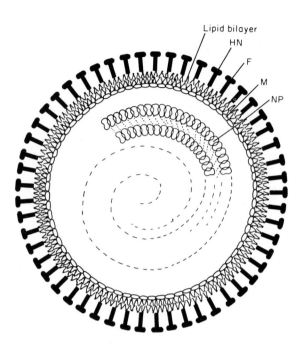

Fig. 8. Schematic diagram of the suggested arrangement of the structural components of paramyxoviruses. The two glycoproteins HN and F are located on the external surface of the lipid bilayer. Their mode of attachment to the lipid and whether they penetrate the bilayer are not certain. Under certain conditions F_0, the precursor to F, is present rather than F. On the internal surface of the bilayer is the nonglycosylated membrane protein M; within the envelope is the helical ribonucleoprotein containing the protein subunit NP and the viral RNA. Also associated with the nucleocapsid in at least some paramyxoviruses is another polypeptide, P. This has not been indicated because the details of its arrangement are unknown. Other polypeptides of unknown function are also present in some paramyxoviruses, but they are not designated here because of the lack of sufficient knowledge of their arrangement (see text for details).

Indeed, it was their common receptor affinity and neuraminidase activity that were major factors in grouping what are now the paramyxoviruses with the influenza viruses in the original myxovirus group (Andrewes *et al.*, 1955).

The subject of adsorption of paramyxoviruses has been extensively reviewed. The early work on this area was covered by Sagik and Levine (1957), Hirst (1959), Cohen (1963), Philipson (1963), and Gottshalk (1965). Recent reviews include Howe and Lee (1970), Dales (1973), and Lonberg-Holm and Philipson (1974). The salient points will be briefly summarized here. Adsorption to receptors on host cells appears to be in principle similar to adsorption to erythrocytes. Adsorption to the neuraminic acid-containing receptors, with the exception of measles virus, is temperature independent, requires cations, and occurs over a broad range of pH. Many of the paramyxoviruses elute rapidly at 37°C, and even at room temperature hemagglutination patterns may be unstable, so that titrations are frequently done in the cold. Treatment of erythrocytes with neuraminidase to an extent which will leave them still agglutinatable by most strains of influenza virus will prevent their agglutination by NDV, mumps virus or SV5. Thus, the influenza viruses can bind to erythrocytes containing fewer neuraminic acid residues than can paramyxoviruses; i.e., paramyxoviruses are above influenza viruses on what was originally called the "receptor gradient" [see Hirst (1959) for review].

One possible factor in the less firm binding of some paramyxoviruses than myxoviruses to erythrocytes at elevated temperatures is the recent finding that the hemagglutinating and neuraminidase activities reside on the same paramyxovirus glycoprotein, in contrast to two proteins in the case of myxoviruses (Scheid *et al.*, 1972; Scheid and Choppin, 1973, 1974*a,b*; Tozawa *et al.*, 1973). It has not yet been established whether the active sites involved are the same, i.e., whether hemagglutination by paramyxoviruses is essentially an enzyme–substrate reaction or whether there are two separate sites on the same protein involved in hemagglutinating and neuraminidase activities. If one active site were involved, the observed elution of the majority of virus at 37°C could be explained, as well as the old observation of the inability to produce "indicator virus" with NDV, in contrast to influenza virus. Indicator virus was the term used for influenza virus whose neuraminidase activity had been inactivated by heat, but which still hemagglutinated, and thus was a sensitive detector of glycoproteins which functioned as competitive inhibitors by virtue of their receptor activity (Francis, 1947; Anderson, 1948).

Although most of the paramyxovirus which adsorbed to erythrocytes in the cold elutes when the temperatures is raised, it was found in early studies that irreversible binding of NDV also occurs (Burnet and Anderson, 1946). Erythrocytes with such adsorbed virus agglutinated fresh red blood cells (RBC) and were agglutinated by antisera to NDV. Further, allowing the virus to adsorb at 4°C and then carrying out repeated resuspension and settling at 37°C results in extension of the hemagglutination titer. In addition, conditions which favor irreversible attachment of virus to RBC also favor hemolysis, and it was suggested that these phenomena were related (Burnet and Lind, 1950). Clavell and Bratt (1972a,b) in a recent extensive study of hemolysis concluded that a single virus particle is capable of causing hemolysis, and that virus which elutes from cells has less capacity to cause hemolysis than the original virus, thus supporting a correlation between irreversible adsorption and hemolysis. In view of these results, the correlation between hemolysis and cell fusion to be mentioned below, and the fact that the paramyxovirus membrane may fuse with erythrocyte membranes under certain conditions (Howe and Morgan, 1969; Bächi et al., 1973; Baker, 1970; Apostolov and Almeida, 1972), it would seem that at least some of the irreversibly adsorbed virus could represent virus whose membranes had fused to those of the erythrocyte membrane.

3.2.2. Adsorption of Measles Virus

Unlike the other paramyxoviruses, viruses of the measles subgroup do not appear to possess the enzyme neuraminidase nor do they adsorb to neuraminic acid-containing receptors (Norrby, 1962; Waterson et al., 1964). Other differences between measles and other paramyxoviruses are that measles virus only agglutinates monkey or baboon cells whereas paramyxoviruses agglutinate fowl, guinea pig, and human cells, higher titers are obtained at 37°C than at 4°C, and the measles virus does not elute (Peries and Chany, 1960; Rosen, 1961). Measles virus also causes hemolysis, and the hemolytic activity has been separated from hemagglutinating activity (Norrby, 1964; Norrby and Hammorskjöld, 1972; Norrby and Gollmar, 1972). The precise chemical nature of the receptor for the measles virus remains to be determined.

3.3. Penetration and Uncoating

As is the case with other enveloped viruses, the mechanism by which the genome of paramyxoviruses gains access to the host cell has not been definitely established. Penetration by "viropexis" or phagocytosis, first proposed by Fazekas de St. Groth (1948), has been observed with paramyxoviruses (Mussgay and Weibel, 1962; Silverstein and Marcus, 1964; Compans et al., 1966). The alternative mechanism of fusion of the viral membrane with the cell membrane, and penetration of the nucleocapsid alone has also been proposed (Adams and Prince,

1957; Meiselman *et al.*, 1967; Morgan and Howe, 1968; Howe and Morgan, 1969). The conclusions of all of these studies depend on the interpretation of electron micrographs, and are inevitably complicated by virus particle-to-infectivity ratios of greater than one, and the high multiplicity of inoculation required to observe a sufficient number of virus particles. This question has recently been extensively and critically reviewed by Dales (1973) and Lonberg-Holm and Philipson (1974), and will not be dealt with in detail here. The reader is referred to these reviews for a thorough discussion of these two alternatives. It is pertinent that among the most impressive examples of fusion of viral and cell membranes was that shown with Sendai virus (Morgan and Howe, 1968; Howe and Morgan, 1969). Neither mechanism has been conclusively demonstrated as the sole means of penetration of the genome, and it is possible that both may be operative.

Very recently observations have been made which bear on this question and do not depend on electron microscopy. As mentioned above, Scheid and Choppin (1974*b*) and Homma and Ohuchi (1973) have found that the activation of hemolysis, cell fusion, and infectivity of Sendai virions were correlated with proteolytic cleavage of a glycoprotein precursor to yield the smaller virion glycoprotein. The finding that hemolysis and cell fusion were activated together in these studies provides evidence that these two activities are expressions of the same biochemical mechanism. This view has been held by many workers since the early studies of Okada (1958). Although it has been questioned at times (Kohn, 1965), the weight of the available evidence suggests a similarity in the two activities, and the recent evidence for activation of both by cleavage of the smaller virion glycoprotein strengthens this argument (Scheid and Choppin, 1974*a,b*). From the standpoint of the question of penetration, it appears to be of particular significance that when the virions acquire the ability to cause cell fusion, they also acquire infectivity, and that the smaller virion glycoprotein is involved in both activities. Since adsorption is due to the larger glycoprotein (HN), which possesses hemagglutinating and neuraminidase activity, the smaller glycoprotein appears to be exerting its action on the process of initiation of infection at a step beyond adsorption. A straightforward explanation would be that this step is penetration and that fusion of the viral and cell membranes is involved. If that were the case, the simultaneous acquisition of the ability to cause cell fusion and infectivity on cleavage of the small protein would be expected. It should be emphasized, however, that these results do not prove that this is the mechanism. One could argue that cleavage of the glycoprotein enhances phagocytosis of the virus or permits the appropriate degradation of the particle within a phagocytic vesicle. These questions are amenable to experimentation, but the present evidence suggests that the ability of the virion to initiate infection is correlated with its ability to induce membrane fusion, and, therefore, this evidence is compatible with the argument that membrane fusion is the mechanism of interiorization of the paramyxovirus nucleocapsid.

Once the nucleocapsid has gained access to the cytoplasmic matrix, either following fusion of viral and cell membranes or by release from a phagocytic vesicle, the viral genome may be transcribed without release from the nucleocapsid. It has been reported that a portion of radioactively labeled paramyxovirus RNA becomes ribonuclease sensitive shortly after infection and then resistant again at 4 hours post-infection (Lerner *et al.*, 1969), an observation which was equated with first uncoating and then a later shift to a double-stranded form. Others also reported that 70% of labeled NDV RNA became ribonuclease sensitive after incubation with chicken cells, and that puromycin inhibited this process (Durand *et al.*, 1970). However, such observations on the bulk of inoculated RNA do not necessarily reflect that RNA which is involved in the initiation of infection, and degradation of nucleocapsid by lysosomal enzymes could lead to these findings. Furthermore, earlier studies found that puromycin did not prevent the initiation of early biosynthetic events (Wheelock, 1962), and more recently it was found that cycloheximide treatment of cells did not prevent transcription (Robinson, 1971*b*). Bukrinskaya *et al.* (1969*b*) also reported evidence suggesting that only partial deproteinization of input nucleocapsid occurred, and that this proceeded very slowly within the cell. In view of the more recent evidence mentioned in Sect. 2.3.2, and described below, which indicates the transcription of the viral RNA within a transcriptive complex containing the nucleocapsid protein, it now appears likely that dissociation of the infecting RNA from the nucleocapsid is not a necessary step in the viral replication cycle.

3.4. Biosynthesis

3.4.1. RNA

3.4.1a. Virion-Associated Transcriptase

The early evidence suggesting that the RNA of paramyxoviruses was complementary to the virion RNA, which will be discussed below, and the lack of infectivity of naked viral RNA suggested that a transcriptase might exist in the virions of paramyxoviruses. After the discovery of a virion-associated polymerase in VS virus, a similar activity was found in NDV virions (Baltimore *et al.*, 1970; Huang *et al.*, 1971). This enzymatic activity, which was much less active than the VS virus enzyme, was demonstrated after treatment of the virion with a nonionic detergent and required all four nucleoside triphoshates, Mg^{2+}, and a reducing agent. The RNA molecules produced sedimented at about 16S and were complementary to the virion RNA. The reaction was sensitive to RNase, but not DNase, was unaffected by actinomycin D, and was sensitive to tryspin. Subsequently, a similar activity was discovered in Sendai virions (Robinson, 1971*c*; Stone *et al.*, 1971) and SV5 (Mountcastle *et al.*, 1971, and unpublished experiments). The Sendai virus enzyme resembled that of NDV in terms of size and complementarity of the product, but was less active, and it sedimented in a gradient with the characteristics of the nucleocapsid (Robinson, 1971*c*).

The first definitive evidence for specific proteins in the transcriptase activity came from analyses of a transcriptive complex isolated from infected cells (Stone *et al.*, 1972). These studies revealed, in addition to the 60,000-dalton nucleocapsid subunit protein, the presence in the complex of the largest virion protein, a nonglycosylated protein with an estimated molecular weight of 69,000–75,000 daltons. More recently (Marx *et al.*, 1974), a transcriptive complex which contained only these two proteins was isolated from Sendai virions disrupted with Triton X-100. The addition of the virion envelope proteins, either the glycoproteins or the nonglycosylated membrane protein, to this complex inhibited the polymerase activity, and brief heating of these proteins before addition abolished their inhibitory activity. Whether the large nonglycosylated protein (P) or the nucleocapsid subunit (NP) is the transcriptase or whether a complex of these two proteins forms the active enzyme is not yet clear (Marx *et al.*, 1974). An interesting question raised by these studies which deserves further study is whether the envelope proteins play a role in regulation of RNA synthesis in the replicative cycle of the virus.

It has not yet been firmly established with other paramyxoviruses which protein(s) are involved in transcription, but there is suggestive evidence with SV5 that a complex analogous to that of Sendai virus is involved. SV5 virions have an active RNA transcriptase when assayed in the presence of Triton X-100 to disrupt the particles; however, purified nucleocapsids lacking the 50,000-dalton protein had no activity (Mountcastle *et al.*, 1971, and unpublished experiments). In contrast, preliminary experiments have indicated that a complex consisting of

SV5 nucleocapsid plus the 50,000-dalton protein does have detectable transcriptase activity (McSharry and Choppin, unpublished experiments). It thus appears likely that in SV5 as well as Sendai virions a nonglycosylated protein in addition to the 60,000-dalton nucleocapsid subunit protein is associated with the nucleocapsid and is necessary for transcriptase activity; however, these proteins differ in size, i.e., approximately 69,000 daltons for the Sendai virus protein and 50,000 for the SV5 protein. As indicated in Sect. 2.3.2 above, the SV5 50,000-dalton protein appears to be more easily dissociable from the complex with high salt than the Sendai virus P protein (Marx *et al.*, 1974). However, by banding in CsCl, Mountcastle *et al.* (1970) were able to isolate nucleocapsid from Sendai virions which contained only a very small amount of protein in the P region of the gel. Meager and Burke (1973) found with NDV that a subviral particle produced by Triton treatment of virions had transcriptase activity, and that purified nucleocapsid did not, suggesting that with this virus also an additional protein other than the nucleocapsid subunit was required for activity, or alternatively that the enzyme had been inactivated in the preparation of nucleocapsids.

It is of interest that in the case of VS virus it has been shown that a large nonglycosylated protein (L) has transcriptase activity when added to a template complex containing the nucleocapsid subunit protein and the viral RNA (Emerson and Wagner, 1972, 1973).

The virion-associated transcriptase of Sendai virus was found to be stimulated by several polyanions, including yeast RNA (Stone and Kingsbury, 1973; Marx *et al.*, 1974). This stimulation was more marked with less active complexes and was independent of the presence of envelope proteins. When a preparation was partially inactivated by mild heat treatment, yeast RNA restored most of the lost activity. These results suggest the stimulating polyanions act at the enzyme-template level and may do so by reversing thermal inactivation of the transcriptase (Marx *et al.*, 1974).

An RNA-dependent DNA polymerase activity has been found in preparations of a mutant of NDV obtained from persistently infected L cells (Furman and Hallum, 1973). This has not yet been confirmed and the significance of this observation in terms of paramyxovirus replication or persistent infection remains to be determined.

3.4.1b. Primary Transcription *In Vivo*

The virion transcriptase which is active *in vitro* also functions intracellularly, and this is presumably the initial step in viral macromolecular synthesis. Such primary transcription can occur in the absence of protein synthesis. When cells were infected at high multiplicity in the presence of cycloheximide (Robinson, 1971b), the species of complementary RNAs which were found were the same as those formed late in infection in the absence of the inhibitor with the significant exception that no 50 S RNA was found. Neither the replication of the genome RNA nor the amplification of the production of complementary RNA which occurs in the absence of inhibitors of protein synthesis occurs in the presence of cycloheximide, indicating the requirement for protein synthesis for the appearance of the RNA replicase function.

The ability to examine primary transcription in the presence of an inhibitor of protein synthesis provides a means for examining early events in virus replication. Indeed, primary transcription provides an explanation for the early studies of Wheelock (1962) which showed that when cells were infected with NDV in the presence of puromycin and the drug was removed after various intervals, as much viral antigen was made in a half-hour period following removal of the drug after four hours in its presence as was normally made in two hours in the absence of the inhibitor. Thus, the early steps in virus multiplication could occur in the presence of the drug. In the light of present knowledge, it would appear that the observed shortening of the latent period with regard to protein synthesis was due to accumulation of primary transcripts which represented messenger RNAs that were subsequently translated when the block in protein synthesis was removed. It has also been proposed that ribosomes form an association with nucleocapsids from infecting virions, presumably associating with nascent RNA (Bukrinskaya et al., 1969a).

3.4.1c. Site of Synthesis

Early studies indicated that neither synthesis nor transcription of cellular DNA was required for paramyxoviruses replication. This was established by the ability of these viruses to replicate in the presence of actinomycin D (Kingsbury, 1962; Barry et al., 1962; Rott and Scholtissek, 1964; Choppin, 1965) and in the presence of inhibitors of DNA synthesis (Simon, 1961; Choppin, 1965). Paramyxoviruses were also found to be capable of replication in UV-irradiated cells (Barry, 1964; Rosenbergová and Rosenberg, 1964). It is pertinent, however, that in those virus–cell systems in which there is a long latent period or in which virus production continues for long periods, actinomycin treatment will eventually cause a reduction in virus yield due to secondary effects on the cell (Granoff and Kingsbury, 1964; Choppin, 1965); thus, inhibition of the production of SV5 begins about 10–12 hours after the addition of actinomycin D (Choppin, 1965; Choppin and Holmes, 1967). Inhibition of mumps and measles viruses by actinomycin have been reported (East and Kingsbury, 1971; Schlueder-berg *et al.*, 1972); however, with these viruses also, RNA transcription is not inhibited by the drug (East and Kingsbury, 1971; Carter *et al.*, 1973; Winston *et al.*, 1973). The mechanism of the inhibition of measles and mumps has not been established, but secondary effects on the cell may play a role in these cases also, particularly since long growth cycles are involved.

In agreement with the lack of a requirement for cellular DNA function during replication of paramyxoviruses, the weight of evidence indicates that the synthesis of viral RNA occurs in the cytoplasm. Early autoradiographic studies (Wheelock, 1963) indicated that the cytoplasm is the site of NDV RNA synthesis. With very short pulses of radioactive precursors, the labeled RNA is found in the cytoplasm (Bratt and Robinson, 1967). Partially double-stranded structures which appear to be replicative and transcriptive intermediates are also found in the cytoplasm of infected cells (Bratt and Robinson, 1971; Robinson, 1971*a*; East and Kingsbury, 1971; Portner and Kingsbury, 1972). There have been reports of nucleolar viral RNA synthesis early in infection (Bukrinskaya *et al.*, 1966) and reports that viral RNA enters the nucleus (Bukrinskaya *et al.*, 1969*b*). A small amount of labeled RNA has also been found associated with nuclei (Kingsbury, 1973*a*); however, the significance of these findings is not clear.

3.4.1d. Species of RNAs in Infected Cells

Early studies indicated that most of the virus-specific RNAs in cells infected with NDV and Sendai viruses were complementary to the genome RNA (Kingsbury, 1966*b*, 1967; Bratt and Robinson, 1967; Blair and Robinson, 1968). These RNAs were hetrogeneous in size and consisted in all cases of a predominant species sedimenting at 18 S, a variable amount of 22 S and 35 S RNA, and a small amount of 50 S RNA which was found to be a mixture of complementary and virion-type RNA. Subsequently, qualitatively similar patterns of virus specific RNAs were found in mumps (East and Kingsbury, 1971) and measles virus-infected cells (Carter *et al.*, 1973; Winston *et al.*, 1973). Variation in the amounts of the different species of RNA occurs among the various types of viruses, and has also been observed with different strains of a single virus, NDV (Bratt, 1969).

Bratt and Robinson (1967) found that the 18 S RNA contained sequences complementary to about half the genome RNA, which indicated heterogeneity of this class of RNA since a single 18 S species could not account for this much of the 50 S genome. In addition, the 35 S RNA was found to be complementary to about 70% of the genome, indicating overlap with sequences contained in the 18 S RNA. Polyacrylamide gel studies of the RNAs from infected cells also suggested heterogeneity of the 18 S RNA (Kingsbury *et al.*, 1970; Lomniczi *et al.*, 1971). Recently Collins and Bratt (Collins and Bratt, 1973; Bratt *et al.*, 1974) have succeeded in separating the 18–22 S NDV RNA into at least 6 or 7 species by polyacrylamide gel electrophoresis. These authors have estimated the sizes of the RNAs on the basis of migration in gels as 5.5–15×10^5 daltons, and have suggested that these values correlate well with the sizes of NDV virion proteins, so that each might represent a specific messenger. This is an attractive hypothesis, which is amenable to testing by *in vitro* protein synthesis experiments. However, it has not yet been shown that each size class separated in the gel is a unique species of RNA, and several questions remain to be clarified, such as: (1) are there no messengers for nonstructural proteins, e.g., a replicase, (2) why was only 50% of the genome found to be represented in the 18 S RNA in earlier studies, and (3) what is the role of the 35 S RNA?

3.4.1e. Proof of the Messenger Function of Complementary RNA

Because of the finding of predominantly complementary RNA in infected cells, and the association of 18–35 S RNA with ribosomes, but not the 50 S RNA, it was thought that this complementary RNA or at least a portion of it represented mRNA (Kingsbury, 1966*b*; Bratt and Robinson, 1967; Blair and Robinson, 1968; 1970). Recently, evidence has been obtained in a cell-free protein-synthesizing system that complementary RNA from Sendai virus-infected cells can act as messenger (Kingsbury, 1973*b*). Using 18 S complementary RNA obtained from infected cells as messenger in a rabbit reticulocyte system, three proteins were synthesized which comigrated in a polyacrylamide gel with three of the virion proteins, and these proteins synthesized *in vitro* were precipitated by antiviral antisera. The most abundant protein produced corresponded to the nucleocapsid protein, and tryptic peptides of this protein comigrated electrophoretically with tryptic peptides of nucleocapsid isolated from virions. Virion 50 S RNA was not active in this protein-synthesizing system. These findings provide direct evidence for the hypothesis that complementary RNAs are the messengers for the synthesis of paramyxovirus proteins.

3.4.1f. Transcription

Polymerases which catalyze the synthesis of RNAs complementary to the viral genome have been isolated from the cytoplasm of cells infected with NDV (Scholtissek and Rott, 1969) and Sendai virus (Mahy *et al.*, 1970; Stone *et al.*, 1971, 1972). The conditions required for the action of these enzymes are similar to those for the virion-associated transcriptase, and, as pointed out above, the same two Sendai virus proteins have been found associated with the complexes obtained from virions and cells, i.e., the large nonglycosylated protein (P) and the nucleocapsid subunit (NP). Whether other proteins may be associated with the transcriptase in the cell and serve a regulatory function is not known. As indicated above, viral envelope proteins do exert an inhibitory effect on the virion-associated transcriptase *in vitro* (Marx *et al.*, 1974), but the biological significance of the finding is not yet clear. The available evidence does suggest that late transcription, as well as primary transcription, may occur on nucleocapsidlike structures (Bukrinskaya *et al.*, 1969a; Robinson, 1971c; Stone *et al.*, 1971; Portner and Kingsbury, 1972). Encapsidation of genome RNA from a pool of nucleocapsid protein subunits appears to occur very rapidly, and there may be no naked genome RNA in cells (Robinson, 1971b). The rate of genome RNA replication probably determines the rate of nucleocapsid formation (Robinson, 1971b; Iinuma *et al.*, 1971).

Partially base-paired structures which are apparently intermediates in transcription and replication have been isolated from cells infected with NDV (Bratt and Robinson, 1971), mumps virus (East and Kingsbury, 1971), and Sendai virus (Portner and Kingsbury, 1972). The presumed transcriptive intermediates of Sendai virus have been found to be heterogeneous in size (Portner and Kingsbury, 1972). Such structures will be discussed further in the next section.

The finding of multiple species of complementary RNAs which can be produced by the virion transcriptase either *in vitro* or *in vivo* by primary transcription in the presence of inhibitors of protein synthesis, and findings of similar species produced late in infection, suggests that the various RNAs are transcribed independently and that there are multiple initiation sites on the genome RNA for the transcriptase.

However, the alternative possibility that the complementary RNA is synthesized as a single large piece and then cleaved to yield the various 18–35 S species cannot yet be completely excluded, although the available evidence is against this hypothesis. On the other hand, there must be a mechanism for formation of 50 S complementary strands since they are found in small amount in infected cells, and are presumably required as templates for the genome RNA. As will be discussed below, the enzyme responsible for such syntheses is not identical to the transcriptase that yields the smaller RNA species. No evidence of ligation of the smaller RNA species to form the larger 50 S structure has been found.

3.4.1g. Replication

A major gap in the knowledge of paramyxovirus replication is the nature of the enzyme(s) responsible for the synthesis of the virion or genome RNA, i.e., the RNA replicase. No *in vitro* replicase activity has been demonstrated. There is convincing evidence that the replicase and transcriptase activities can be separated, most readily by use of inhibitors of protein synthesis. As discussed above, primary transcription in the presence of cycloheximide yields the 18–35 S RNAs, but not the 50 S RNA. Furthermore, in early studies it was shown under conditions of low-multiplicity infection that the addition of inhibitors such as puromycin shut off virus-specific RNA synthesis only if added in the first few hours after infection (Wilson and Lo Gerfo, 1964; Scholtissek and Rott, 1965); later addition allowed RNA synthesis to continue for several hours. Choppin and Holmes (1967) found that when poliovirus was added to SV5-infected cells and cellular protein synthesis was inhibited, on-going virus-specific RNA synthesis not only continued but was significantly increased for up to 12 hours. Subsequently, puromycin and cycloheximide were also found to stimulate SV5 virus-specific RNA synthesis when added to cells already producing virus (Choppin, unpublished experiments). When inhibitors of protein synthesis were added to Sendai and mumps virus-infected cells and the species of virus-specific RNAs were examined, it was found that 18 S complementary RNA continued to be made whereas synthesis of 50 S RNA was inhibited (Robinson, 1971*b*; East and Kingsbury, 1971). These results suggest that protein(s) involved in the replication of genome RNA is relatively unstable, and that continued protein synthesis is required for RNA replication, in contrast to transcription which continues for hours in the absence of protein synthesis.

Further evidence for the discreteness of the replication and transcription processes was obtained by Portner and Kingsbury (1972), who were able to separate by sedimentation what appeared to be replicative and transcriptive intermediates. The replicative intermediates separated relatively homogeneously at around 24 S, accumulated, and, like 50 S RNA, they were labeled less as the interval between the addition of cycloheximide and the label was increased. Transcriptive intermediates sedimented heterogeneously between 26 and 60 S, did not accumulate, and, like 18 S RNA, were labeled long after inhibition of protein synthesis.

The above evidence clearly indicates that the enzymes involved in transcription and replication are not identical, and that replication involves a protein(s) with a short life. It is not yet known whether the enzymes responsible for the synthesis of the 50 S complementary strand and the 50 S genome strand are different, or whether the replicase consists of a protein or proteins which are completely distinct from those involved in transcription or is composed of the transcriptase plus other modifying protein(s); the possibility that it contains a host component has also not been excluded. It is of interest and probably of considerable biological significance that with each of three groups of viruses in which the messenger RNA is complementary to the virion RNA and which contain virion-associated transcriptase, i.e., myxovirus, paramyxoviruses, and rhabdoviruses, the replicase activity appears to be unstable and replication requires continued protein synthesis, but transcription does not. (See Chapts. 1 and 3 in this volume). In each case the nature of the replicase and the details of the replication reaction are not fully understood. Further, where it has been examined, inhibition by defective virus particles appears to operate at the level of replication rather than transcription, another fact compatible with the supply of replicase being a limiting factor in virus multiplication. An understanding of exactly how replication of the genome RNA occurs with any one of these three viruses should shed light on the replication of the others. Conversely, the fact that all three of these "negative-strand" virus groups exhibit the same characteristic may provide an important clue to the eventual solution of the problem.

3.4.1h. Adenylation of Complementary RNAs

As is the case with most mRNAs in eukaryotic cells, adenylate-rich sequences have been found on the complementary RNAs of

Sendai virus (Pridgen and Kingsbury, 1972) and NDV (Weiss and Bratt, 1974; Bratt *et al.*, 1974). Weiss and Bratt (1974) found that all of the 6–7 classes of the 18–22 S RNA extracted from infected cells contained poly A sequences, with an estimated average size of 120–130 nucleotides. Poly A was also found associated with the 35 S and 50 S intracellular species, but the content was more heterogeneous and not analyzed in detail. These authors further found that 18–22 S RNA synthesized *in vitro* by the virion transcriptase also consisted of 6–7 size classes similar to those found in infected cells, and that these RNAs contained covalently linked poly A sequences which were larger and more heterogeneous than those on RNAs obtained from the infected cells.

The mechanism of synthesis of the poly A regions is not yet clear. Since it can be synthesized *in vitro*, a cellular enzyme is not required. On the other hand, Marshall and Gillespie (1972) failed to detect any poly U regions in NDV virion RNA by hybridization with poly A, and Weiss and Bratt (1974) have pointed out that the content of UMP in the virion, though high relative to the other bases, can probably be accounted for in the complementary RNA by AMP which is not contained in poly A regions. This fact, and the finding that the size of the poly A regions synthesized *in vitro* varied with conditions, led Weiss and Bratt (1974) to suggest that the synthesis is probably not transcriptive, but is added without transcription by the transcriptase itself or by another virion-bound enzyme. The function of the poly A on paramyxovirus RNAs, like that on the other mRNA molecules, is unknown. Since the paramyxovirus RNAs are synthesized in the cytoplasm, it is clear that the facilitation of transportation from the nucleus to the cytoplasm is not a factor in this case.

3.4.1i. Regulation of Paramyxovirus RNA Synthesis

It is apparent from the above discussion that regulation of the relative amounts of complementary and genome-type RNA occurs in the infected cell, and that one of the factors in the control of the synthesis of genome RNA may be the limited supply of replicase. On the other hand, there is evidence that control of the amount of transcription may also occur in paramyxovirus-infected cells. With NDV (Granoff and Kingsbury, 1964), SV5 (Holmes and Choppin, 1966; Choppin and Holmes, 1967), and Sendai virus (Blair and Robinson, 1968), only a relatively small fraction of the total RNA synthesis in the infected cells is virus-specific. A striking example is SV5-infected monkey kidney cells, which yield a large amount of virus, i.e., up to 1500 PFU in 24 hours, and in which virus production continues for days, yet the level of virus-induced RNA synthesis does not exceed about 1% of the total cellular synthesis, as indicated by actinomycin D treatment. Since the virus is present and replicates for days in these cells, the maintenance of RNA synthesis at such a low level implies tight control. It is of interest that, as mentioned above, inhibition of protein synthesis in this system *increased* the level of virus-specific RNA, which suggested control by a protein (Choppin and Holmes, 1967). Furthermore, poliovirus was used to turn off host cell protein synthesis, but not SV5 protein synthesis, and this also stimulated SV5 RNA synthesis. These results suggested that a host protein might be involved in control of viral RNA synthesis (Choppin and Holmes, 1967). Although in these early studies the polarity of the viral RNA was not determined, the subsequent studies cited above with Sendai and NDV have indicated that after inhibition of protein synthesis transcription continues but replication ceases; thus an increase in RNA synthesis after inhibition of protein synthesis suggests release from control of transcription. The mechanism of such control is unknown.

The question of temporal control of transcription is also not clear. The similarity of the pattern of complementary RNAs synthesized by primary transcription *in vivo* (Robinson, 1971*b*) and *in vitro* (Bratt *et al.*, 1974) and the pattern of RNAs synthesized late in infection suggests that temporal control may not exist and that the same relative amounts of the various RNAs are synthesized throughout the infective cycle. However, until the question of the uniqueness of each class of RNA is established, the possibility of some temporal control with "early" and "late" mRNAs cannot be excluded.

3.4.2. Proteins

Early studies with fluorescent antibodies indicated that synthesis of paramyxovirus proteins occurred in the cytoplasm of infected cells (Wheelock and Tamm, 1959; 1961*a*; Traver *et al.*, 1960; Cohen *et al.*, 1961). Although antigens, eosinophilic inclusions, and nucleocapsids have been seen in the nuclei of infected cells by a number of workers with various paramyxsoviruses, the weight of evidence obtained in many laboratories has indicated that paramyxovirus proteins are synthesized in the cytoplasm, and that such nuclear accumulations, which are usually seen late in infection, result from transport from the cytoplasm to the nucleus. Studies of the synthesis of specific proteins in paramyxovirus-infected cells have been hindered by the presence of a high background of cellular protein synthesis in most virus–cell systems. However, recently studies have begun to reveal the details of the virus-induced protein synthesis in infected cells (Lomniczi *et al.*, 1971; Alexander and Reeve, 1972; Samson and Fox, 1973; Kaplan and Bratt, 1973; Bratt *et al.*, 1974; Hightower and Bratt, 1974). Most of these studies have employed difference analysis with double labels in order to permit the subtraction of the background of cellular synthesis.

Lomniczi *et al.* (1971) investigated protein synthesis with six different strains of NDV in chick embryo cells and were able to detect three major virion proteins in cells infected with each strain. In the light of present knowledge, these proteins would appear to correspond to the HN, NP, and M proteins. Cells infected with avirulent strains continued to synthesize proteins longer than those infected with virulent strains. In cells infected with three of these NDV strains, an additional protein was found which migrated between the HN protein and nucleocapsid protein, which would correspond to a protein with a molecular weight of 62,000–66,000 daltons. Samson and Fox (1973) also found in NDV-infected cells the three major proteins and another protein migrating approximately in the 65,000-dalton region. In pulse-chase experiments this protein appeared to be converted to a protein migrating with a mobility similar to that of the nucleocapsid. These authors suggested that the nucleocapsid, or alternatively a minor protein with the same electrophoretic mobility, was derived from this precursor. It is pertinent to recall here that the smaller glycoprotein of NDV was previously shown to comigrate with the nucleocapsid protein (Mountcastle *et al.*, 1971). Bratt and his co-workers (Kaplan and Bratt, 1973; Hightower and Bratt, 1974; Bratt *et al.*, 1974) also found evidence for processing of a similar protein; however they further showed that the *ca.* 65,000-precursor was a glycoprotein, that it was found in association with membranes, and that it appeared to be the precursor of the small virion glycoprotein. These observations fit nicely with the findings of Homma (Homma and Ohuchi, 1973; Homma, 1974) and Scheid and Choppin (1974*a,b*) that the smaller virion glycoprotein of Sendai virus is derived by proteolytic cleavage from *ca.* 65, 000-dalton precursor, and that depending on the host cell, this cleavage may not occur. In the NDV–chick embryo system cleavage apparently usually occurs before virus maturation, although, as discussed in Sect. 2.2 above, small amounts of this protein have been detected in virions. The small glycoprotein is the only paramyxovirus protein which has been shown to undergo post-translational processing.

Bratt *et al.* (1974) and Hightower and Bratt (1974) found that all the other NDV virion proteins were found in approximately the same proportion early and late after infection, suggesting that the rates of accumulation give a reasonably accurate reflection of the relative rates of synthesis. These authors also found a protein in infected cells migrating with an estimated molecular weight of 36,000 which is not a virion protein and whose nature and function are not clear.

In each of these studies of NDV proteins in infected cells, the proteins were not found in equimolar amounts in cells, but rather the relative amounts of the various proteins in infected cells resembled in general those found in virions. Thus, some control of protein synthesis is clearly operative. Whether this is transcriptional or translational or both has not yet been established.

Choppin and Holmes (1967) showed that addition of puromycin to infected cells which were continually producing SV5 caused a rapid inhibition of the release of virus, even if the inhibitor was added 24 hours after infection, thus indicating that continuous protein synthesis is necessary for continuous maturation of virus. Iinuma *et al.* (1971) also found that addition of inhibitors of protein synthesis late in infection, when large amounts of virus proteins were present in infected cells, inhibited further virion production. They found that when radioactive label was added late after infection, the virions subsequently harvested had a lower specific activity than virions harvested after a pulse label earlier in infection. These authors raised the question of the requirement for a maturation protein. Subsequently, Iinuma *et al.*, (1973) found that arginine was required for the production of NDV, and that in the absence of arginine, nucleocapsid and hemagglutinin, and neuraminidase activities were present in cells, but hemadsorption and release of virus did not occur. Addition of arginine to such cultures resulted in rapid release of virus, but when arginine and cycloheximide were added together no virus release occurred. These results suggest that arginine is required for the synthesis of a protein(s) necessary for virus maturation.

In the opinion of these reviewers the most likley candidate for such a protein is the nonglycosylated membrane protein (M). This conclusion is based on an analogy to the influenza virus system, where evidence was first obtained that the M protein was present in relatively small amounts in infected cells although it was the most abundant virion protein, and that it was incorporated efficiently into the plasma membrane soon after synthesis (Lazarowitz *et al.*, 1971). It was therefore suggested that synthesis of the protein was tightly controlled so that it was the rate-limiting step in virus maturation. Subsequently, it was found that the relative rates of synthesis of this protein increased with time after infection (Skehel, 1972; Meier-Ewert and Compans, 1974) and that the M protein incorporated into influenza B virions was synthesized late in infection, after the nucleocapsid (Choppin *et al.*, 1974). Experiments to test this hypothesis with paramyxoviruses are in progress.

Although several recent studies describe the effect of inhibitors of glycosylation such as 2-deoxy-glucose and glucosamine on protein synthesis and assembly of influenza virus (see Chapt. 2 in this volume), there has been less such work on paramyxoviruses. It was first reported that NDV was inhibited very little by such inhibitors (Kaluza *et al.*, 1972). However, the inhibition of NDV replication and the inhibition of cell fusion by NDV were subsequently described (Gallaher *et al.*, 1973). More recently it was shown that the elimination of all glucose from the medium was necessary for inhibition of NDV by 2-deoxy-glucose (Scholtissek *et al.*, 1974).

3.4.3. Lipids

As discussed in Sect. 2.2, there is extensive evidence that the lipid composition of paramyxoviruses largely reflects that of the plasma membrane, and thus there is no evidence for the synthesis of virus-specific lipids in infected cells. Relatively little work has been done on lipid synthesis in cells infected by these viruses. The finding of Scheid and Choppin (Scheid and Choppin, 1971; and unpublished experiments; Choppin *et al.*, 1972) that SV5 infection of MDBK cells caused an increase in the synthesis of sphingomyelin and the corresponding progressive changes in the lipid composition of virions harvested at intervals has been discussed in detail in Sect. 2.2 and will not be repeated here. It indicates a virus-induced alteration in lipid metabolism, but appears to be an exaggeration of a trend toward glycosphingolipid synthesis at the expense of sphingomyelin synthesis which occurs normally in ageing confluent monolayers (Scheid and Choppin, 1971; Choppin *et al.*, 1972).

A general increase in the incorporation of ^{32}P into cells infected with Sendai virus has been reported (Shibuta *et al.*, 1971; Blair and Brennan, 1972). On the other hand, a decrease in overall phospholipid synthesis in cells infected with NDV has also been reported [Gallaher and Blough (1972) which was cited in Blough and Tiffany (1973)], but this decrease occurred late in infection. The significance of these alterations remains to be determined; they may be due to secondary effects of infection. As pointed out above, Scheid and Choppin (1971) found no change in the synthesis of any of the phospholipids except sphingomyelin in SV5-infected cells. These studies included chemical determination of lipid composition at intervals after infection as well as labeling experiments employing ^{32}P and radioactive choline.

3.4.4. Carbohydrate

The origin and possible functions of the carbohydrate in virions have been described in Sect. 2.3. As mentioned there, the available evidence suggests that the compositions of the carbohydrate chains attached to either glycoproteins or glycolipids are in part, if not totally, determined by the host cell. No evidence has been obtained to prove that virus-specific glycosyl transferases are induced by paramyxovirus infection. The use of radioactive precursors such as fucose, glucosamine, and galactose has shown that the sugars are incorporated into newly synthesized carbohydrate chains on glycoproteins and glycolipids. The inhibition of virus production and of cell fusion by 2-deoxyglucose or glucosamine indicates that the synthesis of new carbohydrate chains is important for the incorporation of viral proteins into membranes and the maturation of infective virus.

3.5. Assembly

Many of the features of assembly of the virion components and release from the cell have been mentioned in the various preceding sections. The assembly process has been reviewed recently (Choppin *et al.*, 1971; 1972; Compans and Choppin, 1971, 1973; Lenard and Compans, 1974). The reader is also referred to Chapts. 1 and 3 in this volume on rhabdoviruses and myxoviruses, respectively, where results pertinent to the assembly of paramyxoviruses are described. In addition, a chapter in a subsequent volume in this series will deal with viral membranes and glycoprotein projections (Choppin and Compans, 1975).

3.5.1. Nucleocapsid

As indicated above, the nucleocapsid is synthesized in the cytoplasm and consists of protein subunits of *ca*. 60,000 daltons, the genome of *ca*. 6×10^6 daltons and at least one other protein appears to be associated with this structure in some virions. The details of the self-assembly process of the nucleocapsid are unknown. The nucleocapsid protein binds tightly to the RNA and protects it from ribonuclease digestion. The susceptibility to proteolytic cleavage of the nucleocapsid protein and the possible function of portions of this protein have been discussed in Sect. 2.3. The nucleocapsids may be present as isolated individual units or as a large accumulation (Figs. 21–23), depending on the virus–cell system (c f. Compans *et al.*, 1966). The nucleocapsid does not appear to associate with any intracellular membranes, but it does associate in a specific manner with the underside of the plasma membrane, as described below. This suggests that intracellular membranes lack the recognition site for the nucleocapsid which is present at those areas of plasma membrane which are destined to become the viral membrane.

3.5.2. Formation of Viral Membranes

Little evidence is available on the precise mechanism of formation of viral membranes. Probably due to the background of cellular protein synthesis, there have not been extensive cell-fractionation studies following parainfluenza virus infection, as there have been with influenza and rhabdoviruses (see Chapts. 1 and 3 in this volume). Early work described the isolation of hemagglutinating membraneous structures from NDV-infected cells (Granoff, 1955); this microsomal fraction, subsequently called "viromicrosomes" (Rott *et al.*, 1962), possessed hemagglutinating activity but did not cause hemolysis nor irreversibly bind to erythrocytes. This work suggested that at least the HN virion protein associates with microsomes; however, the progression from rough to smooth membranes with growth of carbohydrate chains as found with influenza virus has not been demonstrated. In the light of the findings discussed above on activation of the hemolyzing and cell-fusing activities of Sendai virus by proteolytic cleavage of a precursor glycoprotein, the failure of these "viromicrosomes" to hemolyze or irreversibly bind to erythrocytes suggests that these structures may contain the uncleaved precursor of the smaller virion glycoprotein.

The possible modes of formation of areas of membrane which become the viral membrane will be discussed in Chapt. 3 in this volume and will be discussed further in a chapter on viral membranes in a subsequent volume in this series (Choppin and Compans, 1975). Briefly, these possibilities include stepwise replacement of cellular protein with viral proteins in an area of preformed membrane, assembly of a new region of membranes about a nucleation site formed by the initial insertion of a viral polypeptide, random incorporation of proteins in the plasma membrane followed by migration in the plane of the membrane until the viral proteins meet and form a patch of virus-specific membrane, and *en bloc* insertion of a vesicle of virus-specific membrane assembled in the Golgi–endoplasmic reticulum complex.

3.5.3. Sequence of Events in Virus Budding

The early studies of Bang (1953) showed that NDV was assembled by a budding process, and subsequently there have been many detailed electron microscopic studies of paramyxovirus replication, e.g., Sendai, Berkaloff (1963); SV5, Compans *et al.* (1966); parainfluenza type 2, Howe *et al.* (1967); NDV, Feller *et al.* (1969); mumps, Duc-Nguyen and Rosenblum (1967); and measles, Nakai *et al.* (1969). The paramyxoviruses provide excellent model systems for studying the assembly process with the electron microscope because the nucleocapsid is readily recognizable in thin sections of the virions (Figs. 9 and 17) and infected cells (Fig. 10).

Although some of the details of the assembly process, including the precise sequence of incorporation of the viral envelope protein into membranes, remain to be elucidated, the existing evidence does permit a reasonably good picture of the maturation of paramyxoviruses. Viral envelope proteins are first incorporated into regions of cell membrane which appear morphologically normal, but which can be shown to contain the viral surface protein by the hemadsorption reaction (Fig. 13) or the use of ferritin-labeled antiviral antibodies (Fig. 14). Although it has not been definitely shown to be the case with paramyxoviruses, the available evidence with influenza virus suggests that the glycoprotein may be associated with membranes before the nonglycosylated membrane protein (M). The nucleocapsid recognizes these areas of membrane which contain viral proteins. As discussed above, on the basis of the presumed location of the M protein on the underside of the membrane and phenotypic mixing experiments (Choppin and Compans, 1970; McSharry *et al.*, 1971), we propose that the M protein provides the recognition site for the nucleocapsid. That specific recognition is occurring is indicated by the regular, ordered arrangement of the nucleocapsid beneath the membrane (Figs. 10 and 11), and by the fact that nucleocapsid associates with only certain areas of plasma membrane, i.e., those which contain envelope proteins. The

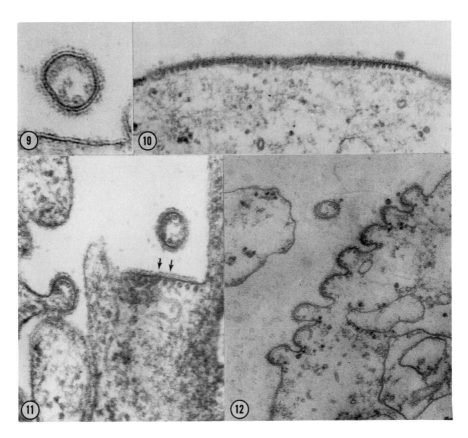

Fig. 9.   Thin section of an SV5 virion adjacent to the surface of a rhesus monkey kidney cell. The unit membrane in the viral envelope is clearly resolved and is morphologically similar to the membrane at the host cell surface. The outer layer of the viral membrane is covered with a layer of projections which are not found on the cell surface. ×147,000. From Compans and Choppin (1973).

Fig. 10.   A region of the surface of an SV5-infected monkey kidney cell showing nucleocapsids, many in cross section, closely aligned under the membrane. A layer of dense projections is present on the outer surface of the membrane. ×73,500. From Compans et al. (1966).

Fig. 11.   SV5 nucleocapsids aligned under a region of the membrane of a BHK21-F cell. A distinct layer of projections (arrows) is present on the outer surface, directly above the nucleocapsid. ×77,000. From Compans et al. (1966).

Fig. 12.   A row of eight particles in the process of budding at the surface of an SV5-infected monkey kidney cell. The nucleocapsid is apparent in cross section in many of the budding particles. ×56,000. From Compans et al. (1966).

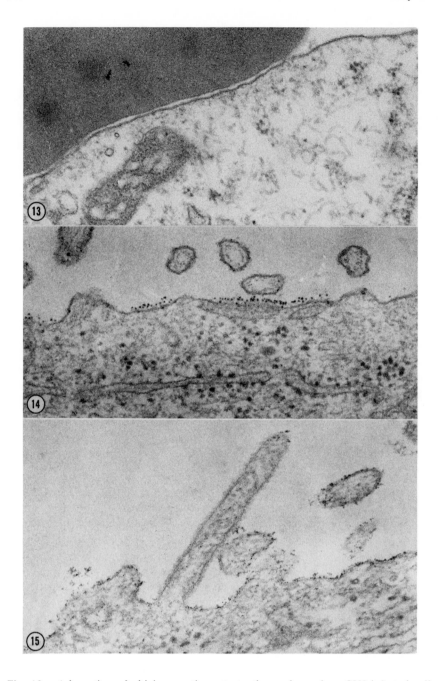

Fig. 13.   Adsorption of chicken erythrocyte to the surface of an SV5-infected cell. Nucleocapsids are present in the cytoplasm, but are not associated with the cell surface in the region where the erythrocyte is attached. ×54,600. From Compans and Choppin (1971).

nature of this recognition is not known; however, the M protein behaves as a hydrophobic protein (McSharry *et al.*, 1972; Scheid *et al.*, 1972; Scheid and Choppin, 1973), and the externally disposed region of the nucleocapsid subunit also appears to be hydrophobic (Mountcastle *et al.*, 1974). Thus the presumed recognition between these proteins may involve hydrophobic interactions.

As pointed out above, the viral surface glycoproteins can be shown to be present in areas of membranes which do not exhibit recognizable spikes on their surface (Figs. 13 and 14). However, in those areas where nucleocapsid is seen in a regular array beneath the cell (Fig. 10 and 11), spikes are seen on the surface. Thus, the arrival of the nucleocapsid may trigger a rearrangement which results in the morphologically detectable appearance of erect spikes. This might result from assembly of oligomeric spikes from protein monomers or from rearrangement of the protein in the membrane, including the possibility of peripheral displacement of proteins which were previously more internally located. The latter might help to explain the apparent dilemma of how recognition occurs between the membrane protein and spike glycoproteins if the spikes do not penetrate through the lipid bilayer of the mature virion. The stimulus for budding is also not clear, but might result from arrival of the nucleocapsid. The hypothesis was put forward above that the M protein might be primarily responsible for maintaining the integrity of the viral membrane as a localized domain within the plasma membrane from which host cell proteins are excluded. The existence of such localized domains has been shown not only by the absence of host proteins in the mature virion, but also by localized labeling with ferritin-labeled antiviral antibodies (Figs. 14 and 16), and by the specific absence of neuraminic acid residues from only those areas of membrane which contain viral proteins (Fig. 15). As discussed above, this absence is due to the incorporation of the viral enzyme neuraminidase into the membrane. It is tempting to speculate that the M protein also demarcates the area of the membrane which participates in budding, and that the arrival of nucleocapsid might in some way precipitate a cooperative interaction involving M-protein molecules such that budding might result.

Fig. 14.   Ferritin-conjugated antiviral antibody tagging areas of the surface of an SV5-infected MDBK cell which are of normal morphology. ×56,000.

Fig. 15.   Absence of neuraminic acid residues on the surface of a budding filamentous SV5 virion. The surface of the cell just adjacent to the virion is stained with colloidal iron hydroxide, indicating the presence of neuraminic acid, but the virion is not stained. ×87,500. From Klenk *et al.* (1970*b*).

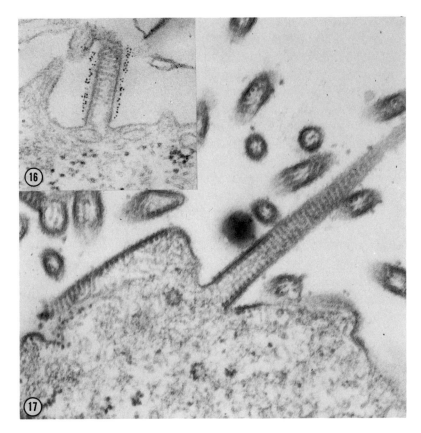

Fig. 16. A filamentous SV5 virion in the process of budding, tagged with ferritin-labeled antiviral antibody. The cell surface just adjacent to the budding particle is devoid of antibody. ×63,000. From Compans and Choppin (1971).

Fig. 17. A region of the cell surface with nucleocapsid closely aligned under the cell membrane, and a long, filamentous virion in the process of budding. The nucleocapsid is coiled in a regular spiral extending the length of the budding particle. ×58,800. From Compans *et al.* (1966).

Marcus (1962), using light microscopy and hemadsorption as an indicator of the presence of virus or hemagglutinin at the surface of the cell, observed that this appeared to occur first at the polar region of the cells. It is of interest that the formation of "patches" of immunoglobulin receptors occurs on the addition to lymphocytes of antibodies and that these patches migrate to form caps at the circumference of cells (Taylor *et al.*, 1971; Mandel, 1972; Yahara and Edelman, 1972). One could view the localized domains represented by regions of virus-specific proteins within the cell membrane as analogous to such patches, and in that event, migration of these domains to the polar region of the cell and budding from that region might be expected. It is perhaps pertinent that Marcus (1962) did observe migration of attached erythrocytes on the surface of the cell.

The phenotypic mixing experiments (Choppin and Compans, 1970; McSharry *et al.*, 1971) discussed above and in Sect. 2.3 in which it was shown that the glycoproteins of SV5 and VS virus could be freely intermixed, but that a specific interaction appeared to be required between the nucleocapsid and M protein, also provided evidence that a specific glycoprotein was not required for maintaining the shape or integrity of the viral envelope, and, further, that if at any stage in assembly recognition or interaction between surface glycoproteins and the internal M protein occurs, then the SV5 glycoprotein must be able to effectively interact with the VS virus membrane protein. Whether such interaction occurs in the assembly process or in the mature virion is not clear. It has been suggested by some workers that in VS virus there is contact between the glycoproteins and the M protein in the virion, but the evidence on this question is not conclusive (see Chapt. 1 in this volume).

During the budding process (Figs. 12, 16–18), the viral and cell membrane are continuous; and following the budding event, the membranes at the base of the protruding particle fuse, completing the formation of the virion. This would result in release of the virion unless it adsorbed to a receptor on the adjacent surface of the cell. The role of neuraminidase in the release of influenza virions from the cell surface has been debated extensively in the literature. As discussed in detail in the accompanying chapter on myxoviruses in this volume (Chapt. 3), the weight of currently available evidence now favors a role of the neuraminidase in release. Little has been done on this question with paramyxoviruses, but if the neuraminidase of influenza does play a role in release, it would seem logical that this would also be the case with paramyxoviruses, particularly since in the latter the neuraminidase and receptor binding functions reside on a single protein and perhaps have the same active site.

3.5.4. Filamentous and Multiploid Virions

As indicated in Sect. 2.1 and 2.3, large virions are occasionally produced which obviously contain several of the 1-μm nucleocapsids and thus presumably contain multiple, non-covalently linkeds copies of the viral genome. Some filamentous particles are shown in Figs. 15–17. The reason for the formation of these large particles is not clear. As

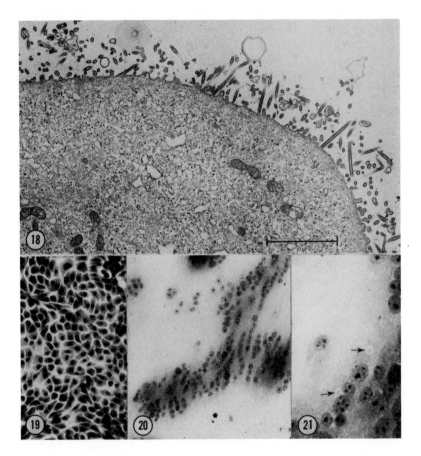

Fig. 18. Low magnification of an SV5-infected monkey kidney cell showing many particles in the process of budding. The cytoplasm appears essentially normal in morphology. ×9,375. From Compans *et al.* (1966).

Fig. 19. SV5-infected rhesus monkey kidney cells 48 hours after inoculation stained with hematoxylin and eosin. Although a very high yield of infective virus has been produced by these cells and virus production is continuing, they appear normal. ×130. From Compans *et al.* (1966).

Figs. 20 and 21. SV5-infected BHK21-F cells 18 hours after inoculation stained with hematoxylin and eosin. All cells have fused into a single, giant syncytium. The nuclei are aligned in rows, and the migration and arrangement of nuclei in such syncytia has been shown to be accomplished by microtubules [see Holmes and Choppin (1968)]. There are large eosinophilic inclusions in the cytoplasm (arrows). Fig. 20, ×130; Fig. 21, ×375). From Compans *et al.* (1966).

described in the accompanying chapter on myxoviruses, the production of large numbers of filamentous influenza virions has been shown to be genetically determined. No good evidence on this point is available with paramyxovirus. The number of filamentous and bizarre-shaped virions produced can be increased by damaging the membrane with agents such as vitamin A (Blough, 1963). There is also genetic evidence for multiploid paramyxovirus particles, and Simon (1972) has recently reviewed this subject.

4. DEFECTIVE VIRUS AND VIRAL INTERFERENCE

4.1. Defective Virions

Defective or incomplete virions have now been recognized with a great many different viruses, and the subject has been recently reviewed by Huang (1973). With paramyxoviruses, noninfectious hemagglutinating particles obtained from infected cells were found in early studies (Granoff *et al.*, 1950). However, these were shown to be microsomal fractions containing viral proteins rather than defective virions (Granoff, 1955; Rott *et al.*, 1962). Subsequently it was found that high-multiplicity infection with Sendai virus resulted in the production of noninfectious virus (Tadokoro, 1958*a,b*; Sokol *et al.*, 1964), a situation resembling the production of incomplete influenza virus particles of the von Magnus type produced by serial undiluted passage (see review in Chapt. 3 in this volume). These noninfectious Sendai virions sedimented in a manner consistent with their being virions, of smaller size than standard virions, rather than being "viromicrosomes" or membrane fragments obtained from infected cells (Tadokoro, 1958*b*).

Kingsbury and co-workers (1970) found virions in populations of Sendai virus particles which contained RNA species smaller than the 50 S RNA that represented the complete viral genome. These were shown to be the defective virions whose presence was enriched by high-multiplicity passage. The virions sedimented at a slower rate than standard infective virions, and the RNAs isolated from these virions sedimented in sucrose gradients at 19 S and 24 S. Annealing studies showed that these RNAs contained sequences similar to those found in the 50 S genome RNA, and that they also self-annealed to a certain extent, as does the 50 S genome RNA as described in Sect. 2.2. The defect in the defective particles has been clearly shown to be in the RNA, and no evidence has yet been obtained that specific proteins are lacking in these virions. There is evidence that defective particles are also formed after infection with other paramyxoviruses such as mumps (Cantell, 1961; East and Kingsbury, 1971), measles (Parfanovich *et al.*, 1971; Schleuderberg, 1971), and SV5 (Choppin, unpublished experiments), and there seems to be little doubt that the production under certain conditions is a general property of this group of viruses, as it is in many other groups (Huang, 1973).

The origin of defective virus appears to be a deletion of a segment of RNA during multiplication and then amplification of this deletion mutant by subsequent replication. The defective particles appear to arise spontaneously, and by cloning of virus stocks (Kingsbury and Portner, 1970) it is possible to obtain a population free of defective particles, a procedure that has been generally successful with defective viruses (Huang, 1973). Passing the virus at high multiplicity enhances the proportion of defective virus, not because of the higher multiplicity of standard virions, but presumably because this increases the probability of a given cell receiving both defective and standard virus particles. The multiplication of the defective particles is dependent on replicative functions supplied by the standard virus (Kingsbury and Portner, 1970).

4.2. Effect of Host Cell

The importance of the host cell in the genesis of defective virions was clearly shown with influenza virus (Choppin, 1969). A high yield of infective influenza virus could be obtained from the MDBK line of bovine kidney cells even after serial passages at high multiplicity, in marked contrast to the results in other cells in which predominantly defective virions are produced under such conditions. Further, virus grown in MDBK cells could be used to inoculate other cell types at high multiplicity, and relatively high infective virus yields were produced, presumably due to the small amount of defective virions in such inocula. With paramyxoviruses, serial high-multiplicity passage of NDV in the chick embryo (Granoff, 1955) or SV5 in primary rhesus monkey kidney cells (Choppin, 1964) or MDBK cells (Choppin, unpublished results) failed to result in the production of significant numbers of defective virions, yet passage of SV5 in the HKCC line of hamster kidney cells yielded largely defective virions after four undiluted passages (Choppin, unpublished results). Kingsbury and Portner (1970) found that defective virions were produced with greater frequency in the embryonated egg than in chick embryo lung cells on serial passage of cloned stocks of Sendai virus. Just as the precise mechanism responsible for the generation of defective virions is not clear, the role of the host in affecting the frequency of such events is also unknown. However, the eventual explanation of the origin of the presumed deletion mutants will have to account for an effect of the host cell on this process.

4.3. Interference by Defective Virions

As in other virus systems [reviewed by Huang (1973)], defective paramyxovirus particles interfere with the replication of standard virions (Portner and Kingsbury, 1971). Such interference is enhanced if the defective virions are added prior to the standard virions, and the interference is abolished by irradiation of the defective virions with ultraviolet light. The interference is specific for the homologous virus, and does not appear to require the production of interferon, although defective virions may induce interferon under certain conditions. With Sendai virus, defective virions does not induce interferon, and inhibition of standard virus by the defective virus is characterized by a greater inhibition of 50 S RNA than of 18 S (Portner and Kingsbury, 1971), whereas interferon causes inhibition of all Sendai virus-induced species of RNA (Richman *et al.*, 1970). Furthermore, the limitation of the interference to the homologous virus and the sensitivity to UV irradiation of the defective virions also argue against a role of interferon. Single-stranded RNAs, which appear to represent the subgenomic RNAs of defective virus, and a unique class of 16 S partially double-stranded RNAs, which may be involved in the replication and transcription of defective virion RNA, have been found in cells in which defective virus is being replicated (Portner and Kingsbury, 1971, 1972). The mechanism of interference of paramyxovirus replication by defective virions has not been firmly established, but the available evidence suggests that interference is most likely at the level of RNA replication and that it involves competition of the defective RNA with the standard RNA for the viral replicase (Portner and Kingsbury, 1971; Kingsbury, 1973*a*).

The availability of defective virions has provided a means of exploring an interesting property of a paramyxovirus, i.e., the ability to inhibit interferon induction or action. SV5 infection of primary rhesus monkey kidney (MK) cells or MDBK cells does not interfere with superinfection by other viruses, and no interferon is produced (Choppin, 1964; Choppin *et al.*, 1968). Furthermore, if SV5-infected cells are superinfected with another virus which is normally capable of inducing interferon, none is produced, and if preformed interferon is added to SV5-infected cells, it does not act (Choppin, unpublished experiments). Thus SV5 infection of either MK or MDBK cells inhibits the induction and action of interferon. On the other hand, if defective SV5 particles produced by serial undiluted passage in HKCC cells are used to infect MK or MDBK cells, interferon is produced, and preformed interferon added to cells inoculated with defective virus does act. These results suggest that the inhibition of interferon induction and action is a positive function of the SV5 genome which has been lost by the defective virions. Further studies are required to determine the nature of this property of SV5 virus which has apparently been lost in the deletion which occurs in the genesis of defective virions.

4.4. Other Forms of Interference

Homologous interference between strains of NDV which does not involve interferon or defective virions has also observed. Interference by UV-irradiated virus at the level of adsorption (Baluda, 1959) and penetration (Bratt and Rubin, 1968) has been described. The exact mechanisms involved in this type of interference are not clear.

A phenomenon termed intrinsic interference has been described by Marcus and Carver (1967). NDV has been used as an indicator for this type of heterologous interference, which was introduced as a means of detecting the presence of and for assaying noncytopathogenic viruses such as rubella. Although the mechanism of this type of interference has not been established, several possibilities have been excluded. As a result of studies using temperature-sensitive mutants of Sindbis virus, it was concluded that the most likely explanation for the phenomenon was that the RNA replicase of the interfering virus interacts with the NDV genome, and thus prevents the replication of the NDV RNA by its own enzyme (Marcus and Zuckerbraun, 1970).

The question of induction of interferon is beyond the scope of this chapter, but it is pertinent to mention that UV-irradiated NDV has been found to be a better inducer of interferon than infective virus (Ho and Breinig, 1965; Younger et al., 1966). Since it was originally assumed that UV-irradiated virus would not generate the synthesis of RNA, this finding was difficult to reconcile with the concept that double-stranded RNA is a more effective inducer of interferon than single-stranded RNA. However, Huppert et al. (1969) reported that UV-irradiated NDV did induce some virus-specific RNA synthesis, and Clavell and Bratt (1971), making use of the discovery of the virion transcriptase, showed that UV-irradiated virus was capable of transcribing RNA in the absence of translation. Thus, double-stranded RNA capable of inducing interferon could be generated in this manner. However, others have found interferon induction apparently in the absence of synthesis of detectable single- or double-stranded RNA in cells inoculated with UV-irradiated virus (Gandhi and Burke, 1970; Gandhi *et al.*, 1970). The production of double-stranded RNA by UV-irradiated virus (Clavell and Bratt, 1971) provides a possible means of explaining interferon production, but does not explain the enhancement of induction by such virus as compared to active virus. This explanation remains obscure; however, one possibility would be that if, as suggested above for SV5, inhibition of interferon induction is a positive function of some paramyxoviruses, then UV irradiation might result in the loss of this function although still allowing some RNA synthesis to occur. Under these conditions enhanced induction of interferon might result.

5. CYTOPATHIC EFFECTS OF PARAMYXOVIRUSES

As one would anticipate from the large number of different paramyxoviruses and cells which they infect, there are a wide variety of paramyxovirus–cell interactions. They span the entire range from rapid cell death to persistent, moderate infection with little evidence of overt cell damage. It is clear from work with several of the paramyxoviruses that some strains are more virulent than others in animals, as well as in cultured cells. For example, although many strains of NDV cause rapid cell death and severe disease in animals, others are less virulent (Hanson and Brandly, 1955; Marcus and Puck, 1958; Wilcox, 1959a; Wheelock and Tamm, 1959; Alexander *et al.*, 1970; Kendal and Allan, 1970; Reeve and Waterson, 1970). Thus, as expected, the virus is a major determinant of the end result of a virus–cell encounter. On the other hand, the cell may also play a prominent role. Different cell types may exhibit marked differences in the degree of cytopathology resulting from infection with the same strain of virus. A striking example of this is provided by SV5 infection of MK cells and the BHK21-F line of baby hamster kidney cells (Choppin, 1964; Holmes and Choppin, 1966; Compans *et al.*, 1966). MK cells produce a very high yield of infective virus, but show little or no morphological or biochemical evidence of cell damage (Figs. 17–19). SV5-infected MK cells divide at normal rates, and they can be superinfected with a variety of other viruses and produce a normal yield of the superinfecting

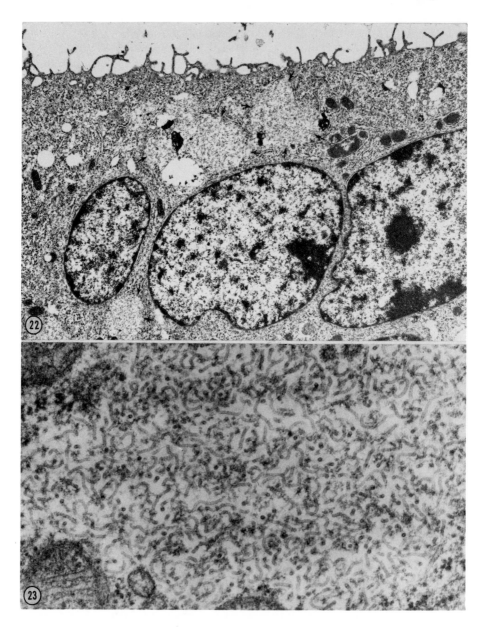

Fig. 22.   A portion of a large syncytium of SV5-infected BHK21-F cells showing five nuclei. Several pale areas in the cytoplasm are large aggregates of SV5 nucleocapsid. The aggregates represent the eosinophilic inclusions seen with the light microscope. ×4,900. From Compans *et al.* (1966).

Fig. 23.   A large collection of SV5 nucleocapsid in the cytoplasm of an SV5-infected BHK21-F cell at higher magnification. ×57,400. From Compans *et al.* (1966).

virus. In marked contrast, BHK21-F cells fuse to form a giant syncytium after 12–24 hours of infection (Figs. 20–22), little virus is produced, and nucleocapsid accumulates to form large aggregates in the cytoplasm due to a block in maturation at the cell membrane (Figs. 21–23). In BHK21-F cells, inhibition of cellular macromolecular synthesis and cell death are apparently secondary to the massive cell fusion (Holmes and Choppin, 1966). In this system the susceptibility of the cell membrane to virus-induced cell fusion appears to determine not only the extent of cytopathology but also virus yield.

The results of the above experiments and those with other virus–cell systems have shown clearly that both the virus and the cell determine the outcome of infection with paramyxoviruses. The precise mechanisms involved in the cell damage induced by paramyxoviruses are still relatively little understood, as they are with most viruses, although much effort has been and is being devoted to this area. Some of the work in this area will be briefly described below; a complete review of the cytopathology of the many paramyxoviruses is not within the scope of this chapter.

6. ALTERATIONS IN CELLULAR MACROMOLECULAR SYNTHESIS

6.1. Nucleic Acid and Protein Synthesis

The rapidity of inhibition of cellular biosynthesis varies considerably with virus and strain, and as pointed out in Sect. 3.4, insufficient inhibition of cellular protein has complicated studies on viral protein synthesis. Nevertheless, inhibition of cellular biosynthesis does occur with some paramyxoviruses, and this has been studied most extensively with NDV. Wheelock and Tamm (1961b) found that cellular DNA and protein synthesis became rapidly inhibited in HeLa cells infected with the Hickman strain of NDV, but that inhibition of RNA synthesis was a later event. The mechanism of inhibition of DNA synthesis has been more extensively studied than that of RNA or proteins. It has been found that the step inhibited is initiation of new DNA chains; chains already begun are completed at a normal rate during infection (Ensminger and Tamm 1970a,b; 1971; Hand et al., 1971; Hand and Tamm, 1972). The inhibition of cellular DNA synthesis in these studies appeared to be secondary to inhibition of the synthesis of cellular proteins which were necessary for the initiation of DNA synthesis. DNA chain elongation apparently does not depend on the continued synthesis of proteins, but initiation does.

The mechanism whereby protein synthesis and RNA synthesis is inhibited by infection is not clear. It has been reported that after infection with NDV, some protein, presumably virus-specific, is synthesized which results in the turnoff of cellular protein and RNA synthesis (Bolognesi and Wilson 1966; Wilson, 1968; Lancz and Johnson, 1971). It has also been suggested that a virus-induced protein is involved in degradation of cellular RNA (Huo and Wilson, 1969).

The inhibition of cellular macromolecular synthesis alone is not sufficient to explain the cytopathic effect in those cases where cell death after infection is rapid since inhibition of cellular RNA and protein synthesis in cells such as HeLa cells will not result in cell lysis as rapidly as does infection (Bablanian et al., 1965). Further, Thacore and Youngner (1970) found that RNA synthesis was depressed less rapidly in chick fibroblasts than in L cells infected with NDV, but morphological cell damage was greater in the chick cells. Moore et al. (1972) did find some indication of a correlation between inhibition of cellular biosynthesis in cells and virulence of NDV in the chicken, but this was not a consistent correlation. A number of factors other than inhibition of cellular biosynthesis, e.g., membrane alterations due to the fusing activity of the virus, neuraminidase activity, and release of lysosomal enzymes, have been suggested as playing a role in cytopathology (Holmes and Choppin, 1966; Bratt and Gallaher, 1969; Poste, 1970, 1971; Alexander et al., 1970; Kendal and Allan, 1970; Reeve and Waterson, 1970; Reeve et al., 1971; Sato et al., 1971), but the precise role of each and the details of the possible interrelationships of these various factors have not yet been sorted out.

6.2. Cellular Lipid and Carbohydrate Synthesis

Alterations in lipid synthesis in paramyxovirus-infected cells have been already mentioned in Sects. 2.2 and 3.4. As discussed there, in those instances where inhibition of lipid synthesis has been observed, it has either been a general decrease late in infection with NDV (Blough and Tiffany, 1973) or a decrease in sphingomyelin synthesis accompanied by an increase in glycolipid synthesis in SV5-infected cells, a system in which cell death does not occur (Scheid and Choppin, 1971). There is no conclusive evidence that inhibition of lipid synthesis is a primary cause of cell damage in paramyxovirus-infected cells.

There is little information available on the effect of paramyxovirus infection on cellular carbohydrate synthesis. As discussed above, glycolipid synthesis may be stimulated under certain conditions; whether there is specific inhibition of the synthesis of cellular carbohydrates as a result of infection with some paramyxoviruses remains to be elucidated.

6.3. Cell Fusion

As has already been discussed, a prominent feature of infection with paramyxoviruses is cell fusion; this is not only an important manifestation of cellular injury, but it is an extremely useful procedure in cytogenetic studies and in the rescue of latent virus or viral functions. There is a very large body of literature in this field which has been reviewed extensively previously (Roizman, 1962; Kohn, 1965; Okada, 1969, 1972; Harris, 1970; Poste, 1970; 1972a; Bratt and Gallaher, 1972). Aspects of cell fusion and hemolysis and the viral components involved in fusion have been discussed in Sects. 2.2 and 2.3 of this chapter, which deal with the viral lipids and viral membrane structure, and in sects. 3.3 and 3.4., which deal with viral penetration and lipid synthesis. In view of this, and the fact that the biochemical mechanism involved in cell fusion is still not clear, this topic will not be discussed in detail here, but some of the salient points in virus-induced fusion will be summarized briefly. The fusion which occurs as a result of infection requires synthesis of viral proteins, is apparently due to the incorporation of virus-specific proteins into the cell membranes, has a pH optimum on the alkaline side, requires energy, and is affected by the divalent cation concentration and by the lipid and carbohydrate composition of the host cell plasma membrane. Fusion may be the important factor in cell death in certain virus–cell systems. The rapid fusion which is induced by high concentrations of virus in the absence of virus replication requires energy, but neither cellular nor viral macromolecular synthesis. The added virus, acting directly on the cell membrane, is capable of causing fusion. Both viral proteins and lipid are required for fusion; the latter may be necessary only to maintain the proper spatial relationship of the viral protein or may be required to interact with cellular lipids. Much work is now going on in many laboratories on this problem; as discussed previously, the ability to reconstitute biologically active systems from lipids and viral proteins, and the finding of the involvement of the smaller virion protein in the fusion reaction, should lead to significant new information on the mechanism of virus-induced cell fusion in the near future.

6.4. Agglutinability of Infected Cells by Plant Lectins

Recent interest in the interaction of plant lectins with cell surfaces has been stimulated by the observation that they cause agglutination of transformed, but not normal, cells (Burger, 1969; Inbar and Sachs, 1969). However, it was subsequently observed that various normal cells infected by enveloped viruses, including the paramyxoviruses NDV and SV5, are also agglutinated by the lectins concanavalin A and wheat germ agglutinin (Becht *et al.*, 1972; Poste, 1972*b*; Poste and Reeve, 1972; Nicolson, 1974). Fusion of BHK21-F cells by infection with SV5 was also completely suppressed by concanavalin A (Rott *et al.*, 1972). Cells infected with influenza virus formed large floccules almost immediately after lectin was added; cells infected with NDV were agglutinated less rapidly and formed aggregates of a more granular appearance (Becht *et al.*, 1972).

Poste (1972*b*) has correlated the agglutinability of NDV-infected cells with a decrease in the thickness of cell coat material measured by ellipsometry, and suggested that digestion by lysosomal enzymes might be important in producing the surface changes responsible for agglutinability. However, it has been demonstrated that the glycoproteins of influenza virus are the sites of lectin binding (Klenk *et al.*, 1972; Klein and Adams, 1972), and it therefore seems likely that the insertion of viral glycoproteins into the plasma membranes of cells infected with paramyxoviruses is primarily responsible for the acquisition of agglutinability to lectins.

7. PERSISTENT INFECTIONS

7.1. In Cultured Cells

As indicated in Sect. 1, an important biological property of paramyxoviruses is their ability to establish persistent infection in cultured cells. Persistent infections have been demonstrated with a sufficient number of paramyxoviruses to establish that the capacity to induce such infections is a general property of this virus group. Examples which have been studied are mumps (Walker and Hinze, 1962; Walker, 1968), measles (Rustigian, 1966*a,b*), parainfluenza 3 (Cole and Hetrick, 1965), Sendai (Maeno *et al.*, 1966), NDV (Henle, 1968; Thacore and Youngner, 1969; Preble and Youngner, 1973*b*), and SV5 (Choppin, 1964; Choppin and Holmes, 1966). Many other workers have also studied cells persistently infected with a variety of paramyxoviruses. The earlier literature on persistent infections has been critically reviewed by Walker (1968), and some points relative to control mechanisms and possible steps in virus production that are blocked in incomplete or abortive infections have already been discussed in previous sections. In addition, persistent infection will be the subject of a chapter by Youngner in a subsequent volume of this series. In view of this, the present comments will be confined to some of the more important general principles that have emerged from studies of paramyxovirus infections. These infections may be of the so-called "carrier culture" type, in which only a few of the cells in the population are infected and producing virus, and the spread of the virus in the culture is limited by genetic resistance of cells in the population or by inhibitory factors such as the presence in the medium of interferon, defective interfering particles, or antibodies (Henle, 1968; Walker, 1968; Thacore and Youngner, 1969). The other type of persistent infection which is very common with paramyxoviruses is the "steady-state" infection, in which essentially all the cells are infected, but they survive. In contrast to the carrier cultures, these infections cannot be "cured" by the presence of antiviral antibodies in the medium. In some systems of this type, virus continues to be produced, although usually at a lower rate than on initial infection (Walker and Hinze, 1962; Walker, 1968; Choppin, 1964; Choppin and Holmes, 1966), whereas in others little or no infective virus is produced (Rustigian, 1966*b*).

As discussed in Section 3.4., dealing with viral biosynthesis, the continued presence of the viral genomes in a surviving cell, with viral macromolecular synthesis representing only a small portion of the total intracellular synthesis, implies tight control of viral biosynthesis. The mechanisms remain to be elucidated and may involve regulatory factors specified not only by the virus, but also by the cell (Choppin and Holmes, 1967; Walker, 1968; Northrop, 1969). Many of the persistent infections are characterized by the lack of production of infective viruses, even though the cell may contain large amounts of viral antigen, including assembled nucleocapsids, and it is therefore apparent that maturation of the virus is blocked in these cells. The characteristics of the persistently infected cells differ considerably; for example, some contain nucleocapsid but do not hemadsorb, others show both characteristics and yet no mature virions are produced. Thus, it is obvious that in the various virus–cell systems there are defects in different steps of virus replication and assembly. A defect in the nonglycosylated membrane protein was postulated above to be responsible for failure of maturation of viruses in systems in which nucleocapsid accumulates although incorporation of functional glyco-protein into the cell membrane has occurred as shown by the hemad-sorption reaction. On the other hand, defects in RNA polymerase activity have been found in virions isolated from cells persistently infected with NDV (Preble and Youngner, 1973a,b). In the case of measles virus, no differences were detected in RNA synthesis between acutely and persistently infected cells (Winston *et al.*, 1973). Thus, some other step seems involved in this system. Investigations of the regulatory mechanisms and defects in virus replication in persistently infected cells are now underway in several laboratories and should eventually shed light on this important, but still little understood, area of paramyxovirus biology.

One of the striking findings that has emerged from studies on persistent infection with paramyxoviruses is that viruses isolated from the persistently infected cells have been found to be temperature sensitive (Preble and Youngner, 1972, 1973a,b; Haspel *et al.*, 1973). In the case of NDV, repeated isolations always yielded *ts* mutants, strongly suggesting that selection of *ts* mutants played a role in the es-tablishment or maintenance of persistent infection. The unravelling of this significant lead will no doubt be of considerable biological im-portance. In addition, the virus isolated from persistently infected cells has differed from the original input virus in characteristics such as vi-rulence for cultured cells or the chick embryo and induction of in-terferon (Henle, 1968; Thacore and Youngner, 1970).

7.2. Persistent Infection in the Whole Animal

As mentioned in Sect. 1, an important proven example of a disease in man produced by persistent infection with a paramyxovirus, measles virus, is subacute sclerosing panencephalitis (SSPE). The ex-tensive literature on SSPE has been reviewed (Sever and Zeman, 1968; ter Meulen *et al.*, 1972b), and much recent work on the disease, on the biology and biochemistry of measles virus, and on its possible role in other chronic diseases of man was presented at a recent Workshop on Measles Viruses (Martin, 1974).

Animal models have been found for persistent infection with paramyxoviruses leading to chronic diseases, and the question has been raised of the involvement of these viruses in other chronic diseases of man, e.g., multiple sclerosis, lupus erythmatosus, and polymyositis. Although a discussion of such findings is not within the scope of this review on virus replication, they increase the importance of a better understanding of the cellular and molecular levels of the mechanisms involved in persistent infections with paramyxoviruses.

8. GENETICS

Knowledge of the genetics of paramyxoviruses is still in a rather rudimentary stage. Extensive early studies failed to yield genetic recombination with NDV (Granoff, 1962), and subsequent attempts have also been unsuccessful. What was originally thought to be successful recombination with NDV was shown subsequently to be due to the presence of complementing heterozygotes (Dahlberg and Simon, 1969), a problem which must be considered with viruses in which the possibility exists of the inclusion of multiple copies of the genome within the virion [reviewed by Simon (1972)].

The isolation, assignment to complementation groups, and characterization of temperature-sensitive mutants of paramyxoviruses have begun with NDV (Dahlberg and Simon, 1969; Pierce and Haywood, 1973; Tsipis and Bratt, 1974), Sendai virus (Portner et al., 1974), and measles virus (Black and Yamazi, 1971). Although the work is still in its early stages, both RNA$^+$ and RNA$^-$ mutants have been recognized, as well as mutants in biological properties such as neuraminidase function and cell fusion. These mutants and those to be isolated in the future should prove very useful in understanding the mechanisms and control of paramyxovirus replication.

ACKNOWLEDGMENTS

The authors wish to thank Drs. Michael A. Bratt, Derek C. Burke, David W. Kingsbury, and Robert A. Lamb for making available preprints of their unpublished work.

Research by the authors was supported by Research Grants AI-05600 and AI-10884 from the National Institute of Allergy and Infectious Diseases.

9. REFERENCES

Adams, J. M., and Imagawa, D. T., 1962, Measles antibodies in multiple sclerosis, *Proc. Soc. Exp. Biol. Med.* **111,** 562.

Adams, W. R., 1965, Extraction of a rapidly sedimenting ribonucleic acid fraction from purified Newcastle disease virus (NDV), *Fed. Proc.* **24,** 159.

Adams, W. R., 1966, Cellular origin of the slowly sedimenting ribonucleic acid (RNA) fraction associated with partially purified Newcastle disease virus (NDV), *Fed. Proc.* **25**, 422.

Adams, W. R., and Prince, A. M., 1957, An electron microscopic study of incomplete virus formation. Infection of Ehrlich ascites tumor cells with "chick embryo-adapted" Newcastle disease virus (NDV), *J. Exp. Med.* **106**, 617.

Alexander, D. J., and Reeve, P., 1972, The proteins of Newcastle disease virus. 2. Virus-induced proteins, *Microbios.* **5**, 247.

Alexander, D. J., Reeve, P., and Allan, W. H., 1970, Characterization and biological properties of the neuraminidase of strains of Newcastle disease virus which differ in virulence, *Microbios.* **1**, 155.

Alexander, D. J., Reeve, P., and Poste, G., 1973a, Studies on the cytopathic effects of Newcastle disease virus: RNA synthesis in infected cells, *J. Gen. Virol.* **18**, 369.

Alexander, D. J., Hewlett, G., Reeve, P., and Poste, G., 1973b, Studies on the cytopathic effects of Newcastle disease virus: The cytopathogenicity of strain Herts 33 in five cell types, *J. Gen. Virol.* **21**, 323.

Anderson, S. G., 1948, Mucins and mucoids in relation to influenza virus action. I. Inactivation by RDE and by viruses of the influenza group, of the serum inhibitor of haemagglutination, *Aust. J. Exp. Biol. Med. Sci.* **26**, 347.

Andrewes, C. H., Bang, F. B., and Burnet, F. M., 1955, A short description of the Myxovirus group (influenza and related viruses), *Virology* **1**, 176.

Apostolov, K., and Almeida, J. D., 1972, Interaction of Sendai (HVJ) virus with human erythrocytes: A morphological study of haemolysis cell fusion, *J. Gen. Virol.* **15**, 227.

Bablanian, R., Eggers, H. J., and Tamm, I., 1965, Studies on the mechanism of poliovirus-induced cell damage. I. The relation between poliovirus-induced metabolic and morphological alterations in cultured cells, *Virology* **26**, 100.

Bächi, T., Aguet, M., and Howe, C., 1973, Fusion of erythrocytes by Sendai virus studied by immuno-freeze-etching, *J. Virol.* **11**, 1004.

Baker, R. F., 1970, Fusion of human red blood cell membranes, *J. Cell Biol.* **53**, 244.

Baltimore, D., Huang, A. S., and Stampfer, M., 1970, Ribonucleic acid synthesis of vesicular stomatitis virus. II. An RNA polymerase in the virion, *Proc. Natl. Acad. Sci. USA* **66**, 572.

Baluda, M. A., 1959, Loss of viral receptors in homologous interference by ultraviolet-irradiated Newcastle disease virus, *Virology* **7**, 315.

Bang, F. B., 1946, Filamentous forms of Newcastle virus, *Proc. Soc. Exp. Biol. Med.* **63**, 5.

Bang, F. B., 1948, Studies on Newcastle disease virus. III. Characters of the virus itself with particular reference to electron microscopy, *J. Exp. Med.* **88**, 251.

Bang, F. B., 1953, The development of Newcastle disease virus in cells of the chorioallantoic membrane as studied by thin sections, *Bull. Johns Hopkins Hosp.* **92**, 309.

Bang, F. B., 1955, Pathology of the cell infected with viruses—Morphological and biochemical aspects, *Fed. Proc.* **14**, 619.

Barry, R. D., 1964, The effects of actinomycin D and ultraviolet irradiation on the production of fowl plague virus, *Virology* **24**, 563.

Barry, R. D., and Bukrinskaya, A. G., 1968, The nucleic acid of Sendai virus and ribonucleic acid synthesis in cells infected by Sendai virus, *J. Gen. Virol.* **2**, 71.

Barry, R. D., and Mahy, B. W. J., eds., 1974, "Negative Strand Viruses," Academic Press, London.

Barry, R. D., Ives, D. R., and Cruickshank, J. G., 1962, Participation of deoxyribonucleic acid in the multiplication of influenza virus, *Nature (Lond.)* **194**, 1139.

Becht, W., Rott, R., and Klenk, H.-D., 1972, Effect of concanavalin A on cells infected with enveloped RNA viruses, *J. Gen. Virol.* **14**, 1.

Berkaloff, A., 1963, Étude au microscope électronique de la morphogènese de la particule du virus sendai, *J. Microscop.* **2**, 633.

Bikel, I., and Duesberg, P. H., 1969, Proteins of Newcastle disease virus and of the viral nucleocapsid, *J. Virol.* **4**, 388.

Black, F. L., and Yamazi, Y., 1971, Temperature sensitive mutants of measles virus, *Bacteriol. Proc.,* 218.

Blair, C. D., and Brennan, P. J., 1972, Effect of Sendai virus infection on lipid metabolism in chick embryo fibroblasts, *J. Virol.* **9**, 813.

Blair, C. D., and Duesberg, P. H., 1970, Myxovirus ribonucleic acids, *Annu. Rev. Microbiol.* **24**, 539.

Blair, C. D., and Robinson, W. S., 1968, Replication of Sendai virus. I. Comparison of the viral RNA and virus-specific RNA synthesis with Newcastle disease virus, *Virology* **35**, 537.

Blair, C. D., and Robinson, W. S., 1970, Replication of Sendai virus. II. Steps in virus assembly, *J. Virol.* **5**, 639.

Blough, H. A., 1963, The effect of vitamin A alcohol on the morphology of myxoviruses. I. The production and comparison of artificially produced filamentous virus, *Virology* **19**, 349.

Blough, H. A., and Lawson, D. E. M., 1968, The lipids of paramyxoviruses: A comparative study of Sendai and Newcastle disease viruses, *Virology* **36**, 286.

Blough, H. A., and Tiffany, J. M., 1973, Lipids in viruses, *Adv. Lipid Res.* **11**, 267.

Bolognesi, D. P., and Wilson, D. E., 1966, Inhibitory proteins in the Newcastle disease virus-induced suppression of cell protein synthesis, *J. Bacteriol.* **91**, 1896.

Bratt, M. A., 1969, RNA synthesis in chick embryo cells infected with different strains of NDV, *Virology* **38**, 485.

Bratt, M. A., and Gallaher, W. R., 1969, Preliminary analysis of the requirements for fusion from within and fusion from without by Newcastle disease virus, *Proc. Natl. Acad. Sci. USA* **64**, 536.

Bratt, M. A., and Gallaher, W. R., 1972, Biological parameters of fusion from within and fusion from without, *in* "Membrane Research" (C. F. Fox, ed.), p. 383, Academic Press, New York.

Bratt, M. A., and Robinson, W. S., 1967, Ribonucleic acid synthesis in cells infected with Newcastle disease virus, *J. Mol. Biol.* **23**, 1.

Bratt, M. A., and Robinson, W. S., 1971, Evidence for an RNA replicative intermediate in cells infected with Newcastle disease virus, *J. Gen. Virol.* **10**, 139.

Bratt, M. A., and Rubin, H., 1968, Specific interference among strains of Newcastle disease virus. III. Mechanisms of interference. *Virology* **35**, 395.

Bratt, M. A., Collins, B. S., Hightower, L. E., Kaplan, J., Tsipis, J. E., and Weiss, S. R., 1974, Transcription and translation of Newcastle disease virus RNA, *in* "Negative Strand Viruses" (R. D. Barry and B. W. J. Mahy, eds.), Academic Press, London.

Brostrom, M. A., Bruening, G., and Bankowski, R. A., 1971, Comparison of neuraminidases of paramyxoviruses with immunologically dissimilar hemagglutinins, *Virology* **46**, 856.

Bukrinskaya, A. G., Burducea, O., and Vorkunova, G. K., 1966, The intracellular site of RNA synthesis of Newcastle disease virus, *Proc. Soc. Exp. Biol. Med.* **123**, 236.

Bukrinskaya, A. G., Bykovsky, A. Ph., and Zhdanov, V. M., 1969a, The participation of Sendai virus ribonucleoprotein in virus-specific polysome formation, *Virology* **39**, 705.

Bukrinskaya, A. G., Zhdanov, V. M., and Vorkunova, G. K., 1969b, Fate of Sendai virus ribonucleoprotein in virus-infected cells, *J. Virol.* **4**, 141.

Burge, B. W., and Huang, A. S., 1970, Comparison of membrane protein glycopeptides of Sindbis virus and vesicular stomatitis virus, *J. Virol.* **6**, 176.

Burger, M. M., 1969, A difference in the architecture of the surface membrane of normal and virally transformed cells, *Proc. Natl. Acad. Sci. USA* **62**, 994.

Burnet, F. M., 1942, The affinity of Newcastle disease virus to the influenza virus group, *Aust. J. Exp. Biol. Med. Sci.* **20**, 81.

Burnet, F. M., and Anderson, S. G., 1946, Modification of human red cells by virus action. II. Agglutination of modified human red cells by sera from cases of infectious mononucleosis, *Brit. J. Exp. Pathol.* **27**, 236.

Burnet, F. M., and Anderson, S. G., 1947, The "T" antigen of guinea-pig and human red cells, *Aust. J. Exp. Biol. Med. Sci.* **25**, 213.

Burnet, F. M., and Lind, P. E., 1950, Haemolysis by Newcastle disease virus. II. General character of haemolytic action, *Aust. J. Exp. Biol. Med. Sci.* **28**, 129.

Calberg-Bacq, C. M., Reginster, M., and Rigo, P., 1967, Alteration of the Newcastle disease virus particle after treatment with pronase or caseinase C, *Acta Virol.* **11**, 52.

Caliguiri, L. A., Klenk, H.-D., and Choppin, P. W., 1969, The proteins of the parainfluenza virus SV5. I. Separation of virion polypeptides by polyacrylamide gel electrophoresis, *Virology* **39**, 460.

Cantell, K., 1961, Mumps virus, *Adv. Virus Res.* **8**, 123.

Carter, C. A., Schluederberg, A., and Black, F. L., 1973, Viral RNA synthesis in measles virus-infected cells, *Virology* **53**, 379.

Chanock, R. M., and Parrott, R. H., 1965, Para-influenza viruses, *in* "Viral and Rickettsial Infections of Man" (F. L. Horsfall, Jr., and I. Tamm, eds.), pp. 741–754, J. B. Lippincott Co., Philadelphia.

Chen, C., Compans, R. W., and Choppin, P. W., 1971, Parainfluenza virus surface projections—Glycoproteins with hemagglutinin and neuraminidase activities, *J. Gen. Virol.* **11**, 53.

Choppin, P. W., 1964, Multiplication of a myxovirus (SV5) with minimal cytopathic effects and without interference, *Virology* **23**, 224.

Choppin, P. W., 1965, Effect of actinomycin D and halogenated deoxyuridines on the replication of simian virus 5, *Proc. Soc. Exp. Biol. Med.* **120**, 699.

Choppin, P. W., 1969, Replication of influenza virus in a continuous cell line: High yield of infective virus from cells inoculated at high multiplicity, *Virology* **39**, 130.

Choppin, P. W., and Compans, R. W., 1970, Phenotypic mixing of envelope proteins of the parainfluenza virus SV5 and vesicular stomatitis virus, *J. Virol.* **5**, 609.

Choppin, P. W., and Compans, R. W., 1975, Viral membranes and surface glycoproteins, *in* "Comprehensive Virology," to be published, (H. Fraenkel-Conrat and R. R. Wagner, eds.), Plenum Press, New York.

Choppin, P. W., and Holmes, K. V., 1967, Replication of SV5 RNA and the effects of superinfection with poliovirus, *Virology* **33**, 442.

Choppin, P. W., and Stoeckenius, W., 1964, The morphology of SV5 virus, *Virology* **23**, 195.

Choppin, P. W., Compans, R. W., and Holmes, K. V., 1968, Replication of the parainfluenza virus SV5 and the effects of superinfection with poliovirus, *in*

"Proceedings of the Second International Symposium, Medical and Applied Virology" (M. Sanders and E. H. Lennette, eds.), pp. 16–30, Warren H. Green, Inc., St. Louis.

Choppin, P. W., Klenk, H.-D., Compans, R. W., and Caliguiri, L. A., 1971, The parainfluenza virus SV5 and its relationship to the cell membrane, *in* "Perspectives in Virology," Vol. VII (M. Pollard, ed.), Chapter 9, From Molecules to Man, pp. 127–158, Academic Press, New York.

Choppin, P. W., Compans, R. W., Scheid, A., McSharry, J. J., and Lazarowitz, S. G., 1972, Structure and assembly of viral membranes, *in* "Membrane Research" (C. F. Fox, ed.), pp. 163–179, Academic Press, New York.

Choppin, P. W., Scheid, A., Lazarowitz, S. G., McSharry, J. J., and Compans, R. W., 1973, Proteins of viral membranes, *in* "Advances in Biosciences," Vol. 11 (G. Raspe, ed.), Workshop on virus–cell interactions, pp. 83–108, Pergamon Press, Vieweg.

Choppin, P. W., Lazarowitz, S. W., and Goldberg, A. R., 1974, Studies on proteolytic cleavage and glycosylation of the hemagglutinin of influenza A and B viruses, in "Negative Strand Viruses" (R. D. Barry and B. M. J. Mahy, eds.), Academic Press, London, in press.

Clavell, L. A., and Bratt, M., 1971, Relationship between the ribonucleic acid-synthesizing capacity of ultraviolet-irradiated Newcastle disease virus and its ability to induce interferon, *J. Virol.* **8**, 500.

Clavell, L. A., and Bratt, M. A., 1972a, Hemolytic interaction of Newcastle disease virus and chicken erythrocytes. II. Determining factors, *Appl. Microbiol.* **23**, 461.

Clavell, L. A., and Bratt, M. A., 1972b, Hemolytic interaction of Newcastle disease virus and chicken erythrocytes. III. Cessation of the reaction as a result of inactivation of hemolytic activity by erythrocytes, *Virology* **44**, 195.

Cohen, A., 1963, Mechanisms of cell infection. I. Virus attachment and penetration, *in* "Mechanisms of Virus Infection" (W. Smith, ed.), pp. 153–190, Academic Press, London.

Cohen, S. M., Bullivant, S., and Edwards, G. A., 1961, A morphologic study of FL cells infected with para-influenza 3 virus, *Arch. Ges. Virusforsch.* **11**, 493.

Cole, F. E., and Hetrick, F. M., 1965, Persistent infection of human conjunctiva cell cultures by myxovirus parainfluenza 3, *Can. J. Microbiol.* **11**, 513.

Collins, B. S., and Bratt, M. A., 1973, Separation of the messenger RNA's of Newcastle disease virus by gel electrophoresis, *Proc. Natl. Acad. Sci. USA* **70**, 2544.

Compans, R. W., and Choppin, P. W., 1967a, Isolation and properties of the helical nucleocapsid of the parainfluenza virus SV5, *Proc. Natl. Acad. Sci. USA* **57**, 949.

Compans, R. W., and Choppin, P. W., 1967b, The length of the helical nucleocapsid of Newcastle disease virus, *Virology* **33**, 344.

Compans, R. W., and Choppin, P. W., 1968, The nucleic acid of the parainfluenza virus SV5, *Virology* **35**, 289.

Compans, R. W., and Choppin, P. W., 1971, The structure and assembly of influenza and parainfluenza viruses, *in* "Comparative Virology" (K. Maramorosch and F. Kurstak, eds.), pp. 407–432, Academic Press, New York.

Compans, R. W., and Choppin, P. W., 1973, Orthomyxoviruses and paramyxoviruses, *in* "Ultrastructure of Animal Viruses and Bacteriophages" (A. J. Dalton and F. Haguenau, eds.), pp. 213–237, Academic Press, New York.

Compans, R. W., Holmes, K. V., Dales, S., and Choppin, P. W., 1966, An electron microscopic study of moderate and virulent virus–cell interactions of the parain-fluenza virus SV5, *Virology* **30,** 411.

Compans, R. W., Harter, D. H., and Choppin, P. W., 1967, Studies on pneumonia virus of mice (PVM) in cell culture. II. Structure and morphogenesis of the virus particle, *J. Exp. Med.* **126,** 267.

Compans, R. W., Klenk, H.-D., Caliguiri, L. A., and Choppin, P. W., 1970, Influenza virus proteins. I. Analysis of polypeptides of the virion and identification of spike glycoproteins, *Virology* **42,** 880.

Compans, R. W., Mountcastle, W. E., and Choppin, P. W., 1972, The sense of the helix of paramyxovirus nucleocapsids, *J. Mol. Biol.* **65,** 167.

Content, J., and Duesberg, P. H., 1970, Electrophoretic distribution of the proteins and glycoproteins of influenza virus and Sendai virus, *J. Virol.* **6,** 707.

Cunha, R., Weil, M. L., Beard, D., Taylor, A. R., Sharp, G., and Beard, J. W., 1947, Purification and characters of the Newcastle disease virus (California strain), *J. Immunol.* **55,** 69.

Dahlberg, J. E., and Simon, E. H., 1969, Recombination in Newcastle disease virus (NDV). The problem of complementing heterozygotes, *Virology* **38,** 490.

Dales, S., 1973, Early events in cell–animal virus interactions, *Bacteriol. Rev.* **37,** 103.

Darlington, R. W., Portner, A., and Kingsbury, D. W., 1970, Sendai virus replication: An ultrastructural comparison of productive and abortive infections in avian cells, *J. Gen. Virol.* **9,** 169.

Dawson, I. M., and Elford, W. J., 1949, The investigation of influenza and related viruses in the electron microscope by a new technique, *J. Gen. Microbiol.* **3,** 298.

Dinter, Z., Hermodsson, S., and Hermodsson, L., 1964, Studies on Yucaipa: Its classification as a member of the paramyxovirus group, *Virology* **22,** 297.

Duc-Nguyen, H., and Rosenblum, E. N., 1967, Immunoelectron microscopy of mumps virus, *J. Virol.* **1,** 415.

Duesberg, P. H., 1968, Physical properties of Rous sarcoma virus RNA, *Proc. Natl. Acad. Sci. USA* **60,** 1511.

Duesberg, P. H., and Robinson, W. S., 1965, Isolation of the nucleic acid of Newcastle disease virus (NDV), *Proc. Natl. Acad. Sci. USA* **54,** 794.

Duesberg, P. H., Robinson, H. L., Robinson, W. S., Huebner, R. J., and Turner, H. C., 1968, Proteins of Rous sarcoma virus, *Virology* **36,** 73.

Durand, D. P., Brotherton, T., Chalgren, S., and Collard, W., 1970, Uncoating of myxoviruses, *in* "The Biology of Large RNA Viruses" (R. D. Barry and B. W. J. Mahy, eds.), pp. 197–206, Academic Press, London.

East, J. L., and Kingsbury, D. W., 1971, Mumps virus replication in chick embryo lung cells: Properties of RNA species in virions and infected cells, *J. Virol.* **8,** 161.

Elford, W. J., Smiles, J., Chu, C. M., and Dudgeon, J. A., 1947, Electronmicrographs of staphylococcus bacteriophage "K" and the viruses of vaccinia and Newcastle disease, *Proc. Biochem. Soc. Biochem. J.* **41,** 25.

Emerson, S. U., and Wagner, R. R., 1972, Dissociation and reconstitution of the transcriptase and template activities of vesicular stomatitis virus B and T virions, *J. Virol.* **10,** 297.

Emerson, S. U., and Wagner, R. R., 1973, L protein requirement for *in vitro* RNA synthesis by vesicular stomatitis virus, *J. Virol.* **10,** 1325.

Enders, J. F., and Peebles, T. C., 1954, Propagation in tissue cultures of cytopatho-genic agents from patients with measles, *Proc. Soc. Exp. Biol. Med.* **86,** 277.

Ensminger, W. D., and Tamm, I., 1970a, The step in cellular DNA synthesis blocked by Newcastle disease or mengovirus infection, *Virology* **40,** 152.

Ensminger, W. D., and Tamm, I., 1970b, Inhibition of synchronized cellular deoxyribonucleic acid synthesis during Newcastle disease virus, mengovirus, or reovirus infection, J. Virol. 5, 672.

Ensminger, W. D., and Tamm, I., 1971, Cellular DNA replication in viral infection, in "Pathobiology Annual" (H. L. Ioachim, ed.), pp. 33–61, Appleton-Century-Crofts, New York.

Evans, M. J., and Kingsbury, D. W., 1969, Separation of Newcastle disease virus proteins by polyacrylamide gel electrophoresis, Virology 37, 597.

Fazekas de St. Groth, S., 1948, Viropexis, the mechanism of influenza virus infection, Nature (Lond.) 162, 294.

Feller, U., Dougherty, R. M., and DeStefano, H. S., 1969, Morphogenesis of Newcastle disease virus in chorioallantoic membrane, J. Virol. 4, 753.

Field, E. J., Cowshall, S., Narang, H. K., and Bell, T. M., 1972, Viruses in multiple sclerosis? Lancet II, 280.

Finch, J. T., and Gibbs, A. J., 1970, Observations on the structure of the nucleocapsids of some paramyxoviruses, J. Gen. Virol. 6, 141.

Francis, T., Jr., 1947, Dissociation of hemagglutinating and antibody-measuring capacities of influenza virus, J. Exp. Med. 85, 1.

Furman, P. A., and Hallum, J. V., 1973, RNA-dependent DNA polymerase activity in preparations of a mutant of Newcastle disease virus arising from persistently infected L cells, J. Virol. 12, 548.

Gallaher, W. R., Levitan, D. B., and Blough, H. A., 1973, Effect of 2-deoxy-D-glucose on cell fusion induced by Newcastle disease and herpes simples viruses, Virology 55, 193.

Gandhi, S. S., and Burke, D. C., 1970, Interferon production by myxoviruses in chick embryo cells, J. Gen. Virol. 6, 95.

Gandhi, S. S., Burke, D. C., and Scholtissek, C., 1970, Virus RNA synthesis by ultraviolet-irradiated Newcastle disease virus and interferon production, J. Gen. Virol. 9, 97.

Gitelman, A. K., and Bukrinskaya, A. G., 1971, Comparison of influenza and parainfluenza RNP properties, Arch. Ges. Virusforsch. 34, 89.

Gottshalk, A., 1965, Interaction between glycoproteins and viruses, in "The Amino Sugars" (E. A. Balazs and R. W. Jeanloz, eds.), p. 337, Academic Press, New York.

Granoff, A., 1955, Noninfectious forms of Newcastle disease and influenza viruses. Studies on noninfectious virus occurring within cells that are producing fully infectious virus, Virology 1, 516.

Granoff, A., 1962, Heterozygosis and phenotypic mixing with Newcastle disease virus, Cold Spring Harbor Symp. Quant. Biol. 27, 319.

Granoff, A., and Kingsbury, D. W., 1964, Effect of actinomycin D on the replication of Newcastle disease and influenza viruses, in "Ciba Foundation Symposium, Cellular Biology of Myxovirus Infections" (G. E. W. Wolstenholme and J. Knight, eds.), Little, Brown and Co., Boston.

Granoff, A., Liu, O. C., and Henle, W., 1950, A small hemagglutinating component in preparations of Newcastle disease virus, Proc. Soc. Exp. Biol. Med. 75, 684.

Hall, W. W., and Martin, S. J., 1973, Purification and characterization of measles virus, J. Gen. Virol. 19, 175.

Hand, R., and Tamm, I., 1972, Rate of DNA chain growth in mammalian cells infected with cytocidal RNA viruses, Virology 47, 331.

Hand, R., Ensminger, W. D., and Tamm, I., 1971, Cellular DNA replication in infections with cytocidal RNA viruses, Virology 44, 527.

Hanson, R. P., and Brandly, C. A., 1955, Identification of vaccine strains of Newcastle disease virus, *Science* (Wash., D.C.) **122**, 156.

Harris, H., 1970, "Cell Fusion, The Dunham Lectures," Harvard University Press, Cambridge, Mass.

Harrison, S. C., David, A., Jumblatt, J., and Darnell, J. E., 1971, Lipid and protein organization in Sindbis virus, *J. Mol. Biol.* **60**, 523.

Haslam, E. A., Cheyne, I. M., and White, D. O., 1969, The structural proteins of Newcastle disease virus, *Virology* **39**, 118.

Haspel, M. V., Knight, P. R., Duff, R. G., and Rapp, F., 1973, Activation of a latent measles virus infection in hamster cells, *J. Virol.* **12**, 690.

Henle, W., 1968, Some aspects of persistent viral infections in cell cultures, *in* "Medical and Applied Virology" (M. Sanders and E. H. Lennette, eds.), pp. 99–110, Warren H. Green, Inc., St. Louis.

Henle, G., Deinhardt, F., and Girardi, A., 1954, Cytolytic effects of mumps virus in tissue cultures of epithelial cells, *Proc. Soc. Exp. Biol. Med.* **87**, 386.

Hightower, L. E., and Bratt, M. A., 1974, Protein synthesis in Newcastle disease virus (NDV)-infected chick embryo cells, *J. Virol.*, **13**, 788.

Hirano, K., Yamaura, K., Shibuta, H., and Matumoto, M., 1971, Lipids of Sendai virus and changes in cellular phospholipid synthesis caused by infection, *Jap. J. Microbiol.* **15**, 383.

Hirst, G. K., 1941, The agglutination of red cells by allantoic fluid of chick embryos infected with influenza virus, *Science* (*Wash., D.C.*) **94**, 22.

Hirst, G. K., 1959, Virus–host cell relation, *in* "Viral and Rickettsial Infections of Man" (T. M. Rivers and F. L. Horsfall, Jr., eds.), 3rd edition, pp. 96–144, Lippincott Co., Philadelphia.

Ho, M., and Breinig, M. K., 1965, Metabolic determinants of interferon formation, *Virology* **25**, 331.

Holmes, K. V., and Choppin, P. W., 1966, On the role of the response of the cell membrane in determining virus virulence. Contrasting effects of the parainfluenza virus SV5 in two cell types, *J. Exp. Med.* **124**, 501.

Holmes, K. V., and Choppin, P. W., 1968, On the role of microtubules in movement and alignment of nuclei in virus-induced syncytia, *J. Cell Biol.* **39**, 526.

Homma, M., 1971, Trypsin action on the growth of Sendai virus in tissue culture cells. I. Restoration of the infectivity for L cells by direct action of trypsin on L cell-borne Sendai virus, *J. Virol.* **8**, 619.

Homma, M., 1972, Trypsin action on the growth of Sendai virus in tissue culture cells. II. Restoration of the hemolytic activity of L cell-borne Sendai virus by trypsin, *J. Virol.* **9**, 829.

Homma, M., 1974, Host-induced modification of Sendai virus, *in* "Negative Strand Viruses" (R. D. Barry and B. W. J. Mahy, eds.), Academic Press, London, in press.

Homma, M., and Ohuchi, M., 1973, Trypsin action on the growth of Sendai virus in tissue culture cells. III. Structural differences of Sendai viruses grown in eggs and tissue culture cells, *J. Virol.* **12**, 1457.

Homma, M., and Tamagawa, S., 1973, Restoration of the fusion activity of L cell-borne Sendai virus by trypsin, *J. Gen. Virol.* **19**, 423.

Horne, R. W., and Waterson, A. P., 1960, A helical structure in mumps, Newcastle disease and Sendai viruses, *J. Mol. Biol.* **2**, 75.

Horne, R. W., and Wildy, P., 1961, Symmetry in virus architecture, *Virology* **15**, 348.

Horne, R. W., Waterson, A. P., Wildy, P., and Farnham, A. E., 1960, The structure and composition of the myxoviruses. I. Electron microscope studies of the structure of myxovirus particles by negative staining techniques, *Virology* **11**, 79.

Hosaka, Y., 1968, Isolation and structure of the nucleocapsid of HVJ, *Virology* **35**, 445.

Hosaka, Y., 1974, Artificial assembly of active envelope particle of HVJ (Sendai virus), *in* "Negative Strand Viruses" (R. D. Barry and B. W. J. Mahy, eds.), Academic Press, London, in press.

Hosaka, Y., and Shimizu, K., 1968, Lengths of the nucleocapsids of Newcastle disease and mumps viruses, *J. Mol. Biol.* **35**, 369.

Hosaka, Y., and Shimizu, K., 1972, Artificial assembly of envelope particles of HVJ (Sendai virus). I. Assembly of hemolytic and fusion factors from envelopes solubilized by Nonidet P_{40}, *Virology* **49**, 627.

Hosaka, Y., Nishi, Y., and Fukai, K., 1961, The structure of HVJ. II. The fine structure of the subunits, *Bikens J.* **4**, 243.

Hosaka, Y., Kitano, H., and Ikeguchi, S., 1966, Studies on the pleomorphism of HVJ virions, *Virology* **29**, 205.

Howe, C., and Lee, L. T., 1970, Virus erythrocyte interactions, *Adv. Virus Res.* **17**, 1.

Howe, C., and Morgan, C., 1969, Interactions between Sendai virus and human erythrocytes, *J. Virol.* **3**, 70.

Howe, C., Morgan, C., deVaux St. Cyr, C., Hsu, K. C., and Rose, H. M., 1967, Morphogenesis of type 2 parainfluenza virus examined by light and electron microscopy, *J. Virol.* **1**, 215.

Hsiung, G. D., 1972, Parainfluenza-5 virus. Infection of man and animal, *Progr. Med. Virol.* **14**, 241.

Huang, A. S., 1973, Defective interfering viruses, *Annu. Rev. Microbiol.* **27**, 101.

Huang, A. S., Baltimore, D., and Bratt, M. A., 1971, Ribonucleic acid polymerase in virions of Newcastle disease virus: Comparison with the vesicular stomatitis virus polymerase, *J. Virol.* **7**, 389.

Huo, W.-H., and Wilson, D. E., 1969, Degradation of cellular ribonucleic acid in Newcastle disease virus-infected cells, *J. Gen. Virol.* **4**, 245.

Huppert, J., Hillova, J., and Gresland, L., 1969, Viral RNA synthesis in chicken cells infected with ultraviolet irradiated Newcastle disease virus, *Nature (Lond.)* **223**, 1015.

Iinuma, M., Nagai, Y., Maeno, K., Yoshida, T., and Matsumoto, T., 1971, Studies on the assembly of Newcastle disease virus: Incorporation of structural proteins into virus particles, *J. Gen. Virol.* **12**, 239.

Iinuma, M., Maeno, K., and Matsumoto, T., 1973, Studies on the assembly of Newcastle disease virus: An argenine-dependent step in virus replication, *Virology* **51**, 205.

Imblum, R. L., and Wagner, R. R., 1974, Protein kinase and phosphoproteins of vesicular stomatitis virus, *J. Virol.* **13**, 113.

Inbar, M., and Sachs, L., 1969, Interaction of the carbohydrate-binding protein concanavalin A with normal and transformed cells, *Proc. Natl. Acad. Sci. USA* **63**, 1418.

Isacson, P., and Koch, A. E., 1965, Association of host antigen with a parainfluenza virus, *Virology* **27**, 129.

Ishida, N., and Homma, M., 1960, A variant Sendai virus, infectious to egg embryos but not to L cells, *Tohoku J. Exp. Med.* **73**, 56.

Ito, Y., Okazaki, H., Sakuma, S., Homma, M., and Ishida, N,. 1969, Specific requirement of serine for the growth of Newcastle disease virus, *Virology* **39**, 277.

Iwai, Y., Iwai, M., Okumoto, M., Hosokawa, Y., and Asai, T., 1966, Properties of the nucleic acid isolated from HVJ, *Bikens J.* **9**, 241.

Joncas, J., Berthiaume, L., and Pavilanis, V., 1969, The structure of respiratory syncytial virus, *Virology* **38**, 493.

Kaplan, J., and Bratt, M. A., 1973, Synthesis and processing of Newcastle disease virus polypeptides, *Abstr. Am. Soc. Microbiol.*, 243.

Kaluza, G., Scholtissek, C., and Rott, R., 1972, Inhibition of the multiplication of enveloped RNA-viruses by glucosamine and 2-deoxy-D-glucose, *J. Gen. Virol.* **14**, 251.

Kates, M., Allison, A. C., Tyrrell, D. A. J., and James, A. T., 1962, Origin of lipids in influenza virus, *Cold Spring Harbor Symp. Quant. Biol.* **27**, 293.

Katz, S. L., and Enders, J. F., 1965, Measles virus, *in* "Viral and Rickettsial Infections of Man" (F. L. Horsfall, Jr. and I. Tamm, eds.), pp. 784–801, J. B. Lippincott, Co., Philadelphia.

Kendal, A. P., and Allan, W. H., 1970, Comparative studies of Newcastle disease virus. 1. Virulence, antigenic specificity and growth kinetics, *Microbios.* **2**, 273.

Kingsbury, D. W., 1962, Use of actinomycin D to unmask RNA synthesis induced by Newcastle disease virus, *Biochem. Biophys. Res. Commun.* **9**, 156.

Kingsbury, D. W., 1966a, Newcastle disease virus RNA. I. Isolation and preliminary characterization of RNA from virus particles, *J. Mol. Biol.* **18**, 195.

Kingsbury, D. W., 1966b, Newcastle disease virus RNA. II. Preferential synthesis of RNA complementary to parental viral RNA by chick embryo cells, *J. Mol. Biol.* **18**, 204.

Kingsbury, D. W., 1967, Newcastle disease virus complementary RNA: Its relationship to the viral genome and its accumulation in the presence or absence of actinomycin D, *Virology* **33**, 227.

Kingsbury, D. W., 1970, Replication and functions of myxovirus ribonucleic acids, *Progr. Med. Virol.* **12**, 49.

Kingsbury, D. W., 1973a, Paramyxovirus replication, *Curr. Top. Microbiol.* **59**, 1.

Kingsbury, D. W., 1973b, Cell-free translation of paramyxovirus messenger RNA, *J. Virol.* **12**, 1020.

Kingsbury, D. W., and Darlington, R. W., 1968, Isolation and properties of Newcastle disease virus nucleocapsid, *J. Virol.* **2**, 248.

Kingsbury, D. W., and Granoff, A., 1970, Studies on mixed infection with Newcastle disease virus. IV. On the structure of heterozygotes, *Virology* **42**, 262.

Kingsbury, D. W., and Portner, A., 1970, On the genesis of incomplete Sendai virions, *Virology* **42**, 872.

Kingsbury, D. W., Portner, A., and Darlington, R. W., 1970, Properties of incomplete Sendai virions and subgenomic viral RNAs, *Virology* **42**, 857.

Klein, P. A., and Adams, W. R., 1972, Location of ferritin-labeled concanavalin A binding to influenza virus and tumor cell surfaces, *J. Virol.* **10**, 844.

Klenk, H.-D., and Choppin, P. W., 1969a, Chemical composition of the parainfluenza virus SV5, *Virology* **37**, 155.

Klenk, H.-D., and Choppin, P. W., 1969b, Lipids of plasma membranes of monkey and hamster kidney cells and of parainfluenza virions grown in these cells, *Virology* **38**, 255.

Klenk, H.-D., and Choppin, P. W., 1970a, Plasma membrane lipids and parainfluenza virus assembly, *Virology* **40**, 939.

Klenk, H.-D., and Choppin, P. W., 1970b, Glycosphingolipids of plasma membranes of cultured cells and an enveloped virus (SV5) grown in these cells, *Proc. Natl. Acad. Sci. USA* **66**, 57.

Klenk, H.-D., and Choppin, P. W., 1971, Glycolipid content of vesicular stomatitis virus grown in baby hamster kidney cells, *J. Virol.* **7**, 416.

Klenk, H.-D., Caliguiri, L. A., and Choppin, P. W., 1970a, The proteins of the parainfluenza virus SV5. II. The carbohydrate content and glycoproteins of the virion, *Virology* **42**, 473.

Klenk, H.-D., Compans, R. W., and Choppin, P. W., 1970b, An electron microscopic study of the presence or absence of neuraminic acid in enveloped viruses, *Virology* **42**, 1158.

Klenk, H.-D., Rott, R., and Becht, H., 1972, On the structure of the influenza virus envelope, *Virology* **47**, 579.

Kohn, A., 1965, Polykaryocytosis induced by Newcastle disease virus in monolayers of animal cells, *Virology* **26**, 228.

Kolakofsky, D., and Bruschi, A., 1973, Molecular weight determination of Sendai RNA by dimethyl sulfoxide gradient sedimentation, *J. Virol.* **11**, 615.

Kolakofsky, D., Boy de la Tour, E., and Delius, H., 1974, Molecular weight determination of Sendai and Newcastle disease virus RNA, *J. Virol.* **13**, 261.

Lamb, R. A., and Mahy, B. W. J., 1974, Characterization of the polypeptides and RNA of Sendai virus, *in* "Negative Strand Viruses" (R. D. Barry and B. W. J. Mahy, eds.), Academic Press, London, in press.

Lancz, G. J., and Johnson, T. C., 1971, Inhibition of protein synthesis in Newcastle disease virus infected L cells, *Proc. Soc. Exp. Biol. Med.* **137**, 1405.

Landsberger, F. R., Lenard, J., Paxton, J., and Compans, R. W., 1971, Spin-label ESR study of the lipid-containing membrane of influenza virus, *Proc. Natl. Acad. Sci. USA* **68**, 2579.

Landsberger, F. R., Compans, R. W., Choppin, P. W., and Lenard, J., 1973, Organization of the lipid phase in viral membranes. Effects of independent variation of the lipid and the protein composition. *Biochemistry* **12**, 4498.

Lazarowitz, S. G., Compans, R. W., and Choppin, P. W., 1971, Influenza virus structural and non-structural proteins in infected cells and their plasma membranes, *Virology* **46**, 830.

Lenard, J., and Compans, R. W., 1974, The membrane structure of lipid-containing viruses, *Biochem. Biophys. Acta* **344**, 51.

Lerner, M. P., Consigli, R. A., Khare, G. P., and Eisenstark, A., 1969, Sequence of events after infection of chicken embryo cells with radioactively labeled Newcastle disease virus, *Am. J. Vet. Res.* **30**, 853.

Levens, J. H., and Enders, J. F., 1945, The hemoagglutinative properties of amniotic fluid from embryonated eggs infected with mumps virus, *Science (Wash., D.C.)* **102**, 117.

Lomniczi, B., Meager, A., and Burke, D. C., 1971, Virus RNA and protein synthesis in cells infected with different strains of Newcastle disease virus, *J. Gen. Virol.* **13**, 111.

Lonberg-Holm, K., and Philipson, L., 1974, Early interactions between animal viruses and cells, *Progr. Med. Virol.*, in press.

McClelland, L., and Hare, R., 1941, The adsorption of influenza virus by red cells and a new *in vitro* method of measuring antibodies for influenza virus, *Can. Pub. Health J.* **32**, 530.

McConnell, H. M., and McFarland, B. L., 1972, The flexibility gradient in biological membranes, *Ann. N.Y. Acad. Sci.* **195**, 207.

McSharry, J. J., and Wagner, R. R., 1971, Carbohydrate composition of vesicular stomatitis virus, *J. Virol.* **7**, 412.

McSharry, J. J., Compans, R. W., and Choppin, P. W., 1971, Proteins of vesicular stomatitis virus (VSV) and of phenotypically-mixed VSV–SV5 virions, *J. Virol.* **8,** 722.

McSharry, J. J., Compans, R. W., Lackland, H., and Choppin, P. W., 1972, Isolation of viral membrane proteins. *Abstr. Am. Soc. Microbiol.,* 215.

Maeno, K., Yoshii, S., Nogata, I., and Matsumoto, T., 1966, Growth of Newcastle disease virus in a HVJ carrier culture of HeLa cells, *Virology* **29,** 255.

Maeno, K., Yoshida, T., Iinuma, M., Nagai, Y., Matsumoto, T., and Asai, J., 1970, Isolation of hemagglutinin and neuraminidase subunits of hemagglutinating virus of Japan, *J. Virol.* **6,** 492.

Mahy, B. W. J., Hutchinson, J. E., and Barry, R. D., 1970, Ribonucleic acid polymerase induced in cells infected with Sendai virus, *J. Virol.* **5,** 663.

Mandel, T. E., 1972, Intramembraneous marker in T lymphocytes, *Nat. New Biol.* **239,** 112.

Marcus, P. I., 1962, Dynamics of surface modification in myxovirus-infected cells, *Cold Spring Harbor Symp. Quant. Biol.* **27,** 351.

Marcus, P. I., and Carver, D. H., 1967, Intrinsic interference: A new type of viral interference, *J. Virol.* **1,** 334.

Marcus, P. I., and Puck, T. T., 1958, Host-cell interaction of animal viruses. I. Titration of cell-killing by viruses, *Virology* **6,** 405.

Marcus, P. I., and Zuckerbraun, H. L., 1970, Viral polymerase proteins as antiviral agents (intrinsic interference), *Ann. N.Y. Acad. Sci.* **173,** 185.

Marshall, S., and Gillespie, D., 1972, Poly U tracts absent from viral RNA, *Nat. New Biol.* **240,** 43.

Martin, S. J., and ter Meulen, V. eds., 1974, Workshop on measles virus, *Med. Microbiol. Immunol.,* in press.

Marx, P. A., Portner, A., and Kingsbury, D. W., 1974, Sendai virion transcriptase complex: Polypeptide composition and inhibition by virion envelope proteins, *J. Virol.* **13,** 298.

Matsumoto, T., and Maeno, K., 1962, A host-induced modification of hemagglutinating virus of Japan (HVJ, Sendai virus) in its hemolytic and cytopathic activity, *Virology* **17,** 563.

Meager, A., and Burke, D. C., 1973, Studies on the structural basis of the RNA polymerase activity of Newcastle disease virus, *J. Gen. Virol.* **18,** 305.

Meier-Ewert, H., and Compans, R. W., 1974, Time course of synthesis and assembly of influenza virus proteins, *J. Virol.,* in press.

Meiselman, N., Kohn, A., and Danon, D., 1967, Electron microscopic study of penetration of Newcastle disease virus into cells leading to formation of polykaryocytes, *J. Cell Sci.* **2,** 71.

Melnick, J. L., 1973, Classification and nomenclature of viruses, *Progr. Med. Virol.* **15,** 380.

Moore, N. F., Lomniczi, B., and Burke, D. C., 1972, The effect of infection with different strains of Newcastle disease virus on cellular RNA and protein synthesis, *J. Gen. Virol.* **14,** 99.

Moore, N., Cheyne, I. M., and Burke, D. C., 1974, The structural polypeptides of Newcastle disease virus, *in* "Negative Strand Viruses" (R.D. Barry and B. W. J. Mahy, eds.), Academic Press, London, in press.

Morgan, C., and Howe, C., 1968, Structure and development of viruses as observed in the electron microscope. IX. Entry of parainfluenza I (Sendai) virus, *J. Virol.* **2,** 1122.

Mountcastle, W. E., Compans, R. W., Caliguiri, L. A., and Choppin, P. W., 1970, Nucleocapsid protein subunits of simian virus 5, Newcastle disease virus, and Sendai virus, *J. Virol.* **6,** 677.

Mountcastle, W. E., Compans, R. W., and Choppin, P. W., 1971, Proteins and glycoproteins of paramyxoviruses: A comparison of simian virus 5, Newcastle disease virus, and Sendai virus, *J. Virol.* **7,** 47.

Mountcastle, W. E., Compans, R. W., Lackland, H., and Choppin, P. W., 1974, Proteolytic cleavage of subunits of the nucleocapsid of the paramyxovirus SV5, *J. Virol.,* in press.

Mussgay, M., and Weibel, J., 1962, Early stages of infection with Newcastle disease virus as revealed by electron microscopy, *Virology* **16,** 506.

Nakai, T., and Shand, F. I., and Howatson, A. F., 1969, Development of measles virus *in vitro, Virology* **38,** 50.

Nakajima, H., and Obara, J., 1967, Physicochemical studies of Newcastle disease virus. III. The content of virus nucleic acid and its sedimentation pattern, *Arch. Ges. Virusforsch.* **20,** 287.

Neurath, A. R., 1965, Study on the adenosine diphosphatase (adenosine triphosphatase) associated with Sendai virus, *Acta Virol.* **9,** 313.

Neurath, A. R., and Sokol, F., 1963, Association of myxoviruses with an adenosine diphosphatase/adenosine triphosphatase/as revealed by chromatography on DEAE-cellulose and by density gradient centrifugation, *Z. Naturforsch.* **18b,** 1050.

Nicolson, G. L., 1974, The interaction of lectins with animal cell surfaces, *Int. Rev. Cytol.,* in press.

Norrby, E., 1962, Hemagglutination by measles virus. II. Properties of the hemagglutinin and of the receptors on the erythrocytes, *Arch. Ges. Virusforsch.* **12,** 164.

Norrby, E., 1964, Separation of measles virus components by equilibrium centrifugation in CsCl gradients, *Arch. Ges. Virusforsch.* **14,** 306.

Norrby, E., and Gollmar, Y., 1972, Appearance and persistence of antibodies against different virus components after regular measles infections, *Infect. Immun.* **6,** 240.

Norrby, E., and Hammarskjöld, B., 1972, Structural components of measles virus, *Microbios.* **5,** 17.

Norrby, E., Marusyk, H., and Orvell, C., 1970, Morphogenesis of respiratory syncytial virus in a green monkey kidney cell line (vero), *J. Virol.* **6,** 237.

Northrop, R. L., 1969, Effect of puromycin and actinomycin D on a persistent mumps virus infection *in vitro, J. Virol.* **4,** 133.

Okada, Y., 1958, The fusion of Ehrlich's tumor cells caused by HVJ virus in vitro, *Bikens J.* **1,** 103.

Okada, Y., 1969, Factors in fusion of cells by HVJ, *Curr. Top. Microbiol. Immunol.* **48,** 102.

Okada, Y., 1972, Fusion of cells by HVJ (Sendai Virus) *in* "Membrane Research" (C. F. Fox, ed.), p. 371, Academic Press, New York.

Parfanovich M., Hammarskjöld, B., and Norrby, E., 1971, Synthesis of virus-specific variants of measles virus, *Arch. Ges. Virusforsch.* **35,** 38.

Peries, J. R., and Chany, C., 1960, Activité hémagglutinante et hémolytique du virus morbilleux, *C. R. Hebd. Seances Acad. Sci. Ser. D Sci. Nat.* **251,** 820.

Philipson, L., 1963, Early interaction of animal viruses and cells *in* "Progress in Medical Virology" (J. L. Melnick, ed.), Vol. 5, p. 43, Karger, New York.

Pierce, J. S., and Haywood, A. M., 1973, Thermal inactivation of Newcastle disease virus, *J. Virol.* **11,** 168.

Portner, A., and Kingsbury, D. W., 1970, Complementary RNAs in paramyxovirions and paramyxovirus-infected cells, *Nature (Lond.)* **228**, 1196.

Portner, A., and Kingsbury, D. W., 1971, Homologous interference by incomplete Sendai virus particles: Changes in virus-specific RNA synthesis, *J. Virol.* **8**,388.

Portner, A., and Kingsbury, D. W., 1972, Identification of transcriptive and replicative intermediates in Sendai virus-infected cells, *Virology* **47**, 711.

Portner, A., Marx, P. A., and Kingsbury, D. W., 1974, Isolation and characterization of Sendai virus temperature-sensitive mutants, *J. Virol.* **13**, 298.

Poste, G., 1970, Virus-induced polykaryocytosis and the mechanism of cell fusion, *Adv. Virus Res.* **16**, 303.

Poste, G., 1971, The role lysosomes in virus-induced cell fusion. 2. Modification of the cell surface, *Microbios.* **3**, 105.

Poste, G., 1972*a*, Mechanisms of virus-induced cell fusion, *Int. Rev. Cytol.* **33**, 157.

Poste, G., 1972*b*, Changes in susceptibility of normal cells to agglutination by plant lectins following modification of cell coat materials, *Exp. Cell Res.* **73**, 319.

Poste, G., and Reeve, P., 1972, Agglutination of normal cells by plant lectins following infection with nononcogenic viruses, *Nat. New Biol.* **237**, 113.

Preble, O. T., and Youngner, J. S., 1972, Temperature-sensitive mutants isolated from L cells persistently infected with Newcastle disease virus, *J. Virol.* **9**, 200.

Preble, O. T., and Youngner, J. S., 1973*a*, Temperature-sensitive defect of mutants isolated from L cells persistently infected with Newcastle disease virus, *J. Virol.* **12**, 472.

Preble, O. T., and Youngner, J. S., 1973*b*, Selection of temperature-sensitive mutants during persistent infection: Role in maintenance of persistent Newcastle disease virus infections of L cells, *J. Virol.* **12**, 481.

Pridgen, C., and Kingsbury, D. W., 1972, Adenylated sequences in Sendai virus transcripts from infected cells, *J. Virol.* **10**, 314.

Prineas, J., 1972, Paramyxovirus-like particles associated with acute demyelination in chronic relapsing multiple sclerosis, *Science (Wash., D.C.)* **178**, 760.

Quigley, J. P., Rifkin, D. B., and Reich, E., 1971, Phospholipid composition of Rous sarcoma virus, host cell membranes, and other enveloped viruses, *Virology* **46**, 106.

Reeve, P., and Waterson, A. P., 1970, The growth cycle of avirulent strains of Newcastle disease virus, *Microbios.* **2**, 5.

Reeve, P., Alexander, D. J., Pope, G., and Poste, G., 1971, Studies on the cytopathic effects of Newcastle disease virus: Metabolic requirements, *J. Gen. Virol.* **11**, 25.

Richman, D. D., Wong, K. T., Robinson, W. S., and Merigan, T. C., 1970, Effect of interferon on the replication of Sendai virus, *J. Gen. Virol.* **9**, 141.

Robinson, W. S., 1970, Self-annealing of subgroup 2 myxovirus RNAs, *Nature (Lond.)* **225**, 944.

Robinson, W. S., 1971*a*, Intracellular structures involved in Sendai virus replication, *Virology* **43**, 90.

Robinson, W. S., 1971*b*, Sendai virus RNA synthesis and nucleocapsid formation in the presence of cycloheximide, *Virology* **44**, 494.

Robinson, W. S., 1971*c*, Ribonucleic acid polymerase activity in Sendai virions and nucleocapsid, *J. Virol.* **8**, 81.

Robinson, W. S., and Duesberg, P. H., 1968, The large RNA viruses. A. The myxoviruses, *in* "Molecular Basis of Virology" (H. Fraenkel-Conrat, ed.), p. 255, Reinhold, New York.

Roizman, B., 1962, Polykaryocytosis, *Cold Spring Harbor Symp. Quant. Biol.* **27**, 327.

Rosen, L., 1961, Hemagglutination and hemagglutination-inhibition with measles virus, *Virology* **13**, 139.

Rosenbergová, M., and Rosenberg, M., 1964, Synthesis of ribonucleic acid and Newcastle disease virus in ultraviolet-irradiated chick embryo cells, *Acta Virol.* **8**, 547.

Rott, R., and Schäfer, W., 1961, Fine structure of subunits isolated from Newcastle disease virus (NDV), *Virology* **14**, 298.

Rott, R., and Scholtissek, C., 1964, Einfluss von Actinomycin auf die Vermehrung von Myxoviren, *Z. Naturforsch.* **19b**, 316.

Rott, R., Reda, I. M., and Schäfer, W., 1962, Isolation and characterization of hemagglutinating noninfectious particles produced during multiplication of Newcastle disease virus (NDV), *Virology* **16**, 207.

Rott, R., Drzeniek, R., Saber, M. S., and Reichert, E., 1966, Blood group substances, Forssman and mononucleosis antigens in lipid-containing RNA viruses, *Arch. Ges. Virusforsch.* **19**, 273.

Rott, R., Becht, H., Klenk, H.-D., and Scholtissek, C., 1972, Interactions of concanavalin A with the membrane of influenza virus-infected cells and with the envelope components of the virus particle, *Z. Naturforsch.* **27b**, 227.

Roux, L., and Kolakofsky, D., 1974, Protein kinase associated with Sendai virions, *J. Virol.* **13**, 545.

Ruddle, F. H., 1974, Somatic cell genetic approaches to problems of mammalian cell regulation, *in* "The Harvey Lectures, 1973–1974," Academic Press, New York.

Rustigian, R., 1966a, Persistent infection of cells in culture by measles virus. I. Development and characteristics of HeLa sublines persistently infected with complete virus, *J. Bacteriol.* **92**, 1792.

Rustigian, R., 1966b, Persistent infection of cells in culture by measles virus. II. Effect of measles antibody on persistently infected HeLa sublines and recovery of a HeLa clonal line persistently infected with incomplete virus, *J. Bacteriol.*, **92**, 1805.

Sagik, B. P., and Levine, S., 1957, The interaction of Newcastle disease virus (NDV) with chicken erythrocytes: Attachment, elution, and hemolysis, *Virology* **3**, 401.

Samson, A. C. R., and Fox, C. F., 1973, Precursor protein for Newcastle disease virus, *J. Virol.* **12**, 579.

Sato, K., Righthand, F., and Karzon, D. T., 1971, Effect of host cell on distribution of a lysosomal enzyme during virus infection, *J. Virol.* **7**, 467.

Schäfer, W., Schramm, G., and Traub, E., 1949, Untersuchungen über das Virus der atypischen Geflügelpest, *Z. Naturforsch.* **4b**, 157.

Scheid, A., and Choppin, P. W., 1971, Synthesis of sphingolipids in bovine kidney (MDBK) cells infected with the parainfluenza virus SV5, *Abstr. Am. Soc. Microbiol.*, 202.

Scheid, A., and Choppin, P. W., 1973, Isolation and purification of the envelope proteins of Newcastle disease virus, *J. Virol.* **11**, 263.

Scheid, A., and Choppin, P. W., 1974a, Identification of biological activities of paramyxovirus glycoproteins. Activation of cell fusion, hemolysis, and infectivity by proteolytic cleavage of an inactive precursor protein of Sendai virus, *Virology* **56**, 475.

Scheid, A., and Choppin, P. W., 1974b, Isolation of paramyxovirus glycoproteins and identification of their biological properties, *in* "Negative Strand Viruses" (R. D. Barry and B. W. J. Mahy, eds.), Academic Press, London, in press.

Scheid, A., Caliguiri, L. A., Compans, R. W., and Choppin, P. W., 1972, Isolation of paramyxovirus glycoproteins. Association of both hemagglutinating and neuraminidase activities with the larger SV5 glycoprotein, *Virology* **50**, 640.

Schluederberg, A., 1971, Measles virus RNA, *Biochem. Biophys. Res. Commun.* **42**, 1012.

Schluederberg, A., Williams, C. A., and Black, F. L., 1972, Inhibition of measles virus replication and RNA synthesis by actinomycin D, *Biochem. Biophys. Res. Commun.* **48**, 657.

Scholtissek, C., and Rott, R., 1965, Metabolic changes in chick fibroblasts after infection with Newcastle disease virus, *Nature (Lond.)* **206**, 729.

Scholtissek, C., and Rott, R., 1969, Ribonucleic acid nucleotidyl transferase induced in chick fibroblasts after infection with Newcastle disease virus, *J. Gen. Virol.* **4**, 565.

Scholtissek, C., Rott, R., Hau, G., and Kaluza, G., 1974, Inhibition of the multiplication of vesicular stomatitis and Newcastle disease virus by 2-deoxy-D-glucose, *J. Virol.* **13**, 1186.

Sever, J. L., and Zeman, W., eds., 1968, Conference on measles virus and subacute sclerosing panencephalitis, *Neurology* **18**, No. 1, part 2, pp. 1–200.

Shibuta, H., Yamaura, K., Hirano, K., and Matumoto, M., 1971, Enhancement of ^{32}P incorporation into phospholipids in cultured cells by Sendai virus of parainfluenza type 1, *Jap. J. Microbiol.* **15**, 185.

Silverstein, S. C., and Marcus, P. I., 1964, Early studies of NDV–HeLa Cell interaction: An electron microscopic study, *Virology* **23**, 370.

Simon, E. H., 1961, Evidence for the nonparticipation of DNA in viral RNA synthesis, *Virology* **13**, 105.

Simon, E. H., 1972, The distribution and significance of multiploid virus particles, *Progr. Med. Virol.* **14**, 36.

Skehel, J. J., 1972, Polypeptide synthesis in influenza virus-infected cells, *Virology* **49**, 23.

Sokol, F., Neurath, A. R., and Vilcek, J., 1964, Formation of incomplete Sendai virus in embryonated eggs, *Acta Virol.* **8**, 59.

Sokol, F., Skačianska, E., and Pivec, L., 1966, Some properties of Newcastle disease virus ribonucleic acid, *Acta Virol.* **10**, 291.

Stone, H. O., and Kingsbury, D. W., 1973, Stimulation of Sendai virion transcriptase by polyanions, *J. Virol.* **11**, 243.

Stone, H. O., Portner, A., and Kingsbury, D. W., 1971, Ribonucleic acid transcriptases in Sendai virions and infected cells, *J. Virol.* **8**, 174.

Stone, H. O., Kingsbury, D. W., and Darlington, R. W., 1972, Sendai virus-induced transcriptase from infected cells: Polypeptides in the transcriptive complex, *J. Virol.* **10**, 1037.

Strauss, J. H., Kelly, R. B., and Sinsheimer, R. L., 1968, Denaturation of RNA with dimethyl sulfoxide, *Biopolymers* **6**, 793.

Tadokoro, J., 1958a, Modified virus particles in undiluted passages of HVJ. I. The production of modified particles, *Bikens J.* **1**, 111.

Tadokoro, J., 1958b, Modified virus particles in undiluted passages of HVJ. II. The characteristics of modified particles, *Bikens J.* **1**, 118.

Taylor, R. B., Duffus, P. H., Raff, M. C., and dePetris, S., 1971, Redistribution and pinocytosis of lymphocyte surface immunoglobulin molecules induced by anti-immunoglobulin antibody, *Nat. New Biol.* **233**, 225.

ter Meulen, V., Koprowski, H., Iwasaki, Y., Käckell, Y. M., and Müller, D., 1972a, Fusion of cultured multiple sclerosis brain cells with indicator cells: Presence of nucleocapsids and virions and isolation of parainfluenza type virus, *Lancet* **II**, 1.

ter Meulen, V., Katz, M., and Müller, D., 1972b, Subacute sclerosing panencephalitis: A review, *Curr. Top. Microbiol. Immunol.* **57**, 1.

Thacore, H., and Youngner, J. S., 1969, Cells persistently infected with Newcastle disease virus. I. Properties of mutants isolated from persistently infected L cells, *Virology* **4**, 244.

Thacore, H., and Youngner, J. S., 1970, Cells persistently infected with Newcastle disease virus. II. Ribonucleic acid and protein synthesis in cells infected with mutants isolated from persistently infected cells, *J. Virol.* **6**, 42.

Tiffany, J. M., and Blough, H. A., 1969a, Myxovirus envelope proteins: A directing influence on the fatty acids of membrane lipids, *Science (Wash., D.C.)* **163**, 573.

Tiffany, J. M., and Blough, H. A., 1969b, Fatty acid composition of three strains of Newcastle disease virus, *Virology* **37**, 492.

Tiffany, J. M., and Blough, H. A., 1970, The interaction of fetuin with phosphatidylcholine monolayers. Characterization of a lipoprotein membrane system suitable for the attachment of myxoviruses, *Biochem. J.* **117**, 377.

Tozawa, H., Watanabe, M., and Ishida, N., 1973, Structural components of Sendai virus. Serological and physicochemical characterization of hemagglutinin subunit associated with neuraminidase activity, *Virology* **55**, 242.

Traver, M. I., Northrop, R. L., and Walker, D. L., 1960, Site of intracellular antigen production by myxo-viruses, *Proc. Soc. Exp. Biol. Med.* **104**, 268.

Tsipis, J. E., and Bratt, M. A., 1974, Temperature sensitive mutants of Newcastle disease virus, *in* "Negative Strand Viruses" (R. D. Barry and B. W. J. Mahy, eds.), Academic Press, London, in press.

Virchow, R., 1858, Reizung und Reizbarkeit, *Virchow's Arch.* **14**, 1.

Walder, R., 1971, Electron microscopic evidence of Nariva virus structure, *J. Gen. Virol.* **11**, 123.

Walker, D. L., 1968, Persistent viral infection in cell cultures, *in* "Medical and Applied Virology" (M. Sanders, and E. H. Lennette, eds.), pp. 99–110, Warren H. Green, Inc., St. Louis.

Walker, D. L., and Hinze, H. C., 1962, A carrier state of mumps virus in human conjunctive cells. I. General characteristics, *J. Exp. Med.* **116**, 739.

Waters, D. J., Hersh, R. T., and Bussell, R. H., 1972, Isolation and characterization of measles nucleocapsid from infected cells, *Virology* **48**, 278.

Waterson, A. P., 1962, Two kinds of myxovirus, *Nature (Lond.)* **193**, 1163.

Waterson, A. P., 1964, Measles virus, *Arch. Ges. Virusforsch.* **16**, 57.

Wecker, E., 1957, Die Verteilung von ^{32}P im Virus der Klassischen Geflügelpest bei verschiedenen Markierungsverfahren, *Z. Naturforsch.* **12b**, 208.

Weiss, S. R., and Bratt, M. A., 1974, Polyadenylate sequences on Newcastle disease virus messenger RNA synthesized *in vivo* and *in vitro, J. Virol.,* **13**, 1220.

Wheelock, E. F., 1962, The role of protein synthesis in the eclipse period of Newcastle disease virus multiplication in HeLa cells as studied with puromycin, *Proc. Natl. Acad. Sci. USA* **48**, 1358.

Wheelock, E. F., 1963, Intracellular site of Newcastle virus nucleic acid synthesis, *Proc. Soc. Exp. Biol. Med.* **114**, 56.

Wheelock, E. F., and Tamm, I., 1959, Mitosis and division in HeLa cells infected with influenza or Newcastle disease virus, *Virology* **8**, 532.

Wheelock, E. F., and Tamm, I., 1961a, Enumeration of cell-infecting particles of Newcastle disease virus by the fluorescent antibody technique, *J. Exp. Med.* **113**, 301.

Wheelock, E. F., and Tamm, I., 1961b, Biochemical basis for alterations in structure and function of HeLa cells infected with Newcastle disease virus, *J. Exp. Med.* **114,** 617.

Wilcox, W. C., 1959*a*, Quantitative aspects of an *in vitro* virus-induced toxic reaction. I. General aspects of the reaction of Newcastle disease virus with L cells, *Virology* **9,** 30.

Wilcox, W. C., 1959*b*, Quantitative aspects of an *in vitro* virus-induced toxic reaction. II. The role of autointerference in the production of cell populations resistant to the cytotoxic effect of Newcastle disease virus, *Virology* **9, 45.**

Wilson, D. E., 1968, Inhibition of host-cell protein nd ribonucleic acid synthesis by Newcastle disease virus, *J. Virol.* **2, 1.**

Wilson, D. E., and Lo Gerfo, P., 1964, Inhibition of ribonucleic acid synthesis in Newcastle disease virus-infected cells by puromycin and 6-azauridine, *J. Bacteriol.* **88,** 1550.

Winston, S. H., Rustigian, R., and Bratt, M. A., 1973, Persistent infection of cells in culture by measles virus. III. Comparison of virus-specific RNA synthesized in primary and persistent infection in HeLa cells, *J. Virol.* **11,** 926.

Yahara, I., and Edelman, G. M., 1972, Restriction of the mobility of lymphocyte immunoglobulin receptors by concanavalin A, *Proc. Natl. Acad. Sci. USA* **69,** 608.

Young, N. P., and Ash, R. J., 1970, Polykaryocyte induction by Newcastle disease virus propagated on different hosts, *J. Gen. Virol.* **7,** 81.

Youngner, J. S., Scott, A. W., Hallum, J. V., and Stinebring, W. R., 1966, Interferon production by inactivated Newcastle disease virus in cell cultures and in mice, *J. Bacteriol.* **92,** 862.

Zakstelskaya, L. V., Almeida, J. D., and Bradstreet, C. M. P., 1967, The morphological characterization of respiratory syncytial virus by a simple electron microscopy technique, *Acta Virol. (Prague)* **11,** 420.

CHAPTER 3

Reproduction of Myxoviruses

Richard W. Compans and Purnell W. Choppin

The Rockefeller University
New York, New York 10021

1. INTRODUCTION

The myxovirus group consists of the influenza viruses of man and animals. The designation was originally suggested (Andrewes *et al.*, 1955) for a group of viruses which exhibited affinity for certain mucoid substances, and included mumps and Newcastle disease viruses (NDV) in addition to influenza viruses. It was recognized subsequently that the former two viruses should be separated into a distinct group because of numerous differences in structure and replication between them and the influenza viruses (Waterson, 1962), and the term paramyxovirus has been adopted for the group which includes these agents. Thus, the myxovirus group (sometimes referred to as orthomyxoviruses; Melnick, 1973) as presently constituted contains only the influenza viruses. As described in sect. 2, among the polypeptides of the influenza virion are two distinct surface polypeptides with hemagglutinin and neuraminidase activities and an internal ribonucleoprotein (RNP). The antigenicity of these polypeptides has provided a basis for the classification of influenza viruses into types, subtypes, and strains. Table 1 indicates the system of classification and lists some of the strains in common use.

Three completely unrelated serological types of influenza virus have been identified, designated A, B, and C. The influenza A viruses are most widespread in nature; they are found in man and a variety of animals, including horses, swine, and birds. Major changes in anti-

TABLE 1

Classification of Influenza Viruses

Species	Type, ribonucleoprotein	Hemagglutinin subtype	Neuraminidase subtype	Common laboratory strains[a]
Human	A	H0	N1	WSN, PR8, BEL
		H1	N1	FM1
		H2	N2	RI/5[+], Jap/305
		H3	N2	Hong Kong 68
	B			Lee
	C			1233
Swine	A	$H_{sw}1$	N1	15
Equine	A	$H_{eq}1$	$N_{eq}1$	
		$H_{eq}2$	$N_{eq}2$	
Avian	A	$H_{av}1$	$N_{eq}1$, $N_{av}3$	Fowl plague
		$H_{av}2$	$N_{eq}1$	
		$H_{av}3$	$N_{av}1$	
		$H_{av}4$	$N_{av}1$	
		$H_{av}5$	$N_{av}2$	
		$H_{av}6$	N2	
		$H_{av}7$	$N_{eq}2$	
		$H_{av}8$	$N_{av}4$	

[a] Prior to 1972, human influenza A strains were placed in subtypes on the basis of their hemagglutinin antigens only, i.e., A_0, A_1, and A_2. These designations have been used for the laboratory strains in the text because of their brevity. Modified from *Bull. World Health Organ.* **45**, 119.

genicity of the hemagglutinin and neuraminidase of influenza A viruses occur periodically in nature, giving rise to new strains of virus which are responsible for pandemics of influenza in man. Thus, subtypes of influenza A viruses exist with completely distinct surface antigens, although the internal nucleoprotein antigens of all type A strains are similar. Within each subtype, numerous strains have been identified with related, but distinguishable surface antigens. Types B and C, which have been isolated only in man, differ from type A viruses in the antigenicity of the internal nucleoprotein, as well as of their hemagglutinin and neuraminidase. With minor exceptions, the various influenza virus strains possess the same structural components, and no major differences in the mechanisms involved in the replication of different strains have been found thus far. Therefore, strain designations are not indicated in this text unless it is thought that differences between strains in a particular aspect of structure or replication are of significance.

2. THE INFLUENZA VIRION

2.1. Morphology

2.1.1. Spherical and Filamentous Virions

Early studies of the structure of influenza virus showed that the majority of the particles are spherical with an average diameter of about 80–100 nm (Elford *et al.*, 1936; Taylor *et al.*, 1943). The application of negative staining demonstrated that the internal component of the virus is helical, and that the surface of the particle is covered with a prominent layer of closely spaced 10-nm projections or spikes (Horne *et al.*, 1960; Hoyle *et al.*, 1961). A typical population of spherical virions is shown in Fig. 1; there is some heterogeneity in particle size, but not the more marked pleiomorphism observed with paramyxoviruses. In shadowed, whole-mount preparations of the Jap/305 strain of influenza A virus, a slightly elongated or bacillary shape is noted, whereas other influenza A_2 strains appear more nearly spherical (Choppin *et al.*, 1960). When seen in thin section, newly formed influenza virions often appear to be elongated, rather than per-

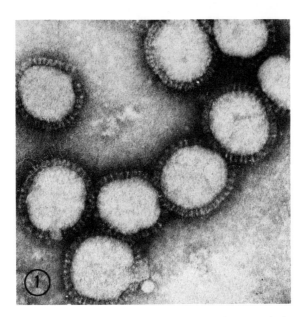

Fig. 1.   Influenza virions (A_0/WSN strain) negatively stained with sodium phosphotungstate. The particles have a diameter of approximately 100 nm, and are covered with spikes 10–12 nm in length. ×160,000. From Compans *et al.*, (1970*a*).

fectly spherical (Compans and Dimmock, 1969; Compans *et al.*, 1969; Bächi *et al.*, 1969). The internal component consists of electron-dense strands arranged parallel to the long axis of the particle, and the envelope consists of a complex membrane with a layer of projections on the outer surface.

In addition to particles with a roughly spherical morphology, many strains of influenza virus produce long filamentous virions (Fig. 2). The diameter of such filaments is similar to that of the spherical particles, and particle lengths up to about 4 μm or greater have been observed. The surface structure of filaments is the same as that of spherical particles (Choppin *et al.*, 1961). The filamentous forms predominate in newly isolated virus strains (Chu *et al.*, 1949; Choppin *et al.*, 1960), and it is possible that these particles occur in human infections of the respiratory tract. With serial passage in culture, particularly in the chick embryo, conversion from filamentous to spherical morphology is observed (Choppin *et al.*, 1960). Probably for this reason, most virus strains which have been studied extensively are now found to be spherical. The specific infectivity of the filamentous particles has been reported to be higher than that of spherical virions, and the filaments have been found to contain more RNA per particle than the spheres (Ada *et al.*, 1958).

The production of filamentous particles is a genetic trait which can be exchanged in recombination experiments (Kilbourne and Murphy, 1960; Kilbourne, 1963; Choppin, 1963). Thus, recombination of spherical A_0 strains with newly isolated filamentous A_2 strains resulted in the production of spherical A_2 and highly filamentous A_0 strains (Kilbourne and Murphy, 1960). Although spontaneous conversion of the A_2 strain from a filamentous to spherical state might have occurred, the spontaneous change in the A_0 virus from a spherical to a highly filamentous form has never been detected. Thus, it was concluded that the change in morphology was a transferable genetic trait, which provided a useful marker for recombination studies. This genetically determined variation in the morphology of the virion suggests a difference in the structure, or rate of synthesis, of a protein, probably an envelope protein. Preliminary studies on spherical and filamentous virions of the same strain have not revealed differences in their overall protein composition (Choppin, unpublished observations); however, further more detailed studies are needed.

When influenza virions were examined by electron microscopy after freeze drying or freeze etching, particles with a high degree of structural regularity were observed (Nermut and Frank, 1971). Some

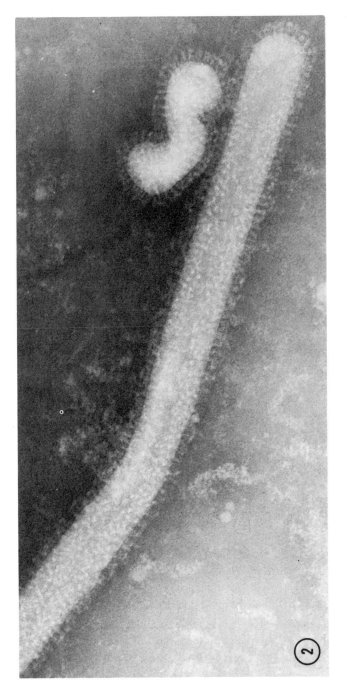

Fig. 2. Influenza virus filament (A_2/RI/4^- strain) negatively stained with sodium phosphotungstate. $\times 280,000$. From Choppin *et al.* (1961).

of the particles cast angular shadows, and it was suggested that they were icosahedral in shape. Regular hexagonal arrangements of surface projections have also been described (Archetti *et al.*, 1967; Almeida and Waterson, 1967, Nermut and Frank, 1971). It has been suggested that a shell of protein beneath the lipid layer in the viral membrane serves as a capsid in the viral envelope structure (Schulze, 1973). There are other examples of formation of icosahedral capsids as well as long tubular arrangements from the same protein subunits, thus raising the possibility that influenza virus spheres and filaments correspond to such structures. However, it should be emphasized that spherical virions in most influenza populations occur in a wide range of sizes, and there is no precedent for packing of identical subunits into icosahedral capsids in a continuum of possible sizes. In addition, it is possible that the spherical particles result from distortion of the elongated particles which are seen in fixed, sectioned material. For these reasons, true icosahedral symmetry in influenza virions seems unlikely. Further information is clearly needed to provide conclusive evidence for or against the existence of such symmetry in the viral membrane.

2.1.2. Subviral Components

The sizes and shapes of subviral components will be described briefly here, and the fine structure of these components and their interactions with each other will be discussed in detail below (Sect. 2.3).

2.1.2a. Surface Projections

In early attempts to separate influenza virus into subviral components, it was observed that treatment with ether resulted in disruption of the virus, and it was possible to isolate a hemagglutinating fraction as well as an internal RNP component (Hoyle, 1952; Schäfer and Zillig, 1954). Later, examination of the isolated hemagglutinin by negative staining revealed rosettelike structures 30–50 nm in diameter in which spikes identical to those on the intact virion were arranged radially; larger fragments of the viral envelope were also observed (Hoyle *et al.*, 1961; Choppin and Stoeckenius, 1964).

Further information on the morphology of the envelope components was obtained with certain virus strains from which it was possible to isolate envelope protein subunits which retained their biological activity after treatment with the detergent sodium dodecyl sulfate (SDS) and purification by electrophoresis on cellulose acetate (Laver and Valentine, 1969). The hemagglutinin subunits of the BEL strain appeared on examination with the electron microscope as rods approximately 14 nm in length and 4 nm in width (Fig. 3). After removal of SDS, a characteristic type of aggregation into clusters of radiating rods was observed. This suggested that one of the ends of the rodlike structure was hydrophobic, and that the spikes aggregated because of affinity of the hydrophobic ends for one another in the absence of detergents. Structures with similar morphology were isolated by Webster and Darlington (1969) using Tween 20 at alkaline pH to disrupt the virus.

Although the hemagglutinin subunits of the BEL strain isolated by detergent treatment did not possess neuraminidase activity, it was possible to isolate a neuraminidase subunit from the X-7F1 strain by SDS treatment (Laver and Valentine, 1969). Such subunits appeared to have oblong heads, approximately 8.5×5 nm, with a centrally attached fiber about 10 nm in length, which appeared to have a small knot about 4 nm in diameter at its end (Fig. 4). In the absence of detergent, the subunits aggregated by the ends of their fibers, suggesting that this was a hydrophobic end which functioned in binding to the viral membrane. In later studies, virions of the B/Lee strain were treated with trypsin, and a subunit with neuraminidase activity was released which appeared to consist of four spheres with a diameters of 4 nm in a coplanar square entry (Wrigley et al., 1973). This tetramer, when viewed end-on, appears to correspond to the 8.5- by 5-nm knob which was seen at the ends of subunits isolated by detergent treatment. Thus, the protease appears to remove the stalk by which the protease-resistant, enzymatically active tetramer is attached to the viral membrane.

These results suggest that the spikes on the surface of the influenza virions are of two morphologically distinct types, one of which is associated with neuraminidase activity, and the other with hemagglutinating activity. It should be noted that it has been possible to resolve clearly the two types of subunit on an intact virus particle. This may be due to the close packing of spikes which is generally observed.

2.1.2b. Other Envelope Components

The viral spikes are attached to a smooth-surfaced membrane. When particles are penetrated by negative stain, this membrane ap-

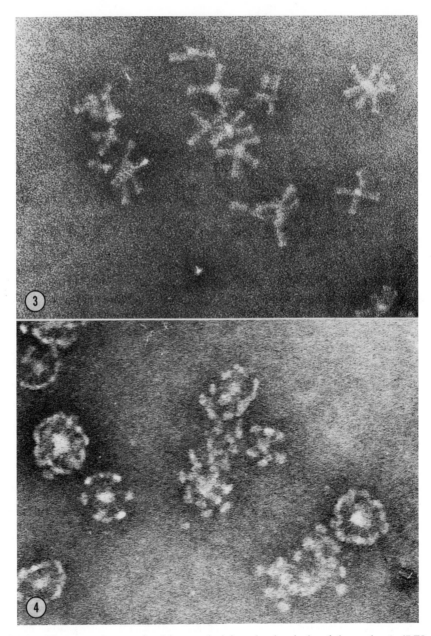

Fig. 3.   Electron micrograph of hemagglutinin subunits, isolated from the A_0/BEL strain of influenza virus, after removal of detergent by precipitation of the subunits with acetone. The rodlike subunits form characteristic rosettelike aggregates. ×400,000. From Laver and Valentine (1969), courtesy of Dr. W. G. Laver.

Fig. 4.   Electron micrograph of isolated A_2 neuraminidase subunits after removal of detergent by precipitation with acetone. ×400,000. From Laver and Valentine (1969), courtesy of Dr. W. G. Laver.

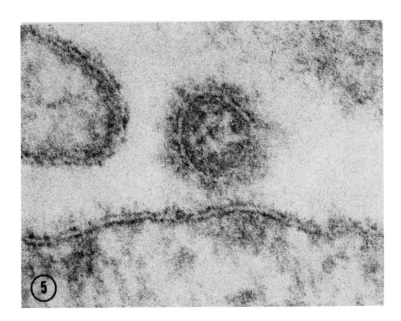

Fig. 5. Thin section of an influenza virion adjacent to the surface of a bovine kidney cell. The viral envelope contains a unit membrane similar to that of the host cell, with an additional dense layer on the inner surface and an outer fringe corresponding to the surface projections. ×320,000. From Compans and Choppin (1973).

pears as an electron-lucent layer about 10 nm in thickness. In thin section, the envelope is seen to contain a unit membrane similar in morphology to the unit membrane on the surface of host cells (Fig. 5). As described below (Sect. 3.4), virus particles are formed by a process of budding at the cell surface during which there is continuity of the unit membranes of the cell surface and viral envelope. However, an additional electron-dense layer which is not present in the normal cellular plasma membranes can be resolved on the inner surface of the viral envelope (Apostolov and Flewett, 1969; Compans and Dimmock, 1969; Bächi *et al.*, 1969). As described below, this layer appears to consist of a shell composed of the most plentiful polypeptide of the virus particle.

2.1.2c. Ribonucleoprotein (RNP) Component

The purified RNP internal components isolated from ether-disrupted influenza virus particles were found to be elongated structures of about 9–10 nm in diameter and of variable length, with a mean length of about 60 nm (Hoyle *et al.*, 1961). The appearance of the strands suggested that they possessed helical symmetry. Strands of similar appearance have been isolated from detergent-disrupted virions, although in recent publications the diameters of the strands were reported to be closer to 15 nm (Pons *et al.*, 1969; Compans *et al.*, 1972*a*). The periodic distribution of alternate deep and shallow grooves along the strands suggests that the nucleoprotein is a double helix, and the presence of loops at one end suggests that it is a strand folded back on itself (Schulze *et al.*, 1970; Compans *et al.*, 1972*a*).

2.2. Composition

There is still considerable uncertainty about the weight of the influenza virus particle, as well as its exact chemical composition. Since there is variation in the particle size of influenza virions, any estimate of particle weight necessarily applies only to a particular size of particle, and not to all virions in a population.

Based on sedimentation properties and electron microscopic measurements, influenza A viruses were estimated to have a particle weight in the range of $270-290 \times 10^6$ daltons (Lauffer and Stanley, 1944; Sharp *et al.*, 1945; Schramm, 1954). However, a much lower value of 151×10^6 was obtained for fowl plague virus based on sedimentation and diffusion coefficients (Schäfer *et al.*, 1952; Schramm, 1954). A particle weight of about 360×10^6 was obtained based on a protein determination and electron microscopic particle counts (Reimer *et al.*, 1966; Blough and Tiffany, 1973).

The approximate composition of populations of virus particles, the purity and homogeneity of which were not conclusively established, was found to be 0.8–1.0% RNA, *ca.* 70% protein, *ca.* 20% lipid, and 5–8% carbohydrate (Ada and Perry, 1954; Frommhagen *et al.*, 1959; Blough *et al.*, 1967). Since most populations of influenza virions consist largely of noninfectious particles, these data may not accurately reflect the composition of a single infectious particle. With the introduction of cell culture systems which produce a high yield of infectious virus and relatively little incomplete virus (Choppin, 1969), it would be of value to determine the chemical composition of such virions after purification by the procedures now available. Despite the uncertainty in the quantitative analysis of the composition of virus particles, there is good agreement in recent results from many laboratories concerning the qualitative analysis of viral RNA and polypeptide species.

2.2.1. RNA

The demonstration by Ada and Perry (1954) that influenza virus contained 0.8–1% RNA, and no DNA, provided one of the first demonstrations that an animal virus contained RNA. Twenty years later, there is still uncertainty about the total weight of the viral RNA genome. Early estimates based on chemical composition gave a result of about 2.0×10^6 daltons per particle (Frisch-Niggemeyer and Hoyle, 1956), whereas more recent estimates based on analysis of RNA by polyacrylamide gel electrophoresis yielded values in the range of 4–5×10^6 daltons (Skehel, 1971a; Bishop et al., 1971b; Lewandowski et al., 1971). If the virion contains the genetic information to code for all of the structural polypeptides and virus-specific non-structural polypeptides, a genome of at least 4×10^6 daltons is required. The base composition of several influenza virus strains has been summarized by Bellett (1967), and a common finding is the unusually high content of 30–34% uridine. The base composition, RNase sensitivity, and dependence of the sedimentation coefficient on salt concentration (Duesberg and Robinson, 1967) indicate that influenza viral RNA is single-stranded.

A number of biological properties of influenza virus suggested that its genome might have a segmented structure. Extremely high recombination frequencies were observed in crosses, and it was suggested that these could be explained by reassortment of a segmented genome (Burnet, 1956; Hirst, 1962). Multiplicity reactivation (Barry, 1961) and stepwise inactivation of various viral functions by a chemical agent (Scholtissek and Rott, 1964) or UV (Gandhi and Burke, 1970) were also compatible with a segmented genome in the influenza virion. These early indications have now been confirmed by numerous biochemical studies demonstrating multiple species of RNA in the virus particle.

Sucrose density gradient analysis of RNA from various strains of influenza virus indicated that the extracted species sedimented heterogeneously and that their molecular weight was much lower than that expected for the viral genome (Davies and Barry, 1966; Duesberg and Robinson, 1967; Nayak and Baluda, 1967). Subsequent analysis by polyacrylamide gel electrophoresis showed that viral RNA could be resolved into at least five species (Duesberg, 1968, Pons and Hirst, 1968b; Choppin and Pons, 1970). A representative pattern of RNA species is shown in Fig. 6. Skehel (1971a) has resolved six different species of RNA, which range in size from 3.4 to 9.8×10^5, with an ag-

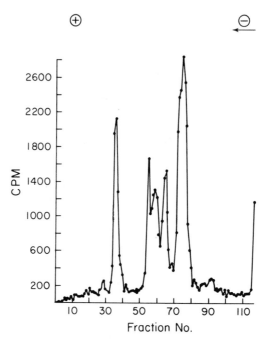

Fig. 6. Polyacrylamide gel electrophoresis of ^{3}H-uridine RNA species extracted from influenza virions grown in MDBK cells. From Choppin and Pons (1970).

gregate weight of approximately 3.9 $\times$ 10^6 daltons. Bishop *et al.* (1971*b*) estimated that a total of seven RNA species, with a total weight of 4.9 $\times$ 10^6, were present in the virion. The fact that a fairly reproducible pattern of viral RNA species is observed using a variety of extraction procedures suggests that the RNA is in separate pieces in the virion, and not fragmented during extraction. Additional support for the existence of a segmented genome within the virion has been obtained by further biochemical characterization of the viral RNA. The 5′ terminus of RNA molecules in each of three size classes obtained by velocity sedimentation has been found to be ATP (Young and Content, 1971). Uridine was found at the 3′ terminus of RNA molecules in all size classes (Lewandowski *et al.*, 1971). These termini would not have been found if cleavage of RNA by RNase had occurred. Cross-hybridization experiments, using three size classes of single-stranded RNA from virions and of double-stranded RNAs from infected cells, indicated that base sequences present in the smallest size class are absent in the larger RNA molecules (Content and Duesberg, 1971). Distinct oligonucleotide sequences have also been identified in the various size classes of viral RNAs (Horst *et al.*, 1972). Thus, all of the available data indicate that the virion RNA exists in the form of segments.

It is uncertain whether there is any specific interaction between the segments of viral RNA in the intact virion. If RNA is extracted in the presence of divalent cations an aggregate with a molecular weight of about 3×10^6 can be obtained (Agrawal and Bruening, 1966; Pons, 1967*a*); such complexes were converted to slower-sedimenting RNA species by heat treatment. Electron microscopic meaurements of viral RNA have revealed a heterogeneous size distribution with a mean length corresponding to a molecular weight of $2.5–3 \times 10^6$ (Li and Seto, 1971). After a brief treatment at pH 3, or prolonged storage, only smaller RNA molecules were observed. These observations do not provide compelling evidence for a specific aggregate formed from the segments of viral RNA. A highly ordered mechanism for incorporation of RNA into the virion appears unlikely in view of recent genetic studies described in Sect. 6.

Influenza RNPs were found to have a low level of infectivity in a plaque assay, but the isolated RNPs had a higher level of biological activity in marker-rescue experiments with a temperature-sensitive mutant (Hirst and Pons, 1972). This activity was markedly reduced by RNase treatment, which had no effect on infectivity of intact virions. However, it has generally not been possible to extract infectious RNA from influenza virions. Ada *et al.* (1959) were unable to demonstrate biological activity of RNA extracted from four different strains when assayed in the mouse brain, chick embryo, or chorioallantoic membrane; marker rescue with the extracted RNA was not observed either. Maassab (1963) observed a RNase-sensitive infective material after cold phenol extraction of chick kidney cells infected with an Asian influenza virus strain, but no biological activity when RNA was extracted from virions. The nature of the infectious component obtained from cells remains to be established. If the virion RNA polymerase which is associated with the RNP (Sect. 3.3) is essential for infectivity, it might be expected that such RNPs, but not the isolated RNA, would be infectious.

2.2.2. Proteins

The polypeptide composition of various strains of influenza virus has been analyzed by polyacrylamide gel electrophoresis in a number of laboratories. While there was some inconsistency in the total number of polypeptide species described in earlier reports, recent results are in good agreement (Haslam *et al.*, 1970; Compans *et al.*, 1970*a*; Schulze, 1970; Skehel and Schild, 1971; Lazarowitz *et al.*, 1971, 1973*a*; Klenk *et al.*, 1972*a*). A typical profile of virus doubly labeled with amino acid and carbohydrate precursors is shown in Fig. 7. Seven polypeptide species are detected, four of which are labeled with the carbohydrate precursor fucose, indicating that these are glycoproteins. Designations for the various viral polypeptides, based on their functions, have been proposed (Kilbourne *et al.*, 1972) and are indicated in Fig. 7. The function and exact location of the highest-molecular-weight polypeptide, P, has not been established; however, it is an internal component of the virion (Compans *et al.*, 1970*a*; Schulze, 1970; Klenk *et al.*, 1972*a*). In some systems, two such polypeptides (P_1, P_2) have been resolved (Skehel and Schild, 1971; Skehel, 1972; Bishop *et al.*, 1972). The largest glycoprotein (HA) possesses hemagglutinating activity. It is synthesized as a single primary gene product but may be cleaved proteolytically into two polypeptides, designated HA_1 and Ha_2 (Lazarowitz *et al.*, 1971, 1973*a,b*; Rifkin *et al.*, 1972; Klenk *et al.*, 1972*b*; Skehel, 1972; Stanley *et al.*, 1973). The extent of this cleavage depends on the host cell, the virus strain, and the presence or absence of serum plasminogen in the medium. The biological

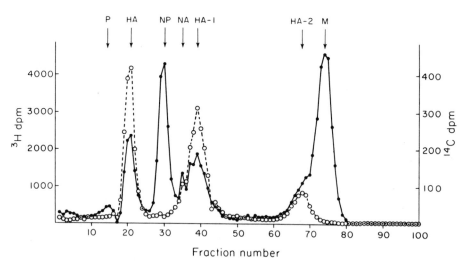

Fig. 7. Polyacrylamide gel electrophoresis of influenza virus polypeptides (WSN strain) double-labeled with ^{3}H-fucose and ^{14}C-amino acid mixture. (●———●) ^{14}C dpm, (O----O) ^{3}H dpm. The designations of the polypeptides are those proposed at Influenza Workshop I (Kilbourne *et al.*, 1972), see text for detailed description. From Compans *et al.* (1970*a*).

TABLE 2

Polypeptide Composition of Influenza Virions[a]

Designation	Mol. wt.	Total protein, %	Approximate number of molecules/virion[b]
P_1, P_2	81,000–94,000	1.5–2.7	30–60
HA	75,000–80,000	0–24	640–930
NP	~60,000	17–26	500–940
NA	~55,000	3.1–6.9	110–240
HA_1	49,000–58,000	0–21	
HA_2	25,000–30,000	0–12	
M	25,000–27,000	33–46	2500–3120

[a] The values represent the ranges obtained in studies by Compans et al. (1970a), Schulze (1970), Skehel and Schild (1971), and Lazarowitz et al. (1973a, b). The great variation in percent of HA reflects differences in the extent of cleavage to HA_1 and HA_2.

[b] The estimate listed for HA represents the sum of uncleaved HA molecules and HA_1 + HA_2 complexes. The estimates are based on a total protein content of 2.0×10^8 daltons per particle.

activity of the hemagglutinin is not affected by the cleavage. The cleavage products HA_1 and HA_2 are linked by disulfide bonds (Laver, 1971). The NP polypeptide is the subunit of the internal RNP component (Pons et al., 1969; Joss et al., 1969). The polypeptide designated NA, which contains carbohydrate, is the subunit of the viral neuraminidase (Webster, 1970; Gregoriades, 1972; Lazdins et al., 1972). The smallest polypeptide, M, which is present in the virion in largest amount, is thought to be associated with the internal surface of the lipid layer in the viral membrane (Compans et al., 1970a; Schulze, 1970, 1972; Klenk et al., 1972a).

Table 2 summarizes the molecular weights of the viral polypeptides, and the percent and estimated number of molecules of each in the virion. These values are only approximations for a number of reasons: The molecular weights of the glycoproteins are uncertain because it is not known how the presence of carbohydrate affects electrophoretic mobilities. Exact values for the number of polypeptide molecules in the virion requires knowledge of the exact total molecular weight and protein content of the virion, data which are not available. Furthermore, any estimate applies only to a specific particle size, whereas, in fact, virus particles are heterogeneous in size.

While the nonglycosylated viral polypeptides are of constant molecular weight in various influenza A viruses grown in different host cells, there is variation in the electrophoretic mobility of the glycoproteins. This may be due in part to the fact that the glycoproteins are the strain-specific antigens. Thus, antigenic differences between various influenza A virus strains are a result of differences in the amino acid sequences of the viral glycoproteins (Webster and Laver, 1971), and some variation in sizes of the polypeptides may also occur. However, in the same strain of virus, host cell-dependent differences in the electrophoretic mobility of viral glycoproteins are also observed (Haslam *et al.*, 1970; Compans *et al.*, 1970*a*; Schulze, 1970). This is presumably due to differences in the carbohydrate which is attached to the glycoproteins by host cell-specific transferases.

Despite the intimate involvement of the host cell membrane in the process of viral assembly (Sect. 3.4), no host cell polypeptides are detected as components of the virus particle. The absence of host cell polypeptides is indicated by failure to detect prelabeled host cell polypeptides in purified virions (Holland and Kiehn, 1970), by the presence of the same polypeptides in the virion when virus is grown in different cell types (Compans *et al.*, 1970*a*; Schulze, 1970), and by the fact that different enveloped viruses can be grown in the same host cell but have no polypeptides in common. All of the virion polypeptides can also be detected as newly synthesized polypeptide species in virus-infected cells (Lazarowitz *et al.*, 1971; Skehel, 1972; Klenk *et al.*, 1972*b*; Compans, 1973*a*).

2.2.3. Correlation of Molecular Weights of Viral RNAs and Polypeptides

The relationships between the estimated molecular weights of viral polypeptides and the sizes of the viral RNA species are indicated in Table 3. A total of 7 RNA species would be required to code for the viral polypeptides which have been definitely identified. These include the 2 high-molecular-weight polypeptides P_1 and P_2, 4 other structural polypeptides, and a non-structural polypeptide, NS, which is present in large amounts in virus-infected cells (Lazarowitz *et al.*, 1971). Virion polypeptides HA_1 and HA_2 are not primary products because they are derived from the HA polypeptide by cleavage. It is obvious that there is a high degree of proportionality between the estimated sizes of viral polypeptides and the RNA segments. Thus, it is a reasonable hypothesis that the two large RNAs contain the genetic information for P_1 and P_2, the 3 intermediate sized RNAs for HA, NP, and NA, and the 2 small RNAs for M and NS. A smaller (*ca.* 11,000 molecular weight), virus-induced polypeptide has also been detected in moderate

TABLE 3

Relationship Between Sizes of Viral RNA and Polypeptide
Species

Polypeptide	Polypeptide mol. wt.[a]	Estimated sizes of virion RNAs[b]
P_1	94,000	9.8×10^5
P_2	81,000	9.3×10^5
HA	75,000	8.2×10^5
NP	60,000	7.0×10^5
NA	55,000	5.8×10^5
M	26,000	3.9×10^5
NS	25,000	3.4×10^5

[a] See Table 2. The contribution of the carbohydrate to the estimated molecular weight of the glycoproteins HA and NA is uncertain.
[b] Data from Skehel (1971a) and Bishop et al. (1971b).

amounts at late times in virus-infected cells (Skehel, 1972). No viral RNA species has yet been identified which would code for this component.

2.2.4. Lipids

About 20% of the mass of the influenza virion consists of lipid (Frommhagen et al., 1959; Kates et al., 1961; Blough and Merlie, 1970). Most of this is in the form of phospholipids and cholesterol, although at least 1–2% of the total is present as glycolipid. In general, the lipid composition of the virion is determined by the cell in which the virus is grown. Early studies showed that prelabeled host cell lipids are incorporated into influenza virus particles (Wecker, 1957), and that influenza virus grown in different cells showed host-specific differences in lipid composition (Kates et al., 1962). Subsequently, detailed analyses of the phospholipid, cholesterol, glycolipid, and fatty acid content of enveloped virus particles, and of the plasma membranes of host cells, have been carried out. These studies have shown that, although some minor differences have been found in some systems, the lipid composition of virions closely reflects that of the host cell (Klenk and Choppin 1969; 1970a,b; Choppin et al., 1971; Renkonen et al., 1971; Laine et al., 1972; McSharry and Wagner, 1971; Quigley et al., 1971).

Blough and co-workers (see Blough and Tiffany, 1973) have analyzed the fatty acid composition of lipids of several strains of influenza virus grown *in ovo*, as well as of fragments of chorioallantoic membrane. In general, the fatty acid compositions of the polar lipids were similar, and a high degree of similarity was noted when fatty acid compositions of each phospholipid class were compared in two strains of virus (Blough, 1971). However, some differences were observed, particularly in the fatty acids of neutral lipids, and such differences have led Blough and co-workers to conclude that lipid incorporation is directed by the viral protein. However, neutral lipids other than cholesterol are a very minor fraction of the total viral lipid. In addition, it is difficult to evaluate data on different viruses grown at different times in the chick embryo under multiple-cycle conditions. Such viruses may differ in growth cycles and effects on cellular metabolism, and there is no knowledge of the lipid composition of the allantoic cell membrane at the time virus was produced. Further, it has been shown that the fatty acid composition of viral envelopes reflects closely that of the serum used in the cell culture, and that the fatty acid composition of a given strain of virus can be varied greatly by using a different serum, or by growing virus in the presence or absence of an essential fatty acid (Klenk and Choppin, 1970a). These results indicate that the viral protein does not have a major determining effect on fatty acid composition.

2.2.5. Carbohydrate

About 5–8% of the mass of the influenza virion is carbohydrate, which is bound either to protein or lipid; there is no evidence for the presence of a pure polysaccharide component in the virion. The covalent attachment of carbohydrate, which is newly synthesized during infection, to viral glycoproteins is demonstrated by the incorporation of the radioactive precursors glucosamine or fucose into viral glycoproteins (Haslam *et al.*, 1970; Content and Duesberg, 1970; Compans *et al.*, 1970a; Schulze, 1970; Klenk *et al.*, 1972a). Galactose, mannose, glucosamine, and fucose are found in influenza virus by chemical analysis, and the overall composition of the carbohydrate is similar to that of the host cell (Ada and Gottschalk, 1956; Frommhagen *et al.*, 1959). All of these sugars have also been found in the purified HA_1 polypeptide, which contains a total of 17% carbohydrate (Laver, 1971). The presence of glycolipid in the virus has also been demonstrated by the use of specific lectins (Klenk *et al.*, 1972a).

It seems likely that the sequence and size of viral carbohydrate moieties are specified by the host cell. At least four specific transferases would appear to be required for biosynthesis of the carbohydrate chains, and it does not appear that the virus possesses sufficient genetic information to code for all these transferases. In addition, host cell-dependent differences in the electrophoretic mobility of viral glycoproteins, described above, suggest that the amount of carbohydrate per protein molecule may be host cell determined. Finally, a host cell antigen has been detected in highly purified virus preparations (Smith *et al.*, 1953; Knight, 1946; Harboe, 1963*a,b;* Laver and Webster, 1966). This antigen has been shown to be carbohydrate in nature and to be linked covalently to the viral hemagglutinin (Harboe 1963*b*; Laver and Webster, 1966; Lee *et al.*, 1969). Thus, viral and cellular carbohydrate moieties are antigenically similar, supporting the view that the sequence of sugar residues is host specified, at least in part.

Viruses which contain neuraminidases do differ from cellular constituents in their carbohydrate composition in that neuraminic acid residues are absent from such virions. This has been shown by chemical analysis (Klenk and Choppin, 1970*a,b*) and also by electron microscopy. The latter evidence for the absence of neuraminic acid in influenza virions was obtained by staining of infected cells with colloidal iron hydroxide (Klenk *et al.*, 1970). This stain, which is specific for neuraminic acid residues, was present over the entire surface of the infected cell, but was absent on the envelopes of budding influenza and parainfluenza virus particles, indicating the localized nature of the loss of these residues. The lack of neuraminic acid in the virion is not essential for viral infectivity. Schulze (1974) has used a sialyl transferase from colostrum to attach neuraminic acid to influenza virions, and observed that approximately 1200 residues were incorporated per virion with no loss of infectivity.

2.3. Fine Structure and Arrangement of Viral Components

The arrangement of the structural components of the influenza virion is depicted schematically in Fig. 8. The surface of the virion is thought to be covered with spikes of two morphological types, corresponding to the hemagglutinin and neuraminidase subunits (Laver and Valentine, 1969), which are composed of viral glycoproteins. The spikes are attached on the outer surface of a continuous lipid bilayer which has a layer of protein located immediately beneath it. Within

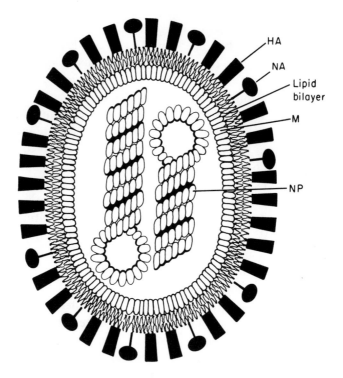

Fig. 8. Schematic diagram of the arrangement suggested for the structural components in the influenza virion. The two types of surface projections, hemagglutinin subunits consisting of HA polypeptides and neuraminidase subunits consisting of NA polypeptides, are on the external surface of a lipid bilayer; the mode of their attachment to the bilayer is unknown. On the internal surface of the bilayer is a layer of the membrane polypeptide M, and within this the ribonucleoprotein composed of NP polypeptides and the viral RNA. The location of the P polypeptides is uncertain.

this complex envelope is the internal RNP. Some of the evidence in support of this model is summarized below.

2.3.1. Spike Structure

The shapes of isolated subunits with hemagglutinin and neuraminidase activities have already been described. Evidence that these structures are composed of the glycoproteins of the virus was first obtained in studies of the effects of proteolytic enzymes on the viral particle. By treatment with the proteases bromelain, chymotrypsin, or pronase, smooth-surfaced spikeless influenza virus particles were obtained (Compans *et al.*, 1970a; Schulze, 1970). These were found to be noninfectious and to lack hemagglutinin and neuraminidase activities, as well as specific polypeptides of the virion. By treatment with bromelain for 3–4 hours, three glycoprotein species were removed, and only HA_2 was still present (Compans *et al.*, 1970*a*). Extensive treatment with chymotrypsin removed all four glycoproteins (Schulze, 1970). In both cases, the proteins which remained appeared to be unaffected by the protease treatment. These results suggested that spikes composed of the glycoproteins were the components with hemagglutinin and neuraminidase activities, and that the glycoprotein HA_2 by itself possessed neither activity.

As described above, the hemagglutinin is synthesized as a single polypeptide chain (HA) which, depending on the virus strain, host cell, and condition of growth, may be cleaved to yield polypeptides HA_1 and HA_2 which are held together by disulfide bonds. The dimensions of the intact hemagglutinin spike suggest that it has a weight of at least 150,000 daltons (Laver and Valentine, 1969). However, the HA polypeptide has a molecular weight of about 75,000 as does a complex of HA_1 and HA_2; thus, there are at least two HA polypeptides or HA_1 + HA_2 complexes in the intact spike. The spikes have a triangular shape when viewed end-on, and it has been suggested that each spike is a trimer composed of three HA polypeptides or HA_1 and HA_2 complexes (Griffith, 1974).

Because protease-treated particles containing HA_2 could be obtained with neither identifiable spikes nor hemagglutinating activity (Compans *et al.*, 1970*a*), HA_2 is likely to be the part of the spike which is involved in binding to the viral membrane. It has also been suggested, on the basis of the characteristic rosettes formed by isolated hemagglutinin spikes, that they possess a hydrophobic end which functions in binding to the viral membrane (Laver and Valentine, 1969). A comparison of the amino acid analysis of HA_2 with that of HA_1 did not indicate a greater content of hydrophobic amino acids (Laver, 1971). However, with some virus strains it is possible to produce solubilized hemagglutinin spikes by treatment with bromelain; these structures contain HA_1 as well as a polypeptide slightly smaller than HA_2 (Brand and Skehel, 1972). This observation suggests that release of the spike occurs after cleavage of HA_2, and provides further support for the involvement of HA_2 in binding to the viral membrane.

Evidence that the neuraminidase is a tetramer was initially provided by biochemical studies, and subsequently confirmed by the morphological studies of Wrigley *et al.*, (1973) described above. The molecular weight of the native subunit was estimated at 200,000–250,000 daltons by polyacrylamide gel electrophoresis and sedimentation in sucrose gradients (Kendal *et al.*, 1968; Bucher and Kilbourne, 1972). When the neuraminidase is dissociated, protein subunits of about 50, 000–60,000 daltons are obtained, suggesting that the native subunit is a tetramer (Kendal and Eckert, 1972; Bucher and Kilbourne, 1972; Gregoriades, 1972; Lazdins *et al.*, 1972). Bucher and Kilbourne (1972) observed two subunits of 65,000 and 58,000 daltons upon dissociation, and Lazdins *et al.* (1972) observed a major peak of 63,000 daltons and a minor peak of 56,000 daltons in neuraminidase preparations. However, the latter authors observed that exclusively 56,000-dalton subunits were observed in enzyme released by trypsin, suggesting that the original structure was of molecular weight of 63,000 daltons and was cleaved proteolytically to yield the smaller polypeptide.

2.3.2. Lipid Bilayer

Electron spin resonance (ESR) studies have provided evidence that the lipids of influenza virus are arranged in a bilayer structure (Landsberger *et al.*, 1971, 1973). Nitroxide-containing stearic acid derivatives were incorporated into the viral membrane, and it was observed that derivatives closer to the polar head group were in a highly rigid environment, compared with derivatives at greater distances down hydrocarbon side chain. This type of flexibility gradient has been observed to be a characteristic of bilayer structures (McConnell and MacFarland, 1972).

Other models of the influenza virus particle have been proposed (Tiffany and Blough, 1970) in which the lipid is arranged in spherical micelles, rather than a lipid bilayer. The basis for these proposals is primarily a calculation that there is about twice as much lipid as needed to form a bilayer. However, Landsberger *et al.* (1971) have made a similar calculation, and concluded that lipid is present in the right amount to form a continuous bilayer. The discrepancy between these calculations is mainly in the total amount of lipid assumed to be present in a particle of given size. The calculations of Tiffany and Blough depend on the value obtained by Reimer *et al.* (1966) of 4.2×10^{-16} gram of protein per virus particle, based on particle counting and a Lowry protein determination. Based on the observed density of influenza virions, it has also been calculated that a particle with this amount of protein would occupy a sphere of 120-nm diameter (Schulze, 1973). However, the calculations of Tiffany and Blough (1970) assumed that a particle of only 100-nm diameter contained 4.2×10^{-16} gram of protein. The calculations of Landsberger *et al.* (1971), based on the volume, density, and composition of the particle, suggest that a 100-nm particle would contain considerably less protein. It is evident that such calculations are not adequate to prove or disprove the existence of a bilayer, but rather they underscore the inadequacy of existing data on the total mass of a virion of defined size.

Glycolipids are exposed on the outer surface of the viral membrane, and can interact with specific lectins (Klenk *et al.*, 1972*a*). This interaction was not observed with intact virions, but the lectin sites were exposed after removal of spikes with the protease bromelain.

2.3.3. Lipid–Protein Relationships

Several observations suggest that the lipid bilayer in the influenza virion is continuous, and not penetrated deeply by protein. Proteolytic enzymes, which degrade the glycoproteins on the surface, do not cause a detectable change in the lipid layer as measured by spin-labeling experiments (Landsberger *et al.*, 1971) or chemical analysis (Klenk *et al.*, 1972*a*). As yet, no segment of the spike protein has been detected in association with the viral membrane after extensive protease treatment. Spikes are sometimes stripped from the particle by surface-tension effects in negatively stained preparations (Schulze, 1973). These results all suggest that spikes do not penetrate deeply into the bilayer, although the exact mechanism of their attachment has not been established.

Of the internal proteins, both the P and NP polypeptides have been found in association with the RNP component (Bishop *et al.*, 1972), and it has been suggested that the low-molecular-weight polypeptide M is associated with the inner surface of the viral membrane (White *et al.*, 1970; Compans *et al.*, 1970*a*; Schulze, 1970). The distinct electron-dense layer beneath the unit membrane in the viral envelope may therefore be composed of this polypeptide. Iodination using oxidation with chloramine T under certain conditions results in labeling of the M polypeptide but not the RNP, indicating that the M polypeptides are external to the RNP (Stanley and Haslam, 1971). Recent studies have demonstrated fluorescence transfer from internal proteins to a fluorescent probe incorporated into the lipid bilayer of influenza virus (Lenard *et al.*, 1974). These results suggest that there is a maximum distance of 1.1 nm between aromatic residues in internal proteins and the lipid bilayer. It has been calculated that the amount M protein in the virion corresponds to that required to form a shell 4–6 nm thick beneath the lipid bilayer (Compans *et al.*, 1972*b*;

Schulze, 1972). Extraction of the lipid from spikeless particles after fixation yields a smooth-surfaced particle, suggesting that a protein layer is still present around the nucleoprotein (Schulze, 1972). Preliminary results of X-ray diffraction studies on influenza virus particles (S. C. Harrison and R. W. Compans, unpublished) indicate a maximum in the electron-density profile in the position of the electron-dense shell beneath the bilayer. The only component of the virion present in sufficient mass to form such a shell is the M protein.

While these observations all suggest close interaction between the M protein and the bilayer, it appears unlikely that this protein penetrates through to the outer surface of the lipid phase. Lack of such penetration is indicated by the complete resistance of the M protein to a variety of proteolytic enzymes (Compans *et al.*, 1970a; Schulze, 1970; Klenk *et al.*, 1972a) and by failure of the M protein to react with labeling reagents specific for proteins on the outer surfaces of membranes (Stanley and Haslam, 1971; Rifkin *et al.*, 1972). Thus, there is no evidence for direct protein–protein interactions between internal and external proteins of the viral membrane. Freeze-fracture electron microscopy of the influenza virus envelope has also suggested that the lipid bilayer is not interrupted by protein (Bächi *et al.*, 1969). The fracture faces of the viral envelope appeared to lack intramembranous particles, which would have been expected if proteins traversed the bilayer.

2.3.4. Internal Ribonucleoprotein (RNP)

The chemical composition of the RNP has been estimated as 10–12% RNA, with the balance composed of the NP polypeptide (Pons *et al.*, 1969; Krug, 1971). RNPs containing RNA molecules of different sizes can be separated by centrifugation in velocity gradients (Duesberg, 1969; Pons, 1971). These RNPs are of the same diameter but differ in length, and three size classes of 90–110 nm, 60–90 nm, and 30–50 nm have been separated (Compans *et al.*, 1972a). The fine structure of the RNP suggests that it is composed of a strand which is folded back on itself and coiled into a regular double helix (Schulze *et al.*, 1970; Compans *et al.*, 1972a). The dimensions and chemical composition of the RNPs suggest that there are 20–26 protein subunits per turn of the *double* helix, and about 20 nucleotides per protein subunit (Compans *et al.*, 1972a).

Polyvinyl sulfate can displace the RNA from the RNP structure, and the morphology is relatively unaltered by this procedure (Pons *et al.*, 1969; Goldstein and Pons, 1970). This suggests that the NP polypeptides will bind to various negatively charged polymers. Extracted NP protein binds equally well to virion RNA and complementary RNA, but less efficiently to cellular RNA species (Scholtissek and Becht, 1971).

There is no evidence for the existence of a stable, lipid-free, "core" structure, other than the RNP, in the influenza virion. In one strain it was possible to isolate a particle containing the P, NP, and M polypeptides after detergent treatment, but the relative amounts of these polypeptides differed from those observed in intact virions (Skehel, 1971*b*). Electron microscopy showed that these particles had a homogeneous interior, and it revealed none of the structural details visible in thin sections of intact virions. These findings, therefore, do not suggest that a native "core" structure had been obtained. In other strains, unsuccessful attempts to isolate cores have been made using a variety of chemical and enzymatic methods (Nermut, 1972), and only after fixation have lipid-free, spikeless particles been obtained (Schulze, 1972). These observations suggest that the shell of M protein is not stabilized to a high degree by protein–protein interactions of the type found with icosahedral capsids, and that interactions between the M protein and the lipid bilayer are important in determining and maintaining the structure of the virion.

2.4. Biological Functions of Virion Components

The functions of the virion components will be discussed further in the discussion of virus replication which follows, and will be summarized only briefly here.

The *hemagglutinin* binds to neuraminic acid-containing receptors on the surface of susceptible cells, initiating the process of infection. Antibody which is specific for the hemagglutinin neutralizes virus infectivity.

The *neuraminidase* cleaves neuraminic acid residues from glycoproteins and gangliosides. Because of the presence of the neuraminidase, there are no neuraminic acid residues on either the glycoproteins or glycolipids of the virions, and the virus can elute from cell surface receptors or from inhibitory mucoproteins such as those bathing the respiratory tract. The relative importance of these effects in virus multiplication have not been established.

The *lipid bilayer* and the underlying *M protein shell* function as structural components which are essential for assembly and maintenance of the viral structure. It is possible that other functions will be discovered for these components, such as participation in the processes of penetration and uncoating.

The RNP internal component contains the genetic information for virus replication as well as an RNA polymerase which catalyzes the synthesis of RNA which is complementary to virion RNA. Whether the P or the NP polypeptide, or a combination of both, possess the enzymatic activity has not been conclusively established.

3. REPLICATION

The kinetics of multiplication of influenza viruses under single-cycle conditions vary considerably with the virus strain and the host cell. In the most efficient and productive systems, the length of the latent period is between 3 and 4 hours and virus production reaches a plateau within 8–12 hours. In other systems, the latent period may be as long as 6 hours and virus production continues for several days. An example of a single-cycle growth curve of the WSN strain in the MDBK line of bovine kidney cells is shown in Fig. 9. This system has many advantages for biochemical studies in that a high yield of in-

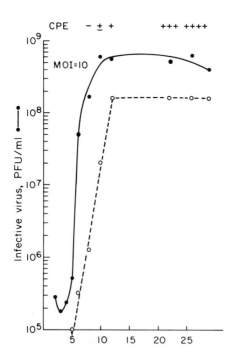

Fig. 9. Single-cycle growth curve of the WSN strain of influenza virus in MDBK cells; the multiplicity of inoculation was 10 PFU/cell From Choppin (1969).

fectious virus is produced under single-cycle conditions by a continuous cell line. Even after inoculation at high multiplicity, there is relatively little incomplete-virus formation (Choppin, 1969). The various steps in the replicative cycle of influenza virus are discussed individually below.

3.1.   Adsorption

The process of infection of susceptible cells is initiated by adsorption of virus particles to receptors on the cell surface. The component of the virion involved in binding is the hemagglutinin protein. The role of viral proteins in initiation of infection has been studied using antibody specific for the two surface proteins, hemagglutinin and neuraminidase, which can be prepared with the use of recombinant viruses. For example, a cross between an A_0 and an A_2 virus yielded a recombinant X-7F1, which possessed the A_0 hemagglutinin and the A_2 neuraminidase (Kilbourne et al., 1968). Antiserum to X-7F1 does not inhibit the neuraminidase of A_0 viruses, but it inhibits hemagglutination and neutralizes the infectivity of the virus. Interaction of the same serum with A_2 viruses does not inhibit hemagglutination or neutralize infectivity, although neutralization of the neuraminidase activity is complete. Thus, the neuraminidase is not involved in initiation of infection.

The study of the interaction of viruses with cell surface receptors was stimulated by the discovery by Hirst (1941) and by McClelland and Hare (1941) that influenza viruses cause agglutination of erythrocytes. Subsequently, the hemagglutinating capacity of a variety of other viruses was identified. In the case of influenza viruses, it was observed that the virus–red cell complex was unstable (Hirst, 1942) and that the receptors on the red cell surface were destroyed by a viral enzyme. This enzyme was later shown to be a neuraminidase which split neuraminic acid residues from mucoproteins (Klenk et al., 1955; Gottschalk, 1957; Rafelson, 1965). This represented the first demonstration of an enzyme as an integral part of a virus particle. Bacterial neuraminidases are also capable of destroying influenza virus receptors (Burnet and Stone, 1947). Thus it has been established that the receptor for influenza virus is a neuraminic acid-containing glycoprotein.

The glycoprotein on the erythrocyte surface which possesses receptor activity has been studied extensively (Marchesi et al., 1972b; Winzler, 1972). It possesses M and N blood group specificities which are also present on glycolipids; whether the latter act as virus receptors has not been established. Trypsin treatment of the erythrocyte surface causes aggregation of the receptor glycoprotein into patches, and it has been demonstrated by electron microscopy that virus binds to such patches (Marchesi *et al.*, 1972*a*).

Numerous soluble sialoglycoproteins possess receptor activity for influenza virions and act as inhibitors of hemagglutination. These include nonspecific serum inhibitors, urinary mucoproteins, and a variety of other mucoproteins. The interactions of influenza viruses with soluble inhibitors have been reviewed previously (Gottshalk, 1965; Choppin and Tamm, 1964; Krizanova and Rathova, 1969). Various strains of influenza virus differ in their affinity for receptors and their sensitivity to such serum inhibitors. Influenza A_2 strains consist of two kinds of virus particles, designated + and −, which differ in their interactions with receptors and antibodies (Choppin and Tamm 1960*a,b;* 1964; Choppin *et al.*, 1960), and their properties have proved to be useful markers in viral genetic studies. The + particles are highly sensitive to antibodies, serum inhibitors, and inhibition by urinary mucoprotein; they elute poorly from human erythrocytes; and are capable of agglutinating erythrocytes treated extensively with *Vibrio cholera* neuraminidase. The − particles are relatively insensitive to inhibition by antibodies and urinary mucoprotein, completely resistant to serum inhibitors, elute rapidly from erythrocytes, and cannot agglutinate erythrocytes treated with *V. cholera* filtrate. Stable homogeneous substrains of + and − particles have been isolated, but the biochemical basis for their different reactivities with receptors has not yet been established. Recent studies have indicated that there are no significant differences in the content of the various envelope polypeptides or in the extent of cleavage of the HA polypeptide (Choppin, unpublished experiments). In addition, no differences in the incorporation of glucosamine or fucose into the hemagglutinin or neuraminidase glycoproteins have been detected, suggesting that there are no gross differences in the glycosylation of these proteins. Thus, the differences between the + and − virions appears to be in the amino acid sequence of the HA polypeptide; further studies are required to resolve this problem.

3.2.   Penetration

There are two main schools of thought concerning the process by which penetration and uncoating occur, not only for influenza viruses but for enveloped viruses in general. Both points of view are supported mainly by electron microscopy studies. In the case of influenza viruses, Fazekas de St. Groth (1948) originally suggested that virus particles enter cells by a process of engulfment, termed "viropexis." Electron microscopic support for this view was obtained by Dales and Choppin (1962) and by Dourmashkin and Tyrrell (1970). Virus particles were observed in direct contact with the cell surface 10 minutes after inoculation, and at 20 minutes particles were observed within cytoplasmic vacuoles. In some cases the particles within vacuoles appeared to be ruptured or had a dense, amorphous appearance, suggesting that partial uncoating might occur within the vesicle.

The contrasting viewpoint has been supported by Morgan and Rose (1968), who studied the entry of virus into chorioallantoic membrane cells. Virus was absorbed in the cold, and samples for electron microscopy were prepared after various periods of incubation at 37°C. Some of the electron micrographs suggested progressive dissolution of the viral and cellular membrane, followed by fusion of the cell membrane and viral envelope, and it was concluded that this was the means of penetration of the viral genome.

At this time there is no general agreement on the mechanism of penetration of influenza virus. Unambiguous conclusions on this subject will not be provided by electron microscopic studies alone since not all virus particles are infectious. Other approaches are needed to establish with certainty the mechanism of penetration. Early virus–cell interactions have been recently reviewed by Dales (1973), and Lonberg-Holm and Philipson (1974).

As described below, influenza virions contain an RNA polymerase associated with their RNP components. Therefore, the process of uncoating is not likely to proceed beyond the release of the RNP into the cytoplasm or nucleus. This step occurs at the cell surface according to the membrane-fusion mechanism of penetration and after phagocytosis in the viropexis mechanism.

3.3. Biosynthesis

3.3.1. RNA Synthesis

The process of influenza viral RNA synthesis has been the subject of a number of investigations, and important new information has been obtained in recent studies. Nevertheless, considerable uncertainty still exists concerning many aspects of this process, including the exact cellular sites and structures involved in synthesis of each type of virus-specific RNA, the role of the nucleus in viral RNA synthesis, and the mechanism by which viral replication is inhibited by drugs such as actinomycin D and α-amanitin.

3.3.1a.   Virion Transcriptase

Following the discovery of a DNA-dependent RNA polymerase in vaccinia virus particles (Kates and McAuslan, 1967), polymerase activities were detected in various other viruses. The presence of an enzyme essential for initiation of replication provided an explanation for the failure to recovery infectious nucleic acids from such viruses. An RNA-dependent RNA polymerase was first described in influenza virions by Chow and Simpson (1971), and soon thereafter by others (Penhoet et al., 1971; Skehel, 1971c). To demonstrate enzyme activity, it was essential to disrupt the viral envelope with a nonionic detergent. The enzyme was not inhibited by actinomycin D, DNase, α-amanitin, or rifampicin, but was sensitive to RNase. Optimal activity required all four ribonucleoside triphosphates at concentrations above certain threshold levels, both Mg^{2+} and Mn^{2+}, and monovalent cations (Bishop et al., 1971a). The virion components with RNA polymerase activity were isolated in sucrose velocity gradients after dissociation of virions with a mixture of detergents, urea, and mercaptoethanol (Bishop et al., 1972). The active structures were RNP complexes containing viral RNA and the NP and P polypeptides.

Studies of the in vitro product RNA have indicated that the viral enzyme is an RNA transcriptase. The in vitro product is at least 95% complementary to the viral RNA species, and it is synthesized in association with virion RNA from which it can be dissociated by heat treatment (Bishop et al., 1971b). Under optimal conditions with the A_0/WS strain of virus, at least 80% of the viral RNA is transcribed, as demonstrated by RNase resistance of ^{3}H-labeled template RNA after annealing (Bishop, personal communication). Initiation of the transcription process starts with the sequence pppGpCp on each strand which is synthesized (Hefti et al., 1974). However, uridine has been found as the 3'-terminal nucleoside of influenza viral RNA species (Lewandowski et al., 1971), whereas cytosine would be expected if transcription were initiated at the 3' termini. If both of these observations are correct, they suggest that transcription is initiated beyond the 3' termini of the virion RNAs. It has been suggested (Hefti et al., 1974) that the entire RNA strand may be copied for replication, but not for transcription into RNA. The change from transcription to replication could result from changing the template-RNA initiation sequence recognized by the enzymes involved.

It is possible to demonstrate synthesis of complementary RNA species in influenza virus-infected cells which have been treated with cycloheximide from the time of infection (Bean and Simpson, 1973). This result indicates that the virion RNA polymerase functions in transcription without a requirement for new protein synthesis.

3.3.1b. Intracellular RNA Polymerase

Virus-induced RNA polymerase activity in influenza virus-infected cells has been described in many laboratories. There is good agreement among studies of the general characteristics of the enzyme, but differences have been found in the nature of the *in vitro* product. Ho and Walters (1966) first described an RNA-dependent RNA polymerase in the microsomal fraction of chorioallantoic membrane cells infected with influenza virus infected with the A_0/PR8 strain. The activity reached a maximum by 3 hours post-infection. Requirements for optimal activity included all four ribonucleoside triphosphates and a divalent cation. The enzyme was inhibited by addition of RNase, but not by actinomycin D or DNase. In contrast to the lack of effect on the RNA polymerase *in vitro*, actinomycin D prevented the appearance of polymerase activity when added to infected cells. If the drug was added 1 hour post-infection, the RNA polymerase activity reached a level of only 15% of that of untreated controls; however, if added 2 hours post-infection or later no inhibition was observed. These observations were confirmed by Scholtissek and Rott (1969), who found that if actinomycin D was added at 2 hours post-infection, RNA polymerase was demonstrable *in vitro* at 6 hours, but the amount of viral RNA synthesized *in vivo* was greatly reduced. The effect of actinomycin on influenza virus replication is discussed further below.

Various cell fractions have been used in assays for RNA polymerase activity, and the highest level was detected in the microsomal fraction (Ho and Walters, 1966; Scholtissek and Rott, 1969; Skehel and Burke, 1969; Ruck et al., 1969; Mahy, 1970). Viral RNA polymerase of lower specific activity was also detected in the nuclear fraction, although in most studies the possibility of cytoplasmic contamination of the nuclear fraction was not ruled out. Recently it was found that highly purified nuclei from influenza virus-infected chick fibroblast cells contain an RNA-dependent RNA polymerase at a level of about 5% that of the cytoplasmic enzyme (Hastie and Mahy,

1973). The induction of the enzyme is prevented by actinomycin D or cycloheximide. Nuclear enzyme activity increases rapidly from 1 hour post-infection and reaches a maximum at 3–4 hours, whereas in the same cells, microsomal fraction activity reaches a maximum at 5–6 hours. The characteristics of the nuclear and cytoplasmic enzymes are similar.

Highly purified preparations of viral RNA polymerase have been obtained from the cytoplasm of influenza virus-infected cells using a combination of equilibrium and velocity centrifugation (Compans and Caliguiri, 1973). The isolated structures with enzyme activity were RNP complexes similar in morphology to the RNP components present in influenza virions, and NP was the only polypeptide detected in the structures, isolated from infected BHK21-F cells labeled from 3 to 4 hours post-infection. However, both the P and NP polypeptides were detected in subsequent studies in which label was added 2 hours post-infection (Caliguiri and Compans, 1974). The RNP complexes sedimented heterogeneously at 50–70 S. A structure sedimenting at 70 S which contained viral RNA polymerase activity was also identified by Skehel and Burke (1969), and was reported to contain polypeptides corresponding to the P, NP, and NS polypeptides. The presence of NS in this region of the gradient was probably due to the presence of cytoplasmic ribosomes, since NS has been found in association with polyribosome-containing fractions (Pons, 1972; Compans, 1973a). The polysomes containing NS can be removed from the RNA polymerase fraction by equilibrium centrifugation (Compans, 1973a; Compans and Caliguiri, 1973). These results indicate that structures with RNA polymerase activity contain the P and NP, but not the NS polypeptide. Whether or not they contain additional minor polypeptides has not been conclusively established. Thus the RNA polymerase activity isolated from infected cells is probably associated with the same RNP structure which is packaged into influenza virions.

The fact that structures sedimenting at 50–70 S with RNA polymerase activity can be isolated from the cytoplasm of infected cells without lysis of membranes by detergent treatment (Skehel and Burke, 1969; Compans and Caliguiri, 1973) suggests that there is no association of the influenza RNA polymerase with cytoplasmic membranes. This is in contrast to the situation in poliovirus-infected cells, in which the bulk of the RNA polymerase is associated with a smooth cytoplasmic-membrane fraction (Caliguiri and Tamm, 1969, 1970). The presence of influenza RNA polymerase activity in the microsomal fraction is probably due to intrinsic sedimentation properties of the

RNP complexes rather than their association with microsomal membranes.

Most reports indicate that the bulk of the *in vitro* product of the cytoplasmic RNA polymerase is complementary to virion RNA (Scholtissek and Rott, 1969; Mahy and Bromley, 1970; Hastie and Mahy, 1973; Caliguiri and Compans, 1974), which further indicates that the cytoplasmic structures are similar to virion RNPs. However, Ruck *et al.* (1969) have described an RNA product similar in nucleotide composition to virion RNA. In this case, enzyme was prepared at a later time in the growth cycle, and an A_2 virus was employed, whereas A_0 viruses have been used in most other studies. Whether these factors account for the differing findings remains to be established.

The inhibition of viral RNA polymerase activity by specific antiserum provides further support for the idea that the enzyme is determined by the viral genome (Scholtissek *et al.*, 1971). Convalescent serum of a chicken infected with fowl plague virus inhibited the polymerase activity of all influenza A viruses, but not of an influenza B virus. A purified γ-globulin fraction from antiserum against the RNP antigen failed to inhibit polymerase activity. Thus, either the antigenic component of the polymerase complex was lost from the RNP antigen preparation, or it failed to stimulate the production in rabbits of antibody which inhibits the reaction.

In summary, there is good evidence that RNP complexes with RNA polymerase activity can be obtained from the cytoplasm of infected cells, and that these structures closely resemble the RNP structures from virions which also possess enzyme activity. *In vitro*, this enzyme synthesizes RNA which is complementary to virion RNA. The components involved in virion-type RNA synthesis *in vivo* have not been identified. An entirely different structure may be involved, or alternatively the activity of the RNP complexes *in vivo* may differ from their *in vitro* activity.

3.3.1c.   Virus-Specific RNA and RNP Species in Infected Cells

Several approaches have been used to identify virus-specific RNA species in influenza virus-infected cells. Actinomycin D, which inhibits cellular DNA-dependent RNA synthesis, has been used to permit radioactive labeling of intracellular RNA species produced by most types of RNA viruses which do not depend on DNA for their replication.

Such experiments have been carried out on influenza virus-infected cells to which the drug has been added approximately 2 hours after infection since viral replication is inhibited if the drug is added earlier. Another approach which has been used to identify RNA species which are complementary to virion RNA is hybridization to virion RNA. Double-stranded RNA species, which may be intermediates in viral replication, have been identified by their resistance to ribonuclease. Finally, RNP structures containing viral RNA have been identified and separated from cellular RNPs based on their physical properties, and the RNA contained in such RNPs has then been analyzed. It is a general finding that the RNA and RNP species in cells correspond in size to the segments of RNA found within virions; no convincing evidence has been obtained for linkage of the segments of the RNA genome during replication.

The earliest detectable synthesis of virus-specific RNA in infected cells involves transcription of the genome of the infecting virus by the virion transcriptase, and has been termed primary transcription (Bean and Simpson, 1973). This was detected by monitoring the conversion of RNA of ^{32}P-labeled virions into a RNase-resistant form in infected cells. Transcription was first detected at a low rate between 40 and 60 minutes of incubation, and accelerated rapidly between 90 and 120 minutes. The initial rate of transcription was unchanged in the presence of cycloheximide, but the rapid increase after 90 minutes of incubation did not occur when protein synthesis was inhibited. Since only about 20% of the virion RNA became RNase-resistant in the presence of cycloheximide, it is uncertain whether all virion RNA segments are being transcribed.

The virus-specific RNA species present in cells at early times post-infection have been analyzed by hybridization experiments (Scholtissek and Rott, 1970) and by isolation of viral RNPs from the nucleus and cytoplasm (Krug, 1972). The peak in rate of synthesis of complementary RNA, as determined by hybridization to virion RNA, was at 2 hours post-infection in fowl plague virus-infected chick fibroblasts, whereas virion RNA synthesis peaked at 3 hours (Scholtissek and Rott, 1970). In MDCK cells infected with the WSN strain, complementary RNA strands were detected in both the nucleus and cytoplasm at 2 hours (Krug, 1972). The amount of complementary RNA in the nucleus remained constant, whereas the amount in the cytoplasm increased until 4 hours, and then remained constant. Thus, it appears that the bulk of the complementary RNA is synthesized early in the growth cycle.

At times in the growth cycle later than 4 hours post-infection, only virion RNA is synthesized and incorporated into cytoplasmic RNPs (Krug, 1972). At these later times it has also been possible to demonstrate synthesis of virus-specific RNA in cells treated with actinomycin D (Duesberg and Robinson, 1967; Nayak, 1970). This RNA sediments heterogeneously with a pattern similar to virion RNA. About 20–25% of the RNA is RNase resistant after self-annealing, and the amount of RNase-resistant radioactivity decreases to 8% when annealed in the presence of unlabeled virion RNA. This decrease indicates that the bulk of the RNA labeled in cells under these conditions corresponds to the viral strand.

The synthesis of RNase-resistant RNA has been identified in infected cells labeled in the presence (Duesberg and Robinson, 1967; Nayak, 1970), or absence (Pons, 1967b), of actinomycin D. This RNA has the characteristics of a base-paired replicative form and can be resolved by polyacrylamide gel electrophoresis into at least 5 species, which may represent replicative forms of each species of virion RNA (Pons and Hirst, 1968b). Most of the radioactivity in the RNase-resistant RNA labeled in the presence of actinomycin D could be displaced by heating and reannealing in the presence of a large excess of virion RNA, indicating that the double strand is asymmetrically labeled, with most of the label in the viral strand (Duesberg and Robinson, 1967; Nayak, 1970).

Virus-specific RNA with the characteristics of a partially double-stranded replicative intermediate has been identified in infected cells labeled in the presence of actinomycin D (Nayak and Baluda, 1969; Nayak, 1970). These RNA species sedimented heterogeneously at approximately 14 S in a sucrose gradient, with a broad tail toward higher S values. Mild RNase treatment converted the 14 S complex to 11 S and 7 S double-stranded RNAs. The 14 S complex was insoluble in 2 M NaCl, whereas the 11 S and 7 S structures were soluble.

RNP structures consisting of viral RNA and the NP polypeptide have been isolated from infected cells by a variety of procedures (Duesberg, 1969; Krug, 1971, 1972; Pons, 1971, 1972; Compans and Caliguiri, 1973). These RNPs from cells have sedimentation properties similar to RNPs obtained from purified virions, which correspond to structures containing the different sizes of viral RNAs. The results of annealing experiments (Pons, 1971) and analyses of base composition (Krug, 1972) indicate that part of the RNA incorporated into RNPs at early times in the growth cycle is complementary to viral RNA. The RNA incorporated into cytoplasmic RNPs labeled from 1 to 3 hours post-infection had a base composition halfway between the viral and complementary strands, whereas the nucleoplasmic RNPs contained predominanttly plus strands (Krug, 1972). The RNPs which contain complementary RNA are not incorporated into virions, and their function is not known. The nucleoplasmic RNPs containing viral RNA are assembled at a slower rate than the cytoplasmic RNPs, suggesting that the nucleoplasmic RNPs are not precursors of the cytoplasmic RNPs (Krug, 1972).

3.3.1d. Effects of Inhibitors

The replication of influenza viruses differs from that of most other RNA viruses in sensitivity to various inhibitors. This was first demonstrated by Barry *et al*. (1962), who observed that actinomycin D inhibited viral replication when added early in the growth cycle but had little effect on virus yield when added later in the growth cycle. Inhibitors of DNA synthesis have no effect on influenza virus multiplication (Barry *et al*., 1962; Scholtissek and Rott, 1961). Replication of influenza virus can also be blocked by UV-irradiation of cells prior to infection and by other inhibitors, including mitomycin and α-amanitin (Rott *et al*., 1965; White and Cheyne, 1965; Nayak and Rasmussen, 1966; Mahy *et al*., 1972). It appears that a host cell function essential for influenza virus replication is blocked by these inhibitors. Most other RNA viruses, including the paramyxoviruses, are insensitive to such inhibitors.

The mechanism by which these inhibitors act to suppress virus multiplication is not clear, although several observations suggest that the synthesis of complementary RNA is blocked in cells treated with actinomycin D, and it now appears likely that this process may involve an actinomycin D-sensitive host cell process *in vivo*. However, as described above, the virion RNA polymerase and the polymerase isolated from infected cells, both of which synthesize complementary RNA *in vitro*, are not inhibited by this drug.

Recently, Bean and Simpson (1973) observed that primary transcription is not observed in the presence of actinomycin D. Thus conversion of parental ^{32}P-labeled RNA into an RNase-resistant form is not observed in the presence of the drug. Both this observation and the 40- to 60-minute delay observed before primary transcription is detected suggest that a host cell function is required before transcription can be initiated *in vivo*. Hybridization experiments indicate that the synthesis of complementary RNA is also inhibited by addition of actinomycin D later in the growth cycle, although such inhibition does not cause a significant reduction in virus yields (Scholtissek and Rott, 1970; Pons, 1973).

The production of virion RNA is not markedly inhibited if actinomycin D is added later than 2–3 hours post-infection. This is indicated by the ability to label virus-specific RNAs in the presence of the drug (Duesberg and Robinson, 1967; Nayak, 1970), by annealing experiments (Scholtissek and Rott, 1970), and by isolation of RNPs containing viral RNA synthesized in the presence of the drug (Pons, 1973). Gregoriades (1970) observed that the overall rate of total RNA synthesis in infected cells was reduced by actinomycin, and that some reduction in virus yield was observed even if the drug was added later in the growth cycle. Synthesis of viral proteins continues in the presence of the drug (Gregoriades, 1970; Pons, 1973). Synthesis of virion RNA is prevented by cycloheximide, indicating that protein synthesis is necessary for formation of the enzymes involved in virion RNA synthesis (Scholtissek and Rott, 1970; Pons, 1973). However, cycloheximide has no effect on primary transcription (Bean and Simpson, 1973), nor does it block the synthesis of complementary RNA when the drug is added later in the growth cycle (Scholtissek and Rott, 1970; Pons, 1973). These observations suggest that the host cell function which may be essential for initiation of complementary RNA synthesis does not involve production of a new polypeptide.

3.3.2. Protein Synthesis

3.3.2a. Viral mRNA and Polysomes

Limited information is available concerning the identification of mRNA and viral polysomes in infected cells, and the available data are not in complete agreement. Nayak (1970) first analyzed the RNA species associated with the polysome region of infected cells after radioactive labeling of RNA in the presence of actinomycin D. The polysome profiles of infected and uninfected chick fibroblast cells were similar. Virus-specific RNA extracted from the polysome region, labeled from 3.5 to 6.5 hours post-infection, had a sedimentation profile similar to virion RNA when analyzed in a sucrose velocity gradient. The results of annealing experiments indicated that both viral and complementary RNA were present in the polysome region.

More recently, Pons (1972, 1973) has obtained evidence that complementary RNA functions as viral messenger. Labeled RNA extracted from the polysome region was found by hybridization to be complementary to virion RNA; in the presence of actinomycin D, which appeared to inhibit the synthesis of complementary RNA, no labeled RNA was found in polysomes. Support for the idea that complementary RNA functions as messenger is also provided by the observations of Kingsbury and Webster (1973), who found that total RNA extracted from infected cells directed the synthesis of virus-specific polypeptides in a cell-free rabbit reticulocyte system. RNA extracted from virions was inactive, indicating that it does not have the capacity to function as messenger. On the other hand, Siegert *et al.* (1973) have recently presented evidence that RNA extracted from influenza virions is translated in a cell-free *Escherichia coli* system. The product when analyzed by gel electrophoresis was markedly heterogeneous; however, some product species appeared to react with antiserum against the virion ribonucleoprotein. Thus, the available information concerning the nature of the mRNA is conflicting, and further information is needed to identify the messenger for each specific polypeptide. Since the rates of synthesis of different viral polypeptides vary during the growth cycle, the relative amounts of different viral mRNAs present in polysomes may depend on the time of harvest. RNAs which function as viral messengers at early times may differ from those found later in the growth cycle, and it is even possible that the synthesis of some polypeptides may be directed by the viral RNA strand, and that of other polypeptides by the complementary RNA strand.

3.3.2b. Identification of Virus-Specific Polypeptides in Infected Cells

A replacement of host-specific by virus-specific polypeptide synthesis is observed in infected cells; the extent and kinetics of this replacement depend on the specific virus–cell system (White *et al.*, 1970; Lazarowitz *et al.*, 1971; Skehel, 1972; Meier-Ewert and Compans, 1974). In some cell types, such as HeLa or BHK21-F, most of the polypeptides labeled at 4 hours post-infection or later are virus-specific, whereas in MDBK cells a high background of host cell polypeptide synthesis is still observed at 6–8 hours. In several early studies, three or four polypeptide peaks were observed in infected cells (Taylor *et al.*, 1969; Joss *et al.*, 1969; Holland and Kiehn, 1970; White *et al.*, 1970). The use of cell-fractionation procedures, and the realization that influenza virions contain as many as 7–8 polypeptides, has led to the identification of additional virus-specific polypeptides. All of the polypeptides of the virion as well as one or two virus-specific non-structural polypeptides have now been identified in infected cells (Lazarowitz *et al.*, 1971; Skehel, 1972; Klenk *et al.*, 1972*b*; Krug and Etkind, 1973). Some of the polypeptides are present in whole cells in small amounts, but are clearly identified in cell fractions. There are marked differences in the rates of synthesis of the different viral polypeptides. Since infecting virus particles presumably contain RNAs in approximately equal numbers with the genetic information to code for the polypeptides, mechanisms must control the rate of transcription or translation of the viral genetic information. Evidence for such control was obtained by Lazarowitz *et al.*, (1971), who found that relatively little of the M protein was present in infected cells despite the fact that it is the most plentiful protein in the virion. This suggested not only that synthesis of the M protein was controlled, but also that it might be a rate-limiting step in virus production. Subsequently, Skehel (1972, 1973) found unequal, and thus controlled, synthesis of the several viral polypeptides. The synthesis of the individual viral proteins is discussed in detail below.

The nucleocapsid subunit, NP, is generally the most abundant species in whole infected cells (Fig. 10). Large amounts of the uncleaved hemagglutinin polypeptide HA, and a *ca.* 25,000-dalton-molecular-weight non-structural polypeptide, NS, are also found in most virus–cell systems. Polypeptides P, NA, and M are usually de-

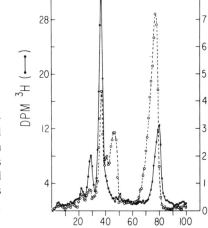

Fig. 10. Polyacrylamide gel electrophoresis of polypeptides synthesized in BHK21-F cells 4 hours after infection with the WSN strain of influenza virus (●——●). Polypeptides of purified virions are included as markers (O----O). From Lazarowitz *et al.* (1971).

tected in lesser amounts; the latter is identified clearly in isolated plasma membranes (Lazarowitz *et al.*, 1971) and smooth cytoplasmic membranes (Compans, 1973*a*). As mentioned above, the extent to which the hemagglutinin polypeptide HA is cleaved to yield HA_2 and HA_1 varies with the virus strain, the host cell type, the extent of cytopathic effect, and the presence or absence of serum in the medium (Lazarowitz *et al.*, 1971, 1973*a,b*; Klenk *et al.*, 1972*b*; Rifkin *et al.*, 1972; Skehel, 1972; Stanley *et al.*, 1973). In the WSN strain–MDBK cell system cleavage occurs at the plasma membrane, and recently it has been shown that the enzyme responsible for cleavage in this system is serum plasminogen activated by an activator produced by host cells (Lazarowitz *et al.*, 1973*b*). In chick embryo fibroblasts infected with fowl plague virus, larger amounts of HA_1 and HA_2 are observed, and it appears that in this system cleavage may occur intracellularly (Skehel, 1972; Klenk *et al.* 1972*b*, 1974).

In coelectrophoresis experiments, it was found that a major polypeptide peak always migrated slightly more rapidly than the M polypeptide of marker virus particles (Lazarowitz *et al.*, 1971). To determine whether the polypeptides from the cell and virion were related, ^{35}S-methionine-labeled polypeptides were isolated by gel filtration in the presence of guanidine and compared by peptide mapping. The results indicated that the two proteins were unrelated (Lazarowitz *et al.*, 1971). Therefore, the *ca.* 25,000-dalton-molecular-weight polypeptide found in large amounts in infected cells has been considered a non-structural polypeptide, and designated NS. A recent study (Gregoriades, 1973) raised some question about the identity of NS as a non-structural polypeptide distinct from virion polypeptide M. It was possible to extract the M polypeptide from virions with acidic chloroform-methanol, and a protein of identical electrophoretic mobility could also be extracted from whole infected cells, nuclei, or polysomes. Previous results (Taylor *et al.*, 1970; Lazarowitz *et al.*, 1971; Pons, 1972; Compans, 1973*a*) had indicated that the NS polypeptide was associated with nuclei and polysomes. Analysis of tryptic digests of the M protein and the nuclear- and polysome-associated proteins extracted by chloroform-methanol revealed many similarities, although some differences in the patterns were evident. These results could be interpreted as indicating that extraction with acidic chloroform-methanol modified either the M or NS polypeptide so that comigration in gels was observed, and they raise the possibility that there is a relationship between M and NS. No comparisons have been made by coelectrophoresis of polypeptides from the same starting material with and without extraction, and it is therefore not possible to determine whether one component is being modified. It is also possible, however, that a mixture of M and NS is being extracted, or that M is being extracted and NS is not. Thus, further information is needed to explain the results obtained by this extraction procedure.

In addition to NS, other non-structural virus-specific polypeptides may exist, although none has been well characterized. Using antiserum directed against non-structural viral antigens, Dimmock and Watson (1969) precipitated radioactively labeled polypeptides from infected cells. Analysis by polyacrylamide gel electrophoresis suggested the presence of three non-structural polypeptides, with the major component corresponding in migration to NS. One of the remaining non-structural components migrated more rapidly, and may correspond to a *ca.* 11,000-dalton-molecular-weight component identified by Skehel (1972) as a non-structural viral polypeptide in cells infected with fowl plague virus. The remaining component found by Dimmock and Watson (1969) may correspond to the uncleaved HA polypeptide, which may not have been present in their purified virions because it was cleaved to HA_1 and HA_2. Because of the absence of HA in fowl plague virions grown in chicken embryo fibroblasts, Skehel (1972) refers to HA as a non-structural polypeptide; however, in most strains of virus HA is clearly a structural component of virions.

The NP and NS polypeptides are generally the first to be detected in infected cells, possibly because they are produced in largest amounts. Skehel (1973) has suggested that the polypeptides P_2, NP, and NS, which were the first to be detected in fowl plague virus-infected cells, are products of RNA species produced by selective transcription of three of the viral genome segments by the virion polymerase. When cells were infected in the presence of cycloheximide and pulse labeled after removal of the drug, only these three polypeptides were detected, suggesting that the messenger RNAs for these components were produced by primary transcription by the input virion transcriptase. From 4 to 6 hours after infection of chick fibro-blasts by fowl plague virus, the rate of synthesis of M increased and that of NS decreased (Skehel, 1972, 1973). Thus, the rates of synthesis of polypeptides may be controlled individually and may vary during the growth cycle.

Apart from the cleavage of HA into HA_1 and HA_2, the extent of which differs with cell type, virus strain, and conditions of incubation (Lazarowitz *et al.*, 1973*a,b*), there is no evidence that influenza virus-specific polypeptides are generated by cleavage of large precursors. Rather, the same polypeptide species are observed with various lengths of pulse labels, and no large precursors were observed when cells were labeled in the presence of amino acid analogues or protease inhibitors (Skehel, 1972; Taylor *et al.*, 1969; Lazarowitz *et al.*, 1971). The observations of Etchison *et al.* (1971) of cleavage of viral polypeptides were probably related to the conversion of HA into HA_1 and HA_2. The results of most investigators suggest that viral polypeptides are direct products of monocistronic mRNAs.

3.3.2c. Intracellular Location of Viral Polypeptides

Early studies of the intracellular location of virus-specific components were carried out by immunofluorescence (Liu, 1955; Breitenfeld and Schäfer, 1957; Holtermann *et al.*, 1960). The internal nucleoprotein antigen was detected in the nucleus at early times in the growth cycle, and at later times also in the cytoplasm. In some virus–cell systems the nuclear fluorescence was lost at later times, suggesting transport of the internal antigen from nucleus to cytoplasm. The antigens of the viral envelope have been detected in the cytoplasm only. These studies have been extended recently by the use of antiserum specific for the hemagglutinin and the neuraminidase, both of which were located in the cytoplasm (Maeno and Kilbourne, 1970). The early observations on the location of the nucleoprotein antigen have been interpreted as indicating nuclear synthesis followed by transport to the cytoplasm. However, it is clear that immunofluorescence detects antigen accumulation, rather than synthesis. New information on the location of viral components in infected cells has been obtained recently using cell-fractionation procedures and gel electrophoresis. The synthesis of all viral polypeptides appears to be cytoplasmic (Taylor *et al.*, 1969, 1970). Several isolated cell fractions have been studied, and will be considered individually.

Nucleus. In pulse-chase experiments, Taylor *et al.* (1969) observed that two virus-specific polypeptides were chased from the cytoplasm to the nucleus. One of these was the NP polypeptide and the other was considered to be the smallest virion polypeptide, M. Upon re-examination of the nuclear fraction in coelectrophoresis experiments (Lazarowitz *et al.* (1971), it became apparent that the smaller polypeptide associated with the nuclei is the non-structural polypeptide NS rather than the M polypeptide. Evidence has also been obtained recently (Krug and Etkind, 1973) that the virion polypeptide P and an 11,000-dalton-molecular-weight non-structural polypeptide (NS_2) are present in isolated nuclei. Upon further subfractionation, it appears that NP is the major component in the nucleoplasm and NS is associated predominantly with the nuclear fraction (Taylor *et al.*, 1970; Krug and Etkind, 1973). Most of the NP polypeptide in the nucleoplasm was present in viral RNPs (Krug and Etkind, 1973). In immunofluorescence studies, Dimmock (1969) observed bright nucleolar staining with antiserum specific for non-structural viral antigens, which probably represented the NS polypeptide. The migration of NS into the nucleus appeared to be much more rapid than that of NP; migration was unaffected by the addition of cycloheximide or actinomycin D (Taylor *et al.*, 1970).

The function of viral polypeptides in the nucleus is not clear, although it is likely that nuclear processes are essential in viral replication. Viral replication does not take place in fragments of cytoplasm from which nuclei have been removed (Cheyne and White, 1969), although paramyxoviruses are able to replicate. The inhibition of influenza virus replication by actinomycin D, mitomycin, α-amanitin, or preirradiation with UV (see above) also suggests that a nuclear function is essential for viral replication. It is possible that viral components in nuclei could be involved in synthesis of viral RNA or inhibition of cellular macromolecular synthesis.

A promising new approach to the study of the role of the nucleus in viral replication is the use of cell fusion. Kelly and Dimmock (1974) observed that the apparently dormant avian erythrocyte nucleus could support the synthesis of viral RNP antigen. In actinomycin D-treated BHK21-F cells, synthesis of RNP antigen was not observed; however, if the drug was removed and the cells fused with avian erythrocytes, RNP antigen was found in the erythrocyte nuclei, but not in the BHK21-F cell nuclei. These results indicate that a nuclear function is necessary for the production of RNP antigen, and that a normally inactive nucleus such as that of the avian erythrocyte is sufficient to provide this function.

Soluble Fraction. The polypeptides remaining in the supernatant after centrifugation at 100,000*g* for 60 minutes, or 200,000*g* for 30 minutes, have been determined (Compans, 1973a; Klenk *et al.*, 1974). With short labeling periods, the NP polypeptide is the most prominent peak. This is not surprising since RNPs have long been designated as "soluble antigen." In longer labeling experiments, Klenk *et al.* (1974) observed a large peak of polypeptide P, and after a 10-minute pulse followed by a 60-minute chase, P was the only detectable virus-specific polypeptide remaining in the supernatant. There is no evidence of a significant amount of the viral envelope proteins, HA, NA, or M being present in the soluble fraction, even after short pulses. Thus, it seems likely that envelope proteins are synthesized in association with membranes or inserted into membranes very rapidly after synthesis.

Cytoplasmic Organelles. The cytoplasmic components which have been analyzed for the presence of viral polypeptides include fractions which have been separated on the basis of differential, equilibrium, or velocity centrifugation. These include microsomal and mitochondrial pellets, smooth and rough endoplasmic reticulum membranes, and polysome-containing fractions. The results indicate that distinct patterns of viral polypeptides are present in different cytoplasmic fractions.

The fractionation procedure of Caliguiri and Tamm (1969, 1970) separates cytoplasmic extracts on the basis of sedimentation to equilibrium in discontinuous sucrose gradients into at least four distinct components: smooth cytoplasmic membranes, an intermediate-density fraction, rough microsomal membranes, and free polysomes. In the smooth membranes isolated by this or other procedures, the hemagglutinin is the major viral component (White *et al.*, 1970; Compans, 1973*a*; Stanley *et al.*, 1973; Klenk *et al.*, 1974). In fowl plague virus-infected cells it is present in the cleaved form as polypeptides HA_1 and HA_2, but in other virus–cell systems it is found as the uncleaved HA polypeptide. The other polypeptides of the viral envelope, NA, and M, can also be detected, although they are present in smaller amounts than HA (Compans, 1973*a*; Klenk *et al.*, 1974).

An intermediate-density fraction, sedimenting between smooth and rough membranes, contains the NP polypeptide as the major component (Compans, 1973*a*; Klenk *et al.*, 1974). This fraction contains the bulk of the viral RNA polymerase activity, which can be further purified by velocity sedimentation. As described above [Sect. 3.3.1.(b)], the enzymatic activity is associated with ribonucleoprotein complexes similar to virion RNPs, which are not bound to cytoplasmic membranes.

The rough microsomal fraction contains polypeptides HA, NP, and NS as major components (Compans, 1973*a*; Klenk *et al.*, 1974). The results of pulse-chase experiments suggest that the HA polypeptide migrates from rough to smooth cytoplasmic membranes. Thus, it seems likely that this viral glycoprotein is synthesized on ribosomes associated with rough endoplasmic reticulum, and that completed chains migrate to the smooth membranes after synthesis.

A polysome fraction has been isolated from infected cells in velocity gradients and found to contain large amounts of the NP and NS polypeptides (Pons, 1972). From an equilibrium gradient, the polysome fractions were generally observed to contain NS as the only prominent polypeptide (Compans, 1973*a*); however, with some conditions of labeling, NP was also observed. In a similar fraction from fowl plague virus-infected cells, polypeptides in free polysomes resembled those in rough membranes (Klenk *et al.*, 1974). These results indicate an association of NS, and possibly NP, with ribosomes and polysomes. The association of NS with ribosomes appears to depend on the ionic strength (Krug and Etkind, 1973). In low-ionic-strength buffers, the polypeptide was found to be absorbed to both ribosomal subunits, whereas it was removed by higher salt. Thus, in these studies NS did not behave as a structural component of the ribosome, and these results do not support the view that this protein in the nucleolus is a precursor of a cytoplasmic ribosomal protein.

Plasma Membranes. It is possible to isolate plasma membranes from infected cells in the form of large cell ghosts by using fluorescein mercuric acetate (FMA) (Warren *et al.*, 1966; Klenk and Choppin, 1969). Such membranes can be analyzed by SDS-polyacrylamide gel electrophoresis, and virus-specific polypeptides can be clearly identified (Lazarowitz *et al.*, 1971; Stanley *et al.*, 1973). All of the virion polypeptides can be detected in association with the plasma membrane, but the non-structural polypeptides are not detected. In BHK21-F cells infected with the WSN strain, the envelope polypeptides HA, NA, and M are the major components detected in a 10-minute pulse (Lazarowitz *et al.*, 1971). After chases, the other virion polypeptides are clearly detected, and in the presence of serum, HA is cleaved into HA_1 and HA_2. Thus, cleavage of HA into HA_1 and HA_2 occurs at the plasma membrane in this system. Most polypeptides are present in approximately the same proportions as in the virion, with the exception of uncleaved HA, which is present in much larger amounts. These observations are compatible with other results (Sect. 3.4), indicating that viral envelope components are the first to arrive at the plasma membrane and that the internal components then associate with areas of modified membrane.

3.3.2d. Effects of Inhibitors

Cleavage of HA into HA_1 and HA_2 can be prevented by the amino acid analogue fluorophenylalanine (Klenk and Rott, 1973) and by protease inhibitors (Klenk and Rott, 1973; Lazarowitz *et al.*, 1973*b*). Hemagglutinating activity is not detected in the presence of fluorophenylalanine (Zimmermann and Schäfer, 1960), although this is not caused by prevention of cleavage (Lazarowitz *et al.*, 1973*a*; Stanley *et al.*, 1973). Rather, it is likely that incorporation of analogue into the HA polypeptide results in an inactive polypeptide, which also is not cleaved. Reduction in temperature appears to cause a specific inhibitory effect on polypeptide synthesis. When infected cells are incubated at 25°C, infectious virus is not produced (Rott and Scholtissek, 1968). This appears to be caused by the lack of production of the M polypeptide, which is not detected at 25°C (Klenk and Rott, 1973). Cleavage of HA to HA_1 and HA_2 occurs at a much slower rate at 25°C, and the hemagglutinin protein is incorporated into the plasma membrane, as demonstrated by hemadsorption.

The effects of high concentrations of glucosamine and the sugar analogue 2-deoxyglucose on polypeptide synthesis are of great interest. Kilbourne (1959) originally observed that 2-deoxyglucose inhibited the production of infectious influenza virus as well as of hemagglutinin. This analogue, as well as high concentrations of the metabolite glucosamine, inhibited the formation of the hemagglutinin polypeptide in infected cells (Gandhi *et al.*, 1972; Kaluza *et al.*, 1972; Klenk *et al.*, 1972*b*). The production of active neuraminidase was also inhibited, whereas no effect was observed on synthesis of nonglycosylated polypeptides. Thus it seemed likely that these inhibitors exerted their effects on the glycosylation of viral glycoproteins. Further evidence for this conclusion was obtained by Klenk *et al.* (1972*b*), who observed a new, apparently unglycosylated, polypeptide in cells treated with these sugars. By pulse-chase experiments and comparison of incorporation of histidine, the new polypeptide appeared to be a precursor of HA, and was therefore designated HA_0 (Klenk *et al.*, 1972*b*). In cell-fractionation experiments, it was observed that HA_0 migrated from rough to smooth membranes, where it was cleaved into two polypeptides, designated HA_{01} and HA_{02} (Klenk *et al.*, 1974). These observations suggest that in the presence of such inhibitors, the polypeptide backbone of viral glycoproteins is synthesized, but glycosylation does not take place. The apparently unglycosylated polypeptide displays the same association with membranes as the normal HA polypeptides, whereas the lack of hemagglutinin activity in infected cells suggests that the unglycosylated protein is unable to bind to receptors.

3.3.3. Lipid Synthesis

Radioactive-labeling experiments with $^{32}PO_4$ first indicated that preformed host cell lipids were incorporated into the influenza virion

(Wecker, 1957). The fact that the lipid composition of influenza virus is generally similar to that of the host cell (Frommhagen *et al.*, 1959; Armbruster and Beiss, 1958; Kates *et al.*, 1961, 1962) also indicates that the viral lipid is derived from that of the host cell. When the lipids of influenza virus grown in two different host cells were compared, it was found that they closely resembled that of the particular cell in which they were grown (Kates *et al.*, 1961, 1962). In general, lipids of viruses which bud at the cell surface reflect closely the lipid composition of the host cell plasma membrane (Klenk and Choppin, 1969, 1970a,b; Choppin *et al.*, 1971; Blough and Tiffany, 1973). The rate of *de novo* synthesis of phospholipids in chick embryo fibroblasts was unchanged up to 7 hours after infection with influenza virus; thereafter all lipid synthesis was depressed (Weinstein and Blough, 1972). This depression is probably not a primary effect, but it may be secondary to inhibition of RNA or protein synthesis or other cytopathic effects. Thus the results obtained to date suggest that synthesis of viral lipids occurs by the normal cellular processes of lipid biosynthesis, and that the viral envelope is formed by incorporation of lipids from the host cell plasma membrane.

3.3.4. Carbohydrate Synthesis

The use of radioactive precursors such as fucose and glucosamine, which are incorporated specifically into viral glycoproteins, has demonstrated that the carbohydrate side chains of these glycoproteins are newly synthesized during infection (Haslam *et al.*, 1970; Compans *et al.*, 1970a; Schulze, 1970; Content and Duesberg, 1970; Klenk *et al.*, 1972a). Cell-fractionation studies have provided further information on the sites of glycosylation of the viral glycoproteins. Glucosamine is associated with the HA polypeptide in both the smooth and rough cytoplasmic membrane fractions; however, fucose is associated with HA in the smooth, but not in the rough membranes (Compans, 1973b). Inhibition of protein synthesis by puromycin stops the incorporation of glucosamine almost immediately, whereas fucose continues to be incorporated for approximately 10–15 minutes (Stanley *et al.*, 1973). These observations suggest that biosynthesis of the carbohydrate side chains of viral glycoproteins occurs in stepwise manner, with different saccharide residues added in distinct cellular compartments. Glucosamine appears to be attached to HA polypeptides in rough membranes very soon after synthesis, whereas fucose appears to be attached later by transferases present in smooth membranes.

Studies of the glycoproteins of the GL/1760 strain of influenza B have revealed that the HA_2 polypeptide of this strain contains glucosamine but no detectable fucose, although the HA_1 polypeptide contains both sugars (Choppin *et al.*, 1974). The lack of fucose, which is usually located distally on the carbohydrate side chains of glycoproteins, is compatible with the evidence cited above that glycosylation is completed sequentially after the association of the HA protein with membranes. In addition, the absence of fucose on the HA_2 polypeptide (which is the portion of the hemagglutinin by which the spike is attached to the viral membrane) and its presence on HA_1 suggests that the intimate relationship of the HA_2 polypeptide with the membrane may interfere with glycosylation. Further, since glucosamine is present on HA_2, the absence of fucose may indicate that the hemagglutinin protein may change its relationship to the membrane as it moves from rough to smooth membranes, with the HA_2 portion becoming more intimately associated with the membrane, so that the addition of the distal sugar fucose does not occur.

Little is known about the biosynthesis of the carbohydrate portion of viral glycolipids. It has not been determined whether preformed or newly synthesized glycolipid is preferentially incorporated into the virion.

3.4. Assembly

3.4.1. Nucleocapsid

Because of the small size of the influenza viral RNPs, it has not been possible to identify them with certainty by electron microscopy of infected cells. Clusters of strands or fibers about 6 nm in diameter, observed in the cytoplasm, may represent the viral RNPs (Apostolov *et al.*, 1970; Compans *et al.*, 1970*b*). However, viral RNPs can be isolated from both the nucleus and cytoplasm (Krug, 1971, 1972). The cytoplasmic RNPs do not appear to be associated with intracellular membranes (Compans and Caliguiri, 1973). Nucleocapsid protein is rapidly incorporated into viral RNPs. In cells exposed to a 5-minute pulse label, incorporation of amino acid into RNPs was maximal after a 5-minute chase (Krug, 1972). On the other hand, RNA may be incorporated into RNPs from a preformed pool. Cytoplasmic RNPs assembled from 3 to 4 hours post-infection in MDCK cells contained newly synthesized viral RNA as well as complementary RNA synthesized at least 1 hour earlier and present as a pool within the cell (Krug, 1972).

3.4.2. The Budding Process

The first demonstration of virus release from cells by a process not involving lysis was provided by Murphy and Bang (1952) in early electron microscopic studies of influenza virus-infected cells. Filaments and spheres were observed to project from the cell surface into the extracellular space. No virus particles were observed in the interior of cells at times when infective virus was produced, and it therefore appeared that the virus particles were formed at the cell surface. Using ferritin-labeled antibody, Morgan *et al.* (1961) observed that the cell surface contained viral antigen in areas where virus was forming. More recent electron microscopic studies have demonstrated that the envelope of the emerging virus contains a unit membrane like that of the host cell, with a layer of projections, corresponding to the viral spikes, on the outer surface (Fig. 11; Bächi *et al.*, 1969; Compans and Dimmock, 1969). On the inner surface of the viral membrane is an addi-

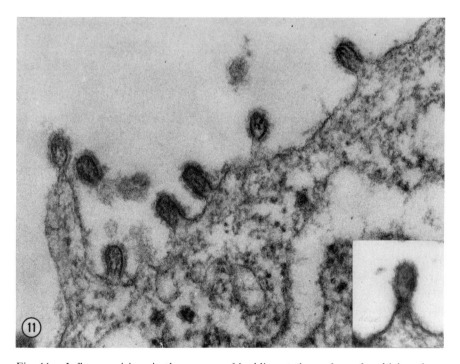

Fig. 11.   Influenza virions in the process of budding at the surface of a chick embryo fibroblast. The particles show electron-dense internal strands and a distinct layer of surface projections, which are absent on the adjacent cell membrane. Inset; budding particle stained in block with uranyl acetate. The unit membrane is resolved, and there is continuity between the layers in the cell membrane and viral envelope. ×112,500. From Compans and Dimmock (1969).

tional electron-dense layer which is not found on the cell surface, and which probably consists of the M polypeptide. This layer has been termed the nanogranular layer (Apostolov *et al.*, 1970) or the viral basic membrane (Compans and Dimmock, 1969).

Electron microscopic observations have provided suggestive evidence for the order in which viral components associate at the cell surface prior to maturation (Compans and Dimmock, 1969; Bächi *et al.*, 1969; Compans *et al.*, 1970b). Viral envelope proteins appear first to be incorporated into areas of membrane which appear to be of normal morphology; however, specific adsorption of erythrocytes is observed to such regions of membrane. The membrane (M) protein then presumably associates with the inner surface of such regions of membranes, forming an electron-dense layer. The RNP then binds specifically to the membrane in such regions, and the process of budding occurs by an out-folding and pinching off of a segment of the membrane, enclosing the associated nucleoprotein. Polyacrylamide gel electrophoresis studies, as described above (Sect. 3.3) also support the idea that envelope proteins associate with the plasma membrane more rapidly than the RNP (Lazarowitz *et al.*, 1971). Host cell polypeptides are excluded from those regions of the membrane which are precursors of the viral envelope, since such polypeptides are not detected in purified virions (see Sect. 2.2).

Neuraminic acid residues, which can be stained with colloidal iron hydroxide, are absent in the envelopes of budding influenza virus particles, but are present in the adjacent cell membrane (Klenk *et al.*, 1970). The lack of neuraminic acid is presumed to be due to viral neuraminidase; vesicular stomatitis virus, which possesses no neuraminidase, was found to contain neuraminic acid bound to both glycoproteins (Burge and Huang, 1970; McSharry and Wagner, 1971) and glycolipids (Klenk and Choppin, 1971). These observations establish that there is an abrupt transition in chemical composition between the envelope of a budding virus particle and the adjacent cell membrane. In an early study of emerging influenza virus filaments using wholemount preparations it was observed that there was a sharp line of demarcation at the base of the filaments (Fig. 12), and this was interpreted at that time as indicating an abrupt transition between the budding virion and the surrounding cell membrane (Choppin, 1963).

The above observations suggest that the precursor to the envelope of a budding virion is a patch of cell membrane containing viral envelope proteins. Various mechanisms are possible for the formation of such patches of membrane, including either insertion of soluble polypeptides directly into the plasma membrane or fusion with the cell surface membrane of preformed cytoplasmic membranes containing

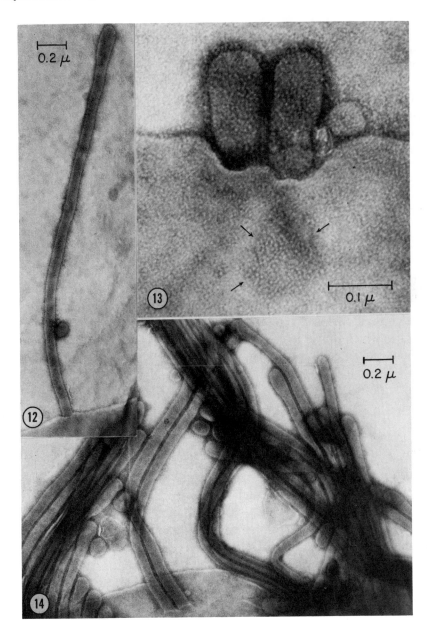

Fig. 12. Whole-mount preparations of influenza virus particles (RI/5+ strain) emerging from rhesus monkey kidney cells. From Choppin (1963). A single filamentous particle emerging from the cell surface. The area around the base is slightly elevated and there is a sharp line of demarcation at the base of the filament. ×38,400.

Fig. 13. Two virus particles emerging in close proximity. The area indicated by arrows shows surface projections and appears to represent a particle that is beginning to emerge. ×168,000.

Fig. 14. Influenza filaments emerging in groups from the cell surface. ×38,400.

viral polypeptides. The fact that all of the viral envelope polypeptides can be found in association with smooth cytoplasmic membranes is compatible with the idea that such membranes may serve as precursors to the viral envelope (Compans, 1973a,b; Klenk *et al.*, 1974). Further information is needed to demonstrate that the components associated with the intracellular membranes do indeed function as virion precursors. More information is also needed to determine the pathway by which the M protein arrives at the membrane, and the mechanism by which the glycoproteins and internal proteins specifically associate prior to the budding process.

3.4.3. Packaging of a Segmented Genome

Extensive biochemical, biophysical, and genetic evidence indicates that the RNA genome in influenza virions exists as 5–7 segments (Sect. 2.2). For an infective particle to be formed it is therefore necessary for one copy of each segment to be present in a virion. Among the possibilities which have been considered for the process of packaging ribonucleoproteins are linkage of the segments by means of interactions between RNAs or protein, or random incorporation of segments into virions. Pons (1970) proposed that the viral RNA segments remain associated during replication by means of a continuous backbone of protein. The finding of complementary RNA associated with intracellular RNPs (Pons, 1971; Krug, 1972) is compatible with this model since they could represent templates for virion RNA synthesis linked together by a protein backbone. To date, however, no evidence for linkage of RNPs during replication has been obtained.

It has alternatively been proposed that RNPs are incorporated randomly into virions from the intracellular pool (Hirst, 1962). The proportion of infective virions in a population may be increased by incorporation of extra pieces of RNA into the average virion (Compans *et al.*, 1970b). For example, if five different pieces of RNA were needed for infectivity, but each virion contained a total of seven pieces incorporated at random, then about 22% of the virions would be infectious. Evidence in favor of random incorporation of RNA segments has been provided by the recent observations of Hirst (1973) that recombination occurs between non-plaque-forming particles in virus populations. The ability of non-plaque-forming particles to undergo recombination can be explained by absence of one or more pieces from the particles, with the missing pieces varying from one particle to another; thus, suitable pairs of defective virus can form recombinants. This concept has been supported further by the experiments of Hirst and Pons (1973) showing that aggregates of influenza virions which either occur normally or are produced with nucleohistone have an enhanced infectivity. Such results are compatible with complementation by two or more virus particles each of which alone contains less than the number of RNA pieces required to induce infection. Random incorporation of RNA into virions is also compatible with the variation in viral RNA profiles at different times of harvest (Barry *et al.*, 1970) and the production of "incomplete" virus which is missing the largest RNA species (Sect. 4.2).

3.5. Release

A number of studies have been carried out on the final process of release of virus from infected cells, i.e., transfer of fully formed virus from a cell-associated state to the culture medium. Cairns and Mason (1953) observed that infectious virus remained at the cell surface for about an hour before it was released into the allantoic fluid. It has been considered likely that the viral neuraminidase might function in this release process. This idea was supported by the ability of antibody specific for neuraminidase to inhibit release of virus (Seto and Rott, 1966; Webster *et al.*, 1968). In addition, such antibody prevents elution of virus from erythrocytes (Brown and Laver, 1968). Bacterial neuraminidase, which is not inhibited by antibody to viral neuraminidase, is able to cause release of virus from antibody-treated cells (Compans *et al.*, 1969; Webster, 1970). However, bivalent antibody to neuraminidase also causes virus aggregation (Seto and Chang, 1969; Compans *et al.*, 1969; Webster, 1970), and Becht *et al.* (1971) have suggested that the primary effect of bivalent antibody was to cross-link virus to antigens present on the cell surface. In support of this, they observed that monovalent antibody obtained by papain treatment did not prevent virus release, although it inhibited over 90% of the neuraminidase activity. Cells infected with mutants defective in neuraminidase produce virus particles containing neuraminic acid which form large aggregates, reducing the yield of released virus (Palese *et al.*, 1974). Thus the viral neuraminidase prevents such aggregation.

4. INCOMPLETE VIRUS FORMATION

4.1. Biological Properties

Noninfectious hemagglutinating particles are produced in most influenza virus–cell systems under conditions of high-multiplicity inoculation, and such particles have been termed "incomplete" virus (von Magnus, 1954). The formation of incomplete virus has also been referred to as the "von Magnus effect." There is a progressive drop in the infectivity-to-hemagglutinin ratio with serial undiluted passages in the egg (von Magnus, 1954). By the third undiluted passage, no increase in infectivity over the inoculum level is observed, although the hemagglutinin titer increases to high levels. The infectivity-to-hemagglutinin ratio of this passage is approximately 10^2, which is 10,000-fold lower than virus yields obtained by low-multiplicity inoculation ("standard" virus). Since hemagglutinin is a measure of the number of physical particles possessing hemagglutinin spikes, these results indicate that undiluted passage causes the production of large numbers of noninfectious particles. On continued passage beyond the fourth serial undiluted passage, the infectivity titer increases for several passages and then declines for several passages in a cyclical pattern. The eventual increase in titer presumably results from a previous passage in which virus yields have declined to a sufficiently low level that low-multiplicity inoculation results.

4.2. Host Cell Dependence

The amount of infectious and noninfectious virus produced in one or several serial passages depends on the particular host cell. In contrast to most cells, it was observed that the MDBK line of bovine kidney cells produces a high yield of infectious virus when inoculated at high multiplicity (Choppin, 1969). Not only the first, but also the second undiluted passage resulted in a high yield. Three serial undiluted passages were required before a marked reduction in the infectivity-to-hemagglutinin ratio was observed. Thus, the von Magnus phenomenon occurs to a much lower degree in MDBK cells.

The yield of virus depends not only on the cell which is producing virus, but on the cell type in which the inoculum virus is grown (Choppin, 1969). Influenza virus stocks grown in MDBK cells produce relatively high yields when used as inoculum at high or low multiplicity in chick fibroblasts, monkey kidney cells, or the allantoic sac of the chick embryo. In contrast, when egg-grown virus is used as inoculum at high multiplicity, much lower yields of infectious virus are produced in these cells, and the infectivity-to-hemagglutinin ratios are about 100-fold lower than those obtained with MDBK-grown virus as inoculum. These results indicate that MDBK cell-grown virus, in addition to containing a high level of infectious virus, contains relatively little incomplete

virus that is capable of causing low yields when the virus is used as inoculum in other cell types.

4.3. Morphological and Biochemical Properties

Early studies suggested that incomplete virus sedimented at about
500 S, whereas standard virus sedimented at 700 S (Von Magnus,
1959). By electron microscopy it was observed that incomplete virus
was markedly pleomorphic (Birch-Andersen and Paucker, 1959;
Morgan *et al.*, 1962; Moore *et al.*, 1962); large particles, with their surface subunits in a square array, were also occasionally observed
(Almeida and Waterson, 1970). In view of the recent evidence that the
neuraminidase has a tetrameric structure (Wrigley *et al.*, 1973), it
seems likely that the surfaces are covered with neuraminidase spikes in
such regions. The relationship of this observation to the von Magnus
phenomenon is not clear.

The most significant biochemical observation on incomplete influenza virus particles concerns the viral RNA. It was observed that
the RNA content per particle was lower, on the average, in incomplete-virus than in standard-virus populations (Ada and Perry, 1956).
Because incomplete virus did not undergo multiplicity reactivation,
Rott and Scholtissek (1963) concluded that a similar RNA defect was
present in each particle. This was confirmed by polyacrylamide gel
electrophoresis studies which indicated that the largest RNA species
were absent from the incomplete virus population and that there was
an increase in the amount of small, heterogeneous RNAs (Duesberg,
1968; Pons and Hirst, 1969; Choppin and Pons, 1970). No differences
have been detected in the proteins of standard and incomplete virus
(Pons and Hirst, 1969).

4.4. Mechanism of Incomplete Virus Formation

A possible mechanism which explains the production and
properties of incomplete virus has been discussed by Choppin and Pons
(1970): If the pieces of influenza viral RNA are replicated independently by the same polymerase, small pieces could be replicated
more rapidly than large pieces. Thus, there would be a tendency to
produce more small RNAs than larger RNAs in an infected cell. If
RNA is incorporated into progeny virions at random, an excess of
smaller pieces would be expected in the virus population. Thus, some

virions might be expected to lack the large RNAs and contain only smaller RNAs. Upon high-multiplicity inoculation, cells will be infected not only with complete, infectious particles, but also with such defective particles. Thus, the initial pool of RNAs to be replicated in such cells will already contain an excess of small RNAs. A successive increase in incomplete virus on serial undiluted passage can be explained by this mechanism. On diluted passage, defective and complete particles would initially infect different cells, and the RNAs of the defective particles would, therefore, not contribute to the pool of RNAs in those cells which give rise to the initial progeny. The precise mechanisms of incomplete virus formation remain to be determined; however, whatever the eventual explanation, it must account not only for the changes that occur in the RNA content, but also for the host cell effects on this process.

4.5.   Abortive Infection

In addition to the incomplete virus formation of the von Magnus type produced by serial passage at high multiplicity, abortive infection has been observed in which noninfective hemagglutinating particles are produced. Examples of such abortive infections with influenza virus are those which have been described in HeLa cells (Henle et al., 1955; Hillis et al., 1960; White et al., 1965) and L cells (Franklin and Breitenfeld, 1959; Rott and Scholtissek, 1963). In these infections, the nucleoprotein antigen is synthesized and accumulates in the nucleus, and noninfective hemagglutinating particles are produced which contain less than the normal amount of viral nucleoprotein. These features of abortive infection are similar to those seen in the von Magnus phenomenon. In addition, Choppin and Pons (1970) found that the noninfective particles produced by HeLa cells show the same defects in their RNA content as incomplete virus, i.e., loss of the largest piece and an increased amount of small, heterogeneous pieces of RNA. Further, it was found that if a virus inoculum was used which had been grown in MDBK cells, and thus contained relatively little incomplete virus, HeLa cells could produce infective virus.

On the basis of the similarities between abortive infection and incomplete-virus formation, it was proposed (Choppin and Pons, 1970) that abortive infection and incomplete virus formation could be considered as a phenomenon which occurs over a spectrum ranging from the relatively "complete" virus produced in MDBK cells, through the incomplete virus produced by serial high-multiplicity passages, to the extreme of the noninfectious virus produced by HeLa or L cells. As indicated above, the mechanism by which the host cell affects the formation of noninfective virions has not yet been elucidated.

5.   VIRUS EFFECTS ON CELLS

5.1.   Alterations in Biosynthesis

Influenza virus infection does not cause a rapid shut off in host cell RNA synthesis; however, several effects of RNA and protein metabolism have been described. An early increase in RNA synthesis and increased DNA-dependent RNA polymerase activity have been observed in chick fibroblasts infected with fowl plague virus (Borland and Mahy, 1968; Mahy, 1970). Using the drug α-amanitin which inhibits nucleoplasmic DNA-dependent RNA polymerase (form II) and not the nucleolar RNA polymerase (form I), Mahy et al. (1972) observed a decrease in RNA polymerase I to less than 20% of that of the controls by 3–4 hours post-infection. In contrast, polymerase II activity was stimulated to 70% above that of the controls after 1.5. hours. These studies, as well as the finding that α-amanitin inhibits virus multiplication (Rott and Scholtissek, 1970; Mahy et al., 1972) suggest that the activity of polymerase II may be essential in virus replication.

A decrease in the labeling of cytoplasmic RNA species after infection was observed by Stephenson and Dimmock (1974). This was observed by decreased incorporation of uridine into ribosomal RNA species resolved by gel electrophoresis. Synthesis of the initial ribosomal transcript in nucleoli was not inhibited, but there appeared to be degradation of the smaller ribosomal RNA precursors in the nucleus. The observation of apparently normal ribosomal RNA transcription is in apparent disagreement with the observation that DNA-dependent RNA polymerase I is inhibited (Mahy et al., 1972). Alterations in ribosome formation may be related to the morphological changes occurring in nucleoli (Sect. 5.2) and the association of the NS polypeptide with the nucleolus (Sect. 3.3).

The gradual replacement of cellular protein synthesis by synthesis of virus-specific proteins has been described above (Sect. 3.3). The basis for the inhibition of cellular protein synthesis is not clear, although the association of the NS polypeptide with cytoplasmic polysomes (Pons, 1972; Compans, 1973a) may be involved. The finding that NS is dissociated from ribosomal subunits by high salt (Krug and Etkind, 1973) does not necessarily exclude such a role for this polypeptide.

5.2. Morphological Changes

Several types of morphological changes specific for influenza virus infection have been observed by light and electron microscopy. The cytopathic effect of influenza viruses in culture generally consists of rounding and eventual detachment of cells. Nucleoli acquire a spotty appearance, gradually enlarge, and disperse through much of the nuclear area (Niven *et al.*, 1962; Compans and Dimmock, 1969). In the cytoplasm, dense inclusions showing periodic striations of about 5 nm are observed by electron microscopy (Kopp *et al.*, 1968; Compans and Dimmock, 1969; Ciampor, 1972). Cytoplasmic inclusions which appear to contain RNP have been described by ter Meulen and Love (1967), and may correspond to the structures observed by electron microscopy. In monkey kidney cells infected with influenza B viruses, basophilic cytoplasmic inclusions were observed which appeared to consist of aggregates of ribosomes (Porebska *et al.*, 1968). Elongated structures with a striated appearance have also been described in influenza virus-infected cells, occurring mainly in the nucleus but also in the cytoplasm (Archetti *et al.*, 1970; Ciampor, 1972).

5.3. Agglutinability by Lectins

Plant lectins such as wheat germ agglutinin and concanavalin A have been observed to agglutinate transformed cells but not normal cells (Burger and Goldberg, 1967; Inbar and Sachs, 1969). However, cells infected with a variety of enveloped viruses, including influenza, are also agglutinated (Becht *et al.*, 1972). Many cell types can be converted from a nonagglutinable to an agglutinable state by influenza virus infection. Recently, evidence has been obtained showing that lectins are bound to transformed cells in clusters, whereas they bind to normal cells in a more dispersed arrangement (Nicolson, 1972). It has already been pointed out that viral envelope proteins are incorporated into patches on the cell surface, and budding virus particles could also represent such patches of glycoprotein. It is also known that the glycoproteins of influenza virus act as receptors for concanavalin A since this lectin will agglutinate intact influenza virions but not protease-treated virions free of glycoproteins (Klenk *et al.*, 1972a). Thus, infection by influenza virus may render cells agglutinable because clusters of lectin sites, in the form of viral glycoproteins, are present on the surfaces of such cells. It is also possible that the cells become agglutinable because the carbohydrate receptors for the lectins are more accessible on the surface of infected cells than uninfected cells by virtue of these sugars being located on the viral spikes which project from the surface of the membrane.

6. INFLUENZA VIRUS GENETICS

A detailed review of genetics is not within the scope of this chapter; however, a brief summary of some of the observations which relate to virus structure and replication will be given. Genetic recombination with influenza viruses was first described by Burnet and Lind (1951), and subsequently by many other workers. It is important to emphasize that the detection of recombinants requires that two mutants give rise to wild-type virus upon mixed infection, but does not indicate the mechanism of this process. The high frequency with which genetic recombination occurs, together with biochemical data suggesting that the viral RNA might be fragmented, led Hirst (1962) to suggest that the viral genome was fragmented, and that recombination might occur by random incorporation of RNA segments from two genetically compatible parents into progeny virions. Although other markers have provided much useful information (Kilbourne, 1963), most recent studies have involved temperature-sensitive mutants (Simpson and Hirst, 1968; Mackenzie, 1970; Sugiura *et al.*, 1972; Hirst, 1973). In recombination studies, such mutants have fallen into groups in which very high levels of recombination were observed between the groups and essentially no recombination occurred within the groups. Five such recombination groups were detected by Simpson and Hirst (1968) and by Sugiura *et al.* (1972).

Hirst (1973) demonstrated that mixed aggregates could give rise to recombinants by a single-hit process, and that recombinant-yielding cells were also generated by a two-hit mechanism in which noninfectious particles were the principal source of recombinants. The recombinants were obtained in cells incubated solely at restrictive temperatures, indicating that they resulted from complementation followed by reassortment of RNA segments during maturation, which yielded wild-type particles in some cases. A total of eight groups was detected, with recombination occurring at high frequency between groups.

Greater reproducibility in recombination tests was reported by Mackenzie (1970) if cells were treated with a receptor-destroying enzyme immediately after adsorption. This effect was thought to result from removal of particles which had not penetrated, leading to greater synchrony of replication. The recombination frequencies obtained were additive and could be ordered into a linear genetic map. However, Sugiura *et al.* (1972) and Hirst (1973) were not able to arrange their data into a linear map.

Most of the recombination data are clearly compatible with a segmented RNA genome in the influenza virion and random incorporation of RNA into progeny virions. Other genetic interactions which are compatible with this idea include cross reactivation (Simpson and Hirst, 1961) and multiplicity reactivation (Barry, 1961). The general failure of incomplete virus to participate in recombination (Hirst, 1973) is explained by the existence of a common defect in such particles, i.e., the lack of the larger RNA segments. However, it would be expected that incomplete virus should yield recombinants with those mutants which occur on the smaller RNA segments.

7. ANTIGENIC VARIATION

The subject of antigenic variation in influenza viruses has recently been reviewed in detail (Webster and Laver, 1971), and will be considered only very briefly here. Two distinct kinds of antigenic variation have been recognized in influenza A viruses. One has been termed antigenic drift (Burnet, 1955), and appears to be due to gradual mutational changes in viral proteins, presumably due to the selection pressure of antibodies in an immune population. This phenomenon can be demonstrated under laboratory conditions as well (Archetti and Horsfall, 1950; Hamre *et al.*, 1958). Laver and Webster (1968) isolated antigenic variants of influenza virus by passage in the presence of sublimiting concentrations of antiviral antibody, and peptide maps of the hemagglutinin proteins of such variants indicated that one or two tryptic peptides differed, but the remainder were unchanged. The phenomenon of antigenic drift in nature occurs with the neuraminidase as well as the hemagglutinin (Paniker, 1968; Schulman and Kilbourne, 1969; Meier-Ewert *et al.*, 1970), and occurs with the influenza type B viruses as well as with type A.

The second type of variation has been found thus far only with type A influenza viruses, and has been termed major antigenic shift. Such changes occur infrequently and involve the appearance of virus strains with surface antigens which are totally unrelated to those found previously in man. The major shifts give rise to the new subtypes of virus which are responsible for pandemics of influenza in man. Some of the shifts, such as the one in 1968 with the Hong Kong strain, involve the hemagglutinin protein only, whereas the 1957 Asian influenza

A_2 viruses possess a neuraminidase as well as a hemagglutinin which are unrelated to previous viral antigens. Two main theories have been proposed to explain the occurrence of major shifts: (1) direct mutation or (2) recombination between a human and an animal strain. Peptide maps of influenza virus hemagglutinin from different subtypes appear to be completely different, indicating that the amino acid sequences of the polypeptides are unrelated (Laver, 1964; Webster and Laver, 1971). It is difficult to envisage a process by which so many mutations, resulting in different amino acid sequences, would all occur at the same time. Direct mutation of a strain from another animal species provides an alternative possibility. The second possibility which has been considered is recombination between a human and animal strain, with the acquisition by the human strain of new surface antigen(s). As described above, influenza viruses are known to undergo recombination with a high frequency, which is probably due to their segmented genome. Only the type A strains of influenza viruses have been found in other animal species, and it has been possible to isolate antigenic hybrids between animal and human strains in the laboratory (Kilbourne, 1968). It has also been possible to detect recombination between different animal virus strains under conditions of natural infection (Webster *et al.*, 1973). These observations suggest that the major changes in the surface antigens of type A influenza viruses which result in pandemics may be caused by a recombination process between human and animal strains.

ACKNOWLEDGMENTS

We thank Dr. W. G. Laver for electron micrographs and Drs. D. H. L. Bishop, N. J. Dimmock, D. W. Kingsbury, H.-D. Klenk, R. M. Krug, I. T. Schulze, R. W. Simpson, and D. O. White for preprints of manuscripts in press. Research by the authors was supported by research grants No. AI 05600 and AI 10884 from the National Institute of Allergy and Infectious Diseases.

8. REFERENCES

Ada, G. L., and Gottschalk, A., 1956, The component sugars of the influenza-virus particle, *Biochem. J.* **62,** 686.

Ada, G. L., and Perry, B. T., 1954, The nucleic acid content of influenza virus, *Aust. J. Exp. Biol. Med. Sci.* **32,** 453.

Ada, G. L., and Perry, B. T., 1956, Influenza virus nucleic acid: Relationship between biological characteristics of the virus particle and properties of the nucleic acid, *J. Gen. Microbiol.* **14,** 623.

Ada, G. L., Perry, B. T., and Abbot, A., 1958, Biological and physical properties of the Ryan strain of filamentous influenza virus, *J. Gen. Microbiol.* **19,** 23.

Ada, G. L., Lind, P. E., Larkin, L., and Burnet, F. M., 1959, Failure to recover infective ribonucleic acid from myxovirus preparations, *Nature (Lond.)* **184,** 360.

Agrawal, H. O., and Bruening, G., 1966, Isolation of high molecular weight P^{32}-labeled influenza virus ribonucleic acid, *Proc. Natl. Acad. Sci. USA* **55,** 3818.

Almeida, J. D., and Waterson, A. P., 1967, Some observations on the envelope of an influenza virus, *J. Gen. Microbiol.* **46,** 107.

Almeida, J. D., and Waterson, A. P., 1970, Two morphological aspects of influenza virus, *in* "The Biology of Large RNA Viruses" (R. D. Barry and B. W. J. Mahy, eds.), pp. 27–51, Academic Press, New York.

Andrewes, C. H., Bang, F. B., and Burnet, F. M., 1955, A short description of the myxovirus group (influenza and related viruses), *Virology* **1,** 176.

Apostolov, K., and Flewett, T. H., 1969, Further observations on the structure of influenza viruses A and C, *J. Gen. Virol.* **4,** 365.

Apostolov, K., Flewett, T. H., and Kendall, A. P., 1970, Morphology of influenza A, B, C, and infectious bronchitis virus (IBV) virions and their replication, *in* "The Biology of Large RNA Viruses" (R. D. Barry and B. W. J. Mahy, eds.), pp. 3–26, Academic Press, New York.

Archetti, I., and Horsfall, F. L., Jr., 1950, Persistent antigenic variation of influenza A viruses after incomplete neutralization *in ovo* with heterologous immune serum, *J. Exp. Med.* **92,** 441.

Archetti, I., Jemolo, A., and Steve-Bocciarelli, D., 1967, On the fine structure of influenza viruses, *Arch. Ges. Virusforsch.* **20,** 133.

Archetti, I., Bereczky, E., Rosati-Valente, F., and Steve-Bocciarelli, D., 1970, Elongated structures present in cells infected with influenza viruses, *Arch. Ges. Virusforsch.* **29,** 275.

Armbruster, O., and Beiss, U., 1958, Die Untersuchungen der Phosphatidkomponenten von Viren der Influenzagruppe, *Z. Naturforsch.* **13b,** 75.

Bächi, T., Gerhard, W., Lindenmann, J., and Mühlethaler, K., 1969, Morphogenesis of influenza A virus in Ehrlich ascites tumor cells as revealed by thin-sectioning and freeze-etching, *J. Virol.* **4,** 769.

Barry, R. D., 1961, The multiplication of influenza virus. II. Multiplicity reactivation of ultraviolet-irradiated virus, *Virology* **14,** 398.

Barry, R. D., Ives, D. R., and Cruickshank, J. G., 1962, Participation of deoxyribonucleic acid in the multiplication of influenza virus, *Nature (Lond.)* **194,** 1139.

Barry, R. D., Bromley, P. A., and Davies, P., 1970, The characterization of influenza virus RNA, *in* "The Biology of Large RNA Viruses" (R. D. Barry and B. W. J. Mahy, eds.), pp. 279–300, Academic Press, New York.

Bean, W. J., and Simpson, R. W., 1973, Primary transcription of the influenza virus genome in permissive cells, *Virology* **56,** 646.

Becht, H., Hämmerling, U., and Rott, R., 1971, Undisturbed release of influenza virus in the presence of univalent antineuraminidase antibodies, *Virology* **46,** 337.

Becht, W., Rott, R., and Klenk, H.-D., 1972, Effect of concanavalin A on cells infected with enveloped RNA viruses, *J. Gen. Virol.* **14,** 1.

Bellett, A. J. D., 1967, Preliminary classification of viruses based on quantitative comparisons of viral nucleic acids, *J. Virol.* **1,** 245.

Birch-Andersen, A., and Paucker, K., 1959, Studies on the structure of influenza virus. II. Ultrathin sections of infectious and noninfectious particles, *Virology* **8,** 21.

Bishop, D. H. L., Obijeski, J. F., and Simpson, R. W., 1971a, Transcription of the influenza ribonucleic acid genome by a virion polymerase. I. Optimal conditions for *in vitro* activity of the ribonucleic acid-dependent ribonucleic acid polymerase, *J. Virol.* **8**, 66.

Bishop, D. H. L., Obijeski, J. F., and Simpson, R. W., 1971b, Transcription of the influenza ribonucleic acid genome by a virion polymerase. II. Nature of the *in vitro* polymerase product, *J. Virol.* **8**, 74.

Bishop, D. H. L., Roy, P., Bean, W. J., Jr., and Simpson, R. W., 1972, Transcription of the influenza ribonucleic acid genome by a virion polymerase. III. Completeness of the transcription process, *J. Virol.* **10**, 689.

Blough, H. A., 1971, Fatty acid composition of individual phospholipids of influenza virus, *J. Gen. Virol.* **12**, 317.

Blough, H. A., and Merlie, J., 1970, The lipids of incomplete influenza virus, *Virology* **40**, 685.

Blough, H. A., and Tiffany, J. M., 1973, Lipids in viruses, *Adv. Lipid Res.* **11**, 267.

Blough, H. A., Weinstein, D. B., Lawson, D. E. M., and Kodicek, E., 1967, The effects of vitamin A on myxoviruses. II. Alterations in the lipids of influenza virus, *Virology* **33**, 459.

Borland, R., and Mahy, B. W. J., 1968, Deoxyribonucleic acid-dependent ribonucleic acid polymerase activity in cells infected with influenza virus, *J. Virol.* **2**, 33.

Brand, C. M., and Skehel, J. J., 1972, Crystalline antigen from the influenza virus envelope, *Nat. New Biol.* **238**, 145.

Breitenfeld, P. M., and Schäfer, W., 1957, The formation of fowl plague virus antigens in infected cells, as studied by fluorescent antibodies, *Virology* **4**, 328.

Brown, J., and Laver, W. G., 1968, The effect of antineuraminidase antibody on the elution of influenza virus from cells, *J. Gen. Virol.* **2**, 291.

Bucher, D. J., and Kilbourne, E. D., 1972, A_2 (N2) neuraminidase of the X-7 influenza virus recombinant: Determination of molecular size and subunit composition of the active unit, *J. Virol.* **10**, 60.

Burge, B. W., and Huang, A. S., 1970, Comparison of membrane protein glycopeptides of Sindbis virus and vesicular stomatitis virus, *J. Virol.* **6**, 176.

Burger, M. M., and Goldberg, A. R., 1967, Identification of tumor-specific determinant on neoplastic cell surfaces, *Proc. Natl. Acad. Sci. U.S.* **57**, 359.

Burnet, F. M., 1955, "Principles of Animal Virology," p. 380, Academic Press, New York.

Burnet, F. M., 1956, Structure of influenza virus, *Science (Wash., D.C.)* **123**, 1101.

Burnet, F. M., and Lind, P. E., 1951, A genetic approach to variation in influenza viruses 4. Recombination of characters between the influenza virus A strain NWS and strains of different serological subtypes, *J. Gen. Microbiol.* **5**, 67.

Burnet, F. M., and Stone, J. D., 1947, The receptor-destroying enzyme of *V. Cholerae, Aust. J. Exp. Biol. Med.* **25**, 227.

Cairns, H. J. F., and Mason, P. J., 1953, Production of influenza virus in cells of the allantois, *J. Immunol.* **71**, 38.

Caliguiri, L. A., and Compans, R. W., 1974, Analysis of the *in vitro* product of an RNA-dependent RNA polymerase isolated from influenza virus-infected cells, *J. Virol.* **14**, 191.

Caliguiri, L. A., and Tamm, I., 1969, Membranous structures associated with translation and transcription of poliovirus RNA, *Science (Wash., D.C.)* **166**, 885.

Caliguiri, L. A., and Tamm, I., 1970, The role of cytoplasmic membranes in poliovirus biosynthesis, *Virology* **42**, 100.

Cheyne, I. M., and White, D. O., 1969, Growth of paramyxoviruses in anucleate cells, *Aust. J. Exp. Biol. Med. Sci.* **47**, 145.

Choppin, P. W., 1963, Multiplication of two kinds of influenza A_2 virus particles in monkey kidney cells, *Virology* **21**, 342.

Choppin, P. W., 1969, Replication of influenza virus in a continuous cell line: High yield of infective virus from cells inoculated at high multiplicity, *Virology* **38**, 130.

Choppin, P. W., and Pons, M. W., 1970, The RNA's of infective and incomplete influenza virions grown in MDBK and HeLa cells, *Virology* **42**, 603.

Choppin, P. W., and Stoeckenius, W., 1964, Interactions of ether-disrupted influenza A_2 virus from erythrocytes, inhibitors, and antibodies, *Virology* **22**, 482.

Choppin, P. W., and Tamm, I., 1960a, Studies of two kinds of virus particles which comprise influenza A_2 virus strains. I. Characterization of stable homogeneous substrains in reactions with specific antibody, mucoprotein inhibitors, and erythrocytes, *J. Exp. Med.* **112**, 895.

Choppin, P. W., and Tamm, I., 1970b, Studies of two kinds of virus particles which comprise influenza A_2 virus strains. II. Reactivity with virus inhibitors in normal sera, *J. Exp. Med.* **112**, 921.

Choppin, P. W., and Tamm, I., 1964, Genetic variants of influenza virus which differ in reactivity with receptors and antibodies, *in* "Ciba Foundation Symposium, Cellular Biology of Myxovirus Infections," Little, Brown and Co., Boston.

Choppin, P. W., Murphy, J. S., and Tamm, I., 1960, Studies of two kinds of virus particles which comprise influenza A_2 virus strains. III. Morphological characteristics: Independence of morphological and functional traits, *J. Exp. Med.* **112**, 945.

Choppin, P. W., Murphy, J. S., and Stoeckenius, W., 1961, The surface structure of influenza virus filaments, *Virology* **13**, 548.

Choppin, P. W., Klenk, H.-D., Compans, R. W., and Caliguiri, L. A., 1971, The parainfluenza virus SV5 and its relationship to the cell membrane, *Perspect. Virol.* **7**, 127.

Choppin, P. W., Lazarowitz, S. G., and Goldberg, A. R., 1974, Studies on proteolytic cleavage and glycosylation of the hemagglutinin of influenza A and B viruses, *in* "Negative Strand Viruses" (R. D. Barry and B. W. J. Mahy, eds.), Academic Press, New York, in press.

Chow, N., and Simpson, R. W., 1971, RNA dependent RNA polymerase activity associated with virions and subviral components of myxoviruses, *Proc. Natl. Acad. Sci. USA* **68**, 752.

Chu, C. M., Dawson, I. M., and Elford, W. J., 1949, Filamentous forms associated with newly isolated influenza virus, *Lancet* **I**, 602.

Ciampor, F., 1972, Electron microscopy of tissue culture cells infected with myxoviruses. I. Nucleo-cytoplasmic changes in A_0/WSN influenza virus-infected chick embryo cells, *Acta Virol.* **16**, 9.

Compans, R. W., 1973a, Influenza virus proteins. II. Association with components of the cytoplasm, *Virology* **51**, 56.

Compans, R. W., 1973b, Distinct carbohydrate components of influenza virus glycoproteins in smooth and rough cytoplasmic membranes, *Virology* **55**, 541.

Compans, R. W., and Caliguiri, L. A., 1973, Isolation and properties of an RNA polymerase from influenza virus-infected cells, *J. Virol.* **11**, 441.

Compans, R. W., and Choppin, P. W., 1971, The structure and assembly of influenza and parainfluenza viruses, *in* "Comparative Virology" (K. Maramorosch and F. Kurstak, eds.), pp. 407–432, Academic Press, New York.

Compans, R. W., and Choppin, P. W., 1973, Orthomyxoviruses and paramyxoviruses, *in* "Ultrastructure of Animal Viruses and Bacteriophages" (A. J. Dalton and F. Haguenau, eds.), pp. 213–237, Academic Press, New York.

Compans, R. W., and Dimmock, N. J., 1969, An electron microscopic study of single-cycle infection of chick embryo fibroblasts by influenza virus, *Virology* **39**, 499.

Compans, R. W., Dimmock, N. J., and Meier-Ewert, H., 1969, Effect of antibody to neuraminidase on the maturation and hemagglutinating activity of an influenza virus A₂, *J. Virol.* **4**, 528.

Compans, R. W., Klenk, H.-D., Caliguiri, L. A., and Choppin, P. W., 1970*a*, Influenza virus proteins. I. Analysis of polypeptides of the virion and identification of spike glycoproteins, *Virology* **42**, 880.

Compans, R. W., Dimmock, N. J., and Meier-Ewert, H., 1970*b*, An electron microscopic study of the influenza virus-infected cell, *in* "The Biology of Large RNA Viruses" (R. D. Barry and B. W. J. Mahy, eds.), pp. 87–108, Academic Press, New York.

Compans, R. W., Content, J., and Duesberg, P. H., 1972*a*, Structure of the ribonucleoprotein of influenza virus, *J. Virol.* **10**, 795.

Compans, R. W., Landsberger, F. R., Lenard, J., and Choppin, P. W., 1972*b*, Structure of the membrane of influenza virus, *in* "International Virology 2" (J. L. Melnick, ed.), pp. 130–132, S. Karger, Basel.

Content, J., and Duesberg, P. H., 1970, Electrophoretic distribution of the proteins and glycoproteins of influenza virus and Sendai virus, *J. Virol.* **6**, 707.

Content, J., and Duesberg, P. H., 1971, Base sequence differences among the ribonucleic acids of influenza virus, *J. Mol. Biol.* **62**, 273.

Dales, S., 1973, Early events in cell–animal virus interactions, *Bacteriol. Rev.* **37**, 103.

Dales, S., and Choppin, P. W., 1962, Attachment and penetration of influenza virus, *Virology* **18**, 489.

Davies, P., and Barry, R. D., 1966, Nucleic acid of influenza virus, *Nature (Lond.)* **211**, 384.

Dimmock, N. J., 1969, New virus-specific antigens in cells infected with influenza virus, *Virology* **39**, 224.

Dimmock, N. J., and Watson, D. H., 1969, Proteins specified by influenza virus in infected cells: Analysis by polyacrylamide gel electrophoresis of antigens not present in the virus particle, *J. Gen. Virol.* **5**, 499.

Dourmashkin, R. R., and Tyrrell, D. A. J., 1970, Attachment of two myxoviruses to ciliated epithelial cells, *J. Gen. Virol.* **9**, 77.

Duesberg, P. H., 1968, The RNA's of influenza virus, *Proc. Natl. Acad. Sci. USA* **59**, 930.

Duesberg, P. H., 1969, Distinct subunits of the ribonucleoprotein of influenza virus, *J. Mol. Biol.* **42**, 485.

Duesberg, P. H., and Robinson, W. S., 1967, On the structure and replication of influenza virus, *J. Mol. Biol.* **25**, 383.

Elford, W. J., Andrewes, C. H., and Tang, F. F., 1936, The sizes of the viruses of human and swine influenza as determined by ultrafiltration, *Brit. J. Exp. Pathol.* **17**, 51.

Etchison, J., Doyle, M., Penhoet, E., and Holland, J., 1971, Synthesis and cleavage of influenza virus proteins, *J. Virol.* **7**, 155.

Fazekas de St. Groth, S., 1948, Viropexis: The mechanism of influenza virus infection, *Nature (Lond.)* **162**, 294.

Franklin, R. M., and Breitenfeld, P. M., 1959, The abortive infection of Earle's L-cells by fowl plague virus, *Virology* **8**, 293.

Frisch-Niggemeyer, W., and Hoyle, L., 1956, The nucleic acid and carbohydrate content of influenza virus A and of virus fractions produced by ether disintegration, *J. Hyg.* **54,** 201.

Frommhagen, L. H., Knight, C. A., and Freeman, N. K., 1959, The ribonucleic acid, lipid and polysaccharide constituents of influenza virus preparations, *Virology* **8,** 176.

Gandhi, S. S., and Burke, D. C., 1970, Viral nucleic acids and interferon formation: Interferon formation by myxoviruses, *in* "The Biology of Large RNA Viruses" (R. D. Barry and B. W. J. Mahy, eds.), pp. 675–683, Academic Press, New York.

Gandhi, S. S., Stanley, P., Taylor, J. M., and White, D. O., 1972, Inhibition of influenza viral glycoprotein synthesis by sugars, *Microbios.* **5,** 41.

Goldstein, E. A., and Pons, M. W., 1970, The effect of polyvinylsulfate on the ribonucleoprotein of influenza virus, *Virology* **41,** 382.

Gottschalk, A., 1957, Neuraminidase: The specific enzyme of influenza virus and *Vibrio cholerae, Biochim. Biophys. Acta* **23,** 645.

Gottschalk, A., 1965, Interaction between glycoproteins and viruses, *in* "The Amino Sugars" (E. A. Balazs and R. W. Jeanloz, eds.), p. 337, Academic Press, New York.

Gregoriades, A., 1970, Actinomycin D and influenza virus multiplication in the chick embryo fibroblast, *Virology* **42,** 905.

Gregoriades, A., 1972, Isolation of neuraminidase from the WSN strain of influenza virus, *Virology* **49,** 333.

Gregoriades, A., 1973, The membrane protein of influenza virus: Extraction from virus and infected cell with acidic chloroform-methanol, *Virology* **54,** 369.

Griffith, I. P., 1974, The fine structure of influenza virus, *in* "Negative Strand Viruses" (R. D. Barry and B. W. J. Mahy, eds.), Academic Press, New York, in press.

Hamre, D., Loosli, C. G., and Gerber, P., 1958, Antigenic variants of influenza A virus (PR8 strain). IV. Serological characteristics of a second line of variants developed in mice given a polyvalent vaccine, *J. Exp. Med.* **107,** 845.

Harboe, A., 1963*a*, The influenza virus hemagglutination inhibition by antibody to host material, *Acta Pathol. Microbiol. Scand.* **57,** 317.

Harboe, A., 1963*b*, The normal allantoic antigen which neutralizes the influenza virus HI-antibody to host material, *Acta Pathol. Microbiol. Scand.* **57,** 488.

Haslam, E. A., Hampson, A. W., Egan, J. A., and White, D. O., 1970, The polypeptides of influenza virus. II. Interpretation of polyacrylamide gel electrophoresis patterns, *Virology* **42,** 555.

Hastie, N. D., and Mahy, B. W. J., 1973, RNA-dependent RNA polymerase in nuclei of cells infected with influenza virus, *J. Virol.* **12,** 951.

Hefti, E., Roy, P., and Bishop, D. H. L., 1974, The initiation of transcription by influenza virion transcriptase, *in* "Negative Strand Viruses" (R. D. Barry and B. W. J. Mahy, eds.), Academic Press, New York, in press.

Henle, G., Girardi, A., and Henle, W., 1955, A non-transmissible cytopathogenic effect of influenza virus in tissue culture accompanied by formation of non-infectious hemagglutinins, *J. Exp. Med.* **101,** 25.

Hillis, W. D., Moffat, M. A. J., and Holtermann, O. A., 1960, The development of soluble (s) and viral (v) antigens of influenza A virus in tissue culture as studied by the fluorescent antibody technique. 3. Studies on the abortive cycle of replication in HeLa cells, *Acta Pathol. Microbiol. Scand.* **50,** 419.

Hirst, G. K., 1941, The agglutination of red cells by allantoic fluid of chick embryos infected with influenza virus, *Science (Wash., D.C.)* **94,** 22.

Hirst, G. K., 1942, Adsorption of influenza hemagglutinins and virus by red blood cells, *J. Exp. Med.* **76,** 195.

Hirst, G. K., 1962, Genetic recombination with Newcastle disease virus, poliovirus and influenza, *Cold Spring Harbor Symp. Quant. Biol.* **27**, 303.

Hirst, G. K., 1973, Mechanism of influenza virus recombination. I. Factor influencing recombination rates between temperature-sensitve mutants of strain WSN and the classification of mutants into complementation-recombination groups, *Virology* **55**, 81.

Hirst, G. K., and Pons, M., 1972, Biological activity in ribonucleoprotein fractions of influenza virus, *Virology* **47**, 546.

Hirst, G. K., and Pons, M. W., 1973, Mechanism of influenza virus recombination. II. Virus aggregation and its effect on plaque formation by so-called noninfectious virus, *Virology* **56**, 620.

Ho, P. P. K., and Walters, C. P., 1966, Influenza virus-induced ribonucleic acid nucleotidyl transferase and the effect of actinomycin D on its formation, *Biochemistry* **5**, 231.

Holland, J. J., and Kiehn, E. D., 1970, Influenza virus effects on cell membrane proteins, *Science (Wash., D.C.)* **167**, 202.

Holtermann, O. A., Hillis, W. D., and Moffat, M. A. J., 1960, The development of soluble (s) and viral (v) antigens of influenza A virus in tissue culture as studied by the fluorescent antibody technique, *Acta Pathol. Microbiol Scand.* **50**, 398.

Horne, R. W., Waterson, A. P., Wildy, P., and Farnham, A. E., 1960, The structure and composition of the myxoviruses. I. Electron microscope studies of the structure of the myxovirus particles by negative staining techniques, *Virology* **11**, 79.

Horst, J., Content, J., Mandeles, S., Fraenkel-Conrat, H., and Duesberg, P., 1972, Distinct oligonucleotide patterns of distinct influenza virus RNA's, *J. Mol. Biol.* **69**, 209.

Hoyle, L., 1952, Structure of influenza virus. The relation between the biological activity and the chemical structure of virus fractions, *J. Hyg.* **50**, 229.

Hoyle, L., Horne, R. W., and Waterson, A. P., 1961, The structure and composition of the myxoviruses. II. Components released from the influenza virus particle by ether, *Virology* **13**, 448.

Inbar, M., and Sachs, L., 1969, Interaction of the carbohydrate-binding protein concanavalin A with normal and transformed cells, *Proc. Natl. Acad. Sci. USA* **63**, 1418.

Joss, A., Gandhi, S. S., Hay, A. J., and Burke, D. C., 1969, Ribonucleic acid and protein synthesis in chick embryo cells infected with fowl plague virus, *J. Virol.* **4**, 816.

Kaluza, G., Scholtissek, C., and Rott, R., 1972, Inhibition of the multiplication of enveloped RNA-viruses by glucosamine and 2-deoxy-D-glucose, *J. Gen. Virol.* **14**, 251.

Kates, J. R., and McAuslan, B. R., 1967, Poxvirus DNA-dependent RNA polymerase, *Proc. Natl. Acad. Sci. USA* **58**, 134.

Kates, M., Allison, A. C., Tyrrell, D. A., and James, A. T., 1961, Lipids of influenza virus and their relation to those of the host cell, *Biochim. Biophys. Acta* **52**, 455.

Kates, M., Allison, A. C., Tyrrell, D. A., and James, A. T., 1962, Origin of lipids in influenza virus, *Cold Spring Harbor Symp. Quant. Biol.* **27**, 293.

Kelly, D. C., and Dimmock, N. J., 1974, Rescue of influenza virus multiplication in actinomycin D-treated cells by fusion with avian erythrocytes, *in* "Negative Strand Viruses" (R. D. Barry and B. W. J. Mahy, eds.), Academic Press, New York, in press.

Kendal, A. P., and Eckert, E. A., 1972, The preparation and properties of ^{14}C-carboxamindomethylated subunits from A2/1957 influenza neuraminidase, *Biochim. Biophys. Acta* **258**, 484.

Kendal, A. P., Biddle, F., and Belyavin, G., 1968, Influenza virus neuraminidase and the viral surface, *Biochim Biophys. Acta* **165**, 419.

Kilbourne, E. D., 1959, Inhibition of influenza virus multiplication with a glucose antimetabolite (2-deoxy-D-glucose), *Nature (Lond.)* **183**, 271.

Kilbourne, E. D., 1963, Influenza virus genetics, *Prog. Med. Virol.* **5**, 79.

Kilbourne, E. D., 1968, Recombination of influenza A viruses of human and animal
origin, *Science (Wash., D.C.)* **160**, 74.

Kilbourne, E. D., and Murphy, J. S., 1960, Genetic studies of influenza virus. I. Viral
morphology and growth capacity as exchangeable genetic traits. Rapid *in ovo*
adaptation of early passage Asian strain isolated by combination with PR8, *J. Exp.
Med.* **111**, 387.

Kilbourne, E. D., Laver, W. G., Schulman, J. L., and Webster, R. G., 1968, Antiviral
activity of antiserum specific for an influenza virus neuraminidase, *J. Virol.* **2**, 281.

Kilbourne, E. D., Choppin, P. W., Schulze, I. T., Scholtissek, C., and Bucher, D. J.,
1972, Influenza virus polypeptides and antigens (Summary of Influenza Workshop
I.), *J. Infect. Dis.* **125**, 447.

Kingsbury, D. W., and Webster, R. G., 1973, Cell-free translation of influenza virus
messenger RNA, *Virology* **56**, 654.

Klenk, E., Faillard, H., and Lempfrid, H., 1955, "Über die enzymatische Wirkung von
Influenzavirus, *Physiol. Chem.* **301**, 235.

Klenk, H.-D., and Choppin, P. W., 1969, Lipids of plasma membranes of monkey and
hamster kidney cells and of parainfluenza virions grown in these cells, *Virology* **38**,
255.

Klenk, H.-D., and Choppin, P. W., 1970*a*, Plasma membrane lipids and parainfluenza
virus assembly, *Virology* **40**, 939.

Klenk, H.-D., and Choppin, P. W., 1970*b*, Glycosphingolipids of plasma membranes
of cultured cells and an enveloped virus (SV5) grown in these cells, *Proc. Natl.
Acad. Sci. USA* **66**, 57.

Klenk, H.-D., and Choppin, P. W., 1971, Glycolipid content of vesicular stomatitis
virus grown in baby hamster kidney cells, *J. Virol.* **7**, 416.

Klenk, H.-D., and Choppin, P. W., 1974, A comparison of the lipids of two strains of
influenza virus with those of infected and uninfected cells, in preparation.

Klenk, H.-D., and Rott, R., 1973, Formation of influenza virus proteins, *J. Virol.* **11**,
823.

Klenk, H.-D., Compans, R. W., and Choppin, P. W., 1970, An electron microscope
study of the presence or absence of neuraminic acid in enveloped viruses, *Virology*
42, 1158.

Klenk, H.-D., Rott, R., and Becht, H., 1972*a*, On the structure of the influenza virus
envelope, *Virology* **47**, 579.

Klenk, H.-D., Scholtissek, C., and Rott, R., 1972*b*, Inhibition of glycoprotein biosynthesis of influenza virus by D-glucosamine and 2-deoxy-D-glucose, *Virology* **49**, 723.

Klenk, H.-D., Wöllert, W., Rott, R., and Scholtissek, C., 1974, Association of influenza virus proteins with cytoplasmic fractions *Virology* **47**, 28.

Knight, C. A., 1946, Precipitin reactions of highly purified influenza viruses and related materials, *J. Exp. Med.* **83**, 281.

Kopp, J. V., Kempf, J. E., and Kroeger, A. V., 1968, Cytoplasmic inclusions observed
by electron microscopy late in influenza virus infection of chicken embryo fibroblasts, *Virology* **36**, 681.

Krizanova, O., and Rathova, V., 1969, Serum inhibitors of myxoviruses, *Curr. Top.
Microbiol. Immunol.* **47**, 125.

Krug, R. M., 1971, Influenza viral RNP's newly synthesized during the latent period
of growth in MDCK cells, *Virology* **44**, 125.

Krug, R. M., 1972, Cytoplasmic and nucleoplasmic viral RNPs in influenza virus-infected MDCK cells, *Virology* **50**, 103.

Krug, R. M. and Etkind, P. R., 1973, Cytoplasmic and nuclear virus-specific proteins in influenza virus-infected MDCK cells, *Virology* **56**, 334.

Laine, R., Kettungen, M.-L., Gahmberg, C. G., Kääräinen, L., and Renkonen, O., 1972, Fatty chains of different lipid classes of Semliki forest virus and host cell membranes, *J. Virol.* **10**, 433.

Landsberger, F. R., Lenard, J., Paxton, J., and Compans, R. W., 1971, Spin label ESR study of the lipid-containing membrane of influenza virus, *Proc. Natl. Acad. Sci. USA* **68**, 2579.

Landsberger, F. R., Compans, R. W., Choppin, P. W., and Lenard, J. L., 1973, Organization of the lipid phase in viral membranes. Effects of independent variation of the lipid and the protein composition, *Biochemistry* **12**, 4498.

Lauffer, M. A., and Stanley, W. M., 1944, Biophysical properties of preparations of PR8 influenza virus, *J. Exp. Med.* **80**, 531.

Laver, W. G., 1964, Structural studies on the protein subunits from three strains of influenza virus, *J. Mol. Biol.* **9**, 109.

Laver, W. G., 1971, Separation of two polypeptide chains from the hemagglutinin subunit of influenza virus, *Virology* **45**, 275.

Laver, W. G., and Valentine, R. C., 1969, Morphology of the isolated hemagglutinin and neuraminidase subunits of influenza virus, *Virology* **38**, 105.

Laver, W. G., and Webster, R. G., 1966, The structure of influenza viruses. IV. Chemical studies of the host antigen, *Virology* **30**, 104.

Laver, W. G., and Webster, R. G., 1968, Selection of antigenic mutants of influenza viruses. Isolation and peptide mapping of their haemagglutinating proteins, *Virology* **34**, 193.

Lazarowitz, S. G., Compans, R. W., and Choppin, P. W., 1971, Influenza virus structural and non-structural proteins in infected cells and their plasma membranes, *Virology* **46**, 830.

Lazarowitz, S. G., Compans, R. W., and Choppin, P. W., 1973*a*, Proteolytic cleavage of the hemagglutinin polypeptide of influenza virus. Function of the uncleaved polypeptide HA, *Virology* **52**, 199.

Lazarowitz, S. G., Goldberg, A. R., and Choppin, P. W., 1973*b*, Proteolytic cleavage by plasmin of the HA polypeptide of influenza virus. Host cell activation of serum plasminogen, *Virology* **56**, 172.

Lazdins, I., Haslam, E. A., and White, D. O., 1972, The polypeptides of influenza virus. VI. Composition of the neuraminidase, *Virology* **49**, 758.

Lee, L. T., Howe, C., Meyer, K., and Choi, H. U., 1969, Quantitative precipitin analysis of influenza virus host antigen and of sulfated polysaccharides of chicken embryonic allantoic fluid, *J. Immunol.* **102**, 1144.

Lenard, J., Wong, C. Y., and Compans, R. W., 1974, Evidence for a close association of the internal membrane protein with the lipid bilayer in influenza virus, *Biochim. Biophys. Acta,* **332**, 341.

Lewandowski, L. J., Content, J., and Leppla, S. H., 1971, Characterization of the subunit structure of the ribonucleic acid genome of influenza virus, *J. Virol.* **8**, 701.

Li, K. K., and Seto, J. T., 1971, Electron microscope study of ribonucleic acid of myxoviruses, *J. Virol.* **7**, 524.

Liu, C., 1955, Studies on influenza infection in ferrets by means of fluorescein-labeled antibody, *J. Exp. Med.* **101**, 677.

Lonberg-Holm, K., and Philipson, L., 1974, Early interactions between animal viruses and cells, *Progr. Med. Virol.,* in press.

Maassab, H. F., 1963, Further studies on the infectivity of ribonucleic acid prepared from influenza virus-infected cells, *J. Immunol.* **90,** 265.

McClelland, L., and Hare, R., 1941, The adsorption of influenza virus by red cells and a new *in vitro* method of measuring antibodies for influenza virus, *Can. Pub. Health J.* **32,** 530.

McConnell, H. M., and McFarland, B. L., 1972, The flexibility gradient in biological membranes, *Ann. N.Y. Acad. Sci.* **195,** 207.

Mackenzie, J. S., 1970, Isolation of temperature-sensitive mutants and the construction of a preliminary genetic map for influenza virus, *J. Gen. Virol.* **6,** 63.

McSharry, J. J., and Wagner, R. R., 1971, Lipid composition of vesicular stomatitis virus, *J. Virol* **7,** 59.

Maeno, K., and Kilbourne, E. D., 1970, Developmental sequence and intracellular sites of synthesis of three structural protein antigens of influenza A_2 virus, *J. Virol.* **5,** 153.

Mahy, B. W. J., 1970, The replication of fowl plague virus RNA, *in* "The Biology of Large RNA Viruses" (R. D. Barry and B. W. J. Mahy, eds.), pp. 392–415, Academic Press, New York.

Mahy, B. W. J., and Bromley, P. A., 1970, *In vitro* product of a ribonucleic acid polymerase induced by influenza virus, *J. Virol.* **6,** 259.

Mahy, B. W. J., Hastie, N. D., and Armstrong, S. J., 1972, Inhibition of influenza virus replication by α-amanitin: Mode of action, *Proc. Natl. Acad. Sci. USA* **69,** 1421.

Marchesi, V. T., Tillack, T. W., and Scott, R. E., 1972*a,* The structure of erythrocyte membranes studies by freeze-etching. II. Localization of receptors for phytohemagglutinin and influenza virus to the intramembranous particles, *J. Exp. Med.* **135,** 1209.

Marchesi, V. T., Segrest, J. P., and Kahane, I., 1972*b,* Molecular features of human erythrocyte glycophorin, *in* "Membrane Research" (C. F. Fox, ed.), p. 41, Academic Press, New York.

Melnick, J. L., 1973, Classification and nomenclature of viruses, *Progr. Med. Virol.* **15,** 380.

Meier-Ewert, H., and Compans, R. W., 1974, Time course of synthesis and assembly of influenza virus proteins, *J. Virol.,* in press.

Meier-Ewert, H., Gibbs, A. J., and Dimmock, N. J., 1970, Studies on antigenic variations of swine influenza virus isolates, *J. Gen. Virol.* **6,** 409.

Moore, D. H., Davies, M. C., Levine, S., and Englert, M. E., 1962, Correlation of structure with infectivity of influenza virus, *Virology* **17,** 470.

Morgan, C., and Rose, H. M., 1968, Structure and development of viruses as observed in the electron microscope. VIII. Entry of influenza virus, *J. Virol.* **2,** 925.

Morgan, C., Hsu, K. C., Rifkind, R. A., Knox, A. W., and Rose, H. M., 1961, The application of ferritin-conjugated antibody to electron microscopic studies of influenza virus in infected cells. I. The cellular surface, *J. Exp. Med.* **114,** 825.

Morgan, C., Hsu, K. C., and Rose, H. M., 1962, Structure and development of viruses as observed in the electron microscope. VII. Incomplete virus formation, *J. Exp. Med.* **116,** 553.

Murphy, J. S. and Bang, F. B., 1952, Observations with the electron microscope on cells of the chick chorio-allantoic membrane infected with influenza virus, *J. Exp. Med.* **95,** 259.

Nayak, D. P., 1970, The replication of influenza virus RNA, *in* "The Biology of Large RNA Viruses" (R. D. Barry and B. W. J. Mahy, eds.), pp. 371–391, Academic Press, New York.

Nayak, D. P., and Baluda, M. A., 1967, Isolation and partial characterization of nucleic acid of influenza virus, *J. Virol.* **1**, 1217.

Nayak, D. P., and Baluda, M. A., 1969, Characterization of influenza virus ribonucleic acid duplex produced by annealing *in vitro, J. Virol.* **3**, 318.

Nayak, D. P., and Rasmussen, A. F., Jr., 1966, Influence of mitomycin C on the replication of influenza virus, *Virology* **30**, 673.

Nermut, M. V., 1972, Further investigation on the fine structure of influenza virus, *J. Gen. Virol.* **17**, 317.

Nermut, M. V. and Frank, H., 1971, Fine structure of influenza A$_2$ (Singapore) as revealed by negative staining, freeze-drying and freeze-etching, *J. Gen. Virol.* **10**, 37.

Nicolson, G. L., 1972, Topography of membrane concanavalin A sites modified by proteolysis, *Nat. New Biol.* **239**, 193.

Niven, J. S. F., Armstrong, J. A., Balfour, B. M., Klemperer, H. G., and Tyrrell, D. A. J., 1962, Cellular changes accompanying the growth of influenza virus in bovine kidney cell cultures, *J. Pathol. Bacteriol.* **84**, 1.

Oxford, J. S., 1973, Polypeptide composition of influenza B viruses and enzymes associated with the purified virus particles, *J. Virol.* **12**, 827.

Palese, P., Tobita, K., Ueda, M., and Compans, R. W., 1974, Characterization of temperature-sensitive influenza virus mutants defective in neuraminidase, *Virology* in press.

Paniker, C. K. J., 1968, Serological relationships between the neuraminidases of influenza viruses, *J. Gen. Virol.* **2**, 385.

Penhoet, E., Miller, H., Doyle, M., and Blatti, S., 1971, RNA-dependent RNA polymerase activity in influenza virions, *Proc. Natl. Acad. Sci. USA* **68**, 1369.

Pons, M. W., 1967*a*, Studies on influenza virus ribonucleic acid, *Virology* **31**, 523.

Pons, M. W., 1967*b*, Some characteristics of double-stranded influenza virus ribonucleic acid, *Arch. Ges. Virusforsch.* **22**, 203.

Pons, M. W., 1970, On the nature of the influenza virus genome, *Curr. Top. Microbiol. Immunol.* **52**, 142.

Pons, M. W., 1971, Isolation of influenza virus ribonucleoprotein from infected cells. Demonstration of the presence of negative-stranded RNA in viral RNP, *Virology* **46**, 149.

Pons, M. W., 1972, Studies on the replication of influenza virus RNA, *Virology* **47**, 823.

Pons, M. W., 1973, The inhibition of influenza virus RNA synthesis by actinomycin D and cycloheximide, *Virology* **51**, 120.

Pons, M., and Hirst, G. K., 1968*a*, Polyacrylamide gel electrophoresis of influenza virus RNA, *Virology* **34**, 386.

Pons, M. W., and Hirst, G. K., 1968*b*, Polyacrylamide gel electrophoresis of the replicative form of influenza virus RNA, *Virology* **35**, 182.

Pons, M. W., and Hirst, G. K., 1969, The single- and double-stranded RNA's and the proteins of incomplete influenza virus, *Virology* **38**, 68.

Pons, M. W., Schulze, I. T., and Hirst, G. K., 1969, Isolation and characterization of the ribonucleoprotein of influenza virus, *Virology* **39**, 250.

Porebska, A., Pereira, H. G., and Armstrong, J. A., 1968, Cytoplasmic inclusions and nuclear changes in cells infected with influenza-B viruses, *J. Med. Microbiol.* **1**, 145.

Quigley, J. P., Rifkin, D. B., and Reich, E., 1971, Phospholipid composition of Rous sarcoma virus, host cell membranes, and other enveloped viruses, *Virology* **46**, 106.

Rafelson, M. E., 1965, Neuraminidases, *in* "The Amino Sugars" (E. A. Balazs and R. W. Jeanloz, eds.), p. 171, Academic Press, New York.

Reimer, C., Baker, R., Newlin, T., and Havens, M. L., 1966, Influenza virus purification with the zonal ultra centrifuge, *Science* (*Wash., D.C.*) **152**, 1379.

Renkonen, O., Kääräinen, L., Simons, K., and Gahmberg, C., 1971, G. The lipid class composition of Semiliki forest virus and of plasma membranes of host cells, *Virology* **46**, 318.

Rifkin, D. B., Compans, R. W., and Reich, E., 1972, A specific labeling procedure for proteins on the outer surface of membranes, *J. Biol. Chem.* **247**, 6432.

Rott, R., and Scholtissek, C., 1963, Investigations about the formation of incomplete forms of fowl plague virus, *J. Gen. Microbiol.* **33**, 303.

Rott, R., and Scholtissek, C., 1968, Biochemical studies on influenza virus multiplication at reduced temperature, *J. Gen. Virol.* **3**, 239.

Rott, R., Saber, S., and Scholtissek, C., 1965, Effect on myxovirus of mitomycin C, actinomycin D, and pretreatment of the host cell with ultra-violet light, *Nature* (*Lond.*) **205**, 1187.

Ruck, B. J., Brammer, K. W., Page, M. G., and Coombes, J. D., 1969, The detection and characterization of an induced RNA polymerase in the chorioallantoic membranes of embryonated eggs infected with influenza A_2 viruses, *Virology* **39**, 31.

Schäfer, W., and Zillig, W., 1954, Uber den Aufbau des Viruselementarteilchens der klassichen Geflügelpest. I. Gewinnung, Physikalisch-chemische und Biologische Eigenschaften einiger Spaltprodukte, *Z. Naturforsch* **96**, 779.

Schäfer, W., Munk, K., and Armbruster, D., 1952, Eigenschaften tierischer Virusarten, untersucht an den Geflügelpest Viren als Modell. III. Mitteilung: Weitere Untersuchungen über die physikochemischen und morphologischen Eigenschaften der Geflügelpest Viren, *Z. Naturforsch.* **7b**, 29.

Scholtissek, C., and Becht, H., 1971, Binding of ribonucleic acids to the RNP-antigen protein of influenza viruses, *J. Gen. Virol.* **10**, 11.

Scholtissek, C., and Rott, R., 1961, Zusammenhänge zwischen der Synthese von Ribonukleinsäure und Protein bei der Vermehung eines Virus der Influenzagruppe (Virus der klassischen Geflügelpest), *Z. Naturfosch.* **16b**, 663.

Scholtissek, C., and Rott, R., 1964, Behavior of virus-specific activities in tissue cultures infected with myxoviruses after chemical changes of the viral ribonucleic acid, *Virology* **22**, 169.

Scholtissek, C., and Rott, R., 1969, Ribonucleic acid nucleotidyl transferase induced in chick fibroblasts after infection with an influenza virus, *J. Gen. Virol.* **4**, 125.

Scholtissek, C., and Rott, R., 1970, Synthesis *in vivo* of influenza virus plus and minus strand RNA and its preferential inhibition by antibiotics, *Virology* **40**, 989.

Scholtissek, C., Becht, H., and Rott, R., 1971, Inhibition of influenza RNA polymerase by specific antiserum, *Virology* **43**, 137.

Schramm, G., 1954, Die Biochemie der Viren, Springer-Verlag, Berlin.

Schulman, J. L., and Kilbourne, E. D., 1969, Independent variation in nature of hemagglutinin and neuraminidase antigens of influenza virus: Distinctiveness of hemagglutinin antigen of Hong Kong/68 virus, *Proc. Natl. Acad. Sci. USA* **63**, 326.

Schulze, I. T., 1970, The structure of influenza virus. I. The polypeptides of the virion, *Virology* **42**, 890.

Schulze, I. T., 1972, The structure of influenza virus. II. A model based on the morphology and composition of subviral particles, *Virology* **47**, 181.

Schulze, I. T., 1973 Structure of the influenza virion, *Adv. Virus Res.* **18**, 1.

Schulze, I. T., 1974, Effects of sialylation on the biological activities of the influenza virions, *in* "Negative Strand Viruses" (R. D. Barry and B. W. J. Mahy, eds.), Academic Press, New York, in press.

Schulze, I. T., Pons, M. W., and Hirst, G. K., 1970, The RNA and proteins of influenza virus, *in* "The Biology of Large RNA Viruses" (R. D. Barry and B. W. J. Mahy, eds.), pp. 324–346, Academic Press, New York.

Seto, J. T., and Chang, F. S., 1969, Functional significance of sialidase during influenza virus multiplication: An electron microscope study, *J. Virol.* **4**, 58.

Seto, J. T., and Rott, R., 1966, Functional significance of sialidase during influenza virus multiplication, *Virology* **30**, 731.

Sharp, D. G., Taylor, A. R., McLean, I. W., Beard, D., and Beard, J. W., 1945, Densities and sizes of the influenza viruses A (PR8 strain) and B (Lee strain) and the swine influenza virus, *J. Biol. Chem.* **159**, 29.

Siegert, W., Bauer, G., and Hofschneider, P. H., 1973, Direct evidence for messenger activity of influenza virion RNA, *Proc. Natl. Acad. Sci. USA* **70**, 2960.

Simpson, R. W., and Hirst, G. K., 1961, Genetic recombination among influenza viruses. I. Cross reactivation of plaque-forming capacity as a method for selecting recombinants from the progeny of crosses between influenza strains, *Virology* **15**, 436.

Simpson, R. W., and Hirst, G. K., 1968, Temperature-sensitive mutants of influenza A virus: Isolation of mutants and preliminary observations on genetic recombination and complementation, *Virology* **35**, 41.

Skehel, J. J., 1971a, Estimations of the molecular weight of the influenza virus genome, *J. Gen. Virol.* **11**, 103.

Skehel, J. J., 1971b, The characterization of subviral particles derived from influenza virus, *Virology* **44**, 409.

Skehel, J. J., 1971c, RNA-dependent RNA polymerase activity of the influenza virus, *Virology* **45**, 793.

Skehel, J. J., 1972, Polypeptide synthesis in influenza virus-infected cells, *Virology* **49**, 23.

Skehel, J. J., 1973, Early polypeptide synthesis in influenza virus-infected cells, *Virology* **56**, 394.

Skehel, J. J., and Burke, D. C., 1969, Ribonucleic acid synthesis in chick embryo cells infected with fowl plague virus, *J. Virol.* **3**, 429.

Skehel, J. J., and Schild, G. C., 1971, The polypeptide composition of influenza A viruses, *Virology* **44**, 396.

Smith, W., Belyavin, G., and Sheffield, F. W., 1953, A host-protein component of influenza viruses, *Nature (Lond.)* **172**, 669.

Stanley, P., and Haslam, E. A., 1971, The polypeptides of influenza virus. V. Localization of polypeptides in the virion by iodination techniques, *Virology* **46**, 764.

Stanley, P., Gandhi, S. S., and White, D. O., 1973, The polypeptides of influenza virus. VII. Synthesis of the haemagglutinin, *Virology* **53**, 92.

Stephenson, J. R., and Dimmock, N. J., 1974, Interaction of influenza virus with the host cell: inhibition of ribosome biosynthesis, *in* "Negative Strand Viruses" (R. D. Barry and B. W. J. Mahy, eds.), Academic Press, New York, in press.

Sugiura, A., Tobita, K., and Kilbourne, E. D., 1972, Isolation and preliminary characterization of temperature-sensitive mutants of influenza virus, *J. Virol.* **10**, 639.

Taylor, A. R., Sharp, D. G., Beard, D., Beard, J. W., Dingle, J. H., and Feller, A. E.,

1943, Isolation and characterization of influenza A virus (PR8 strain), *J. Immunol.* **47**, 261.

Taylor, J. M., Hampson, A. W., and White, D. O., 1969, The polypeptides of influenza virus. I. Cytoplasmic synthesis and nuclear accumulation, *Virology* **39**, 419.

Taylor, J. M., Hampson, A. W., Layton, J. E., and White, D. O., 1970, The polypeptides of influenza virus. IV. An analysis of nuclear accumulation, *Virology* **42**, 744.

ter Meulen, V., and Love, R., 1967, Virological, immunochemical, and cyochemical studies of four HeLa cell lines infected with two strains of influenza virus, *J. Virol.* **1**, 626.

Tiffany, J., and Blough, H., 1970, Models of structure of the envelope of influenza virus, *Proc. Natl. Acad. Sci. USA.* **65**, 1105.

von Magnus, P., 1954, Incomplete forms of influenza virus, *Adv. Virus Res.* **2**, 59.

Warren, L., Glick, M. C., and Nass, M. K., 1966, I. Methods of isolation of the surface membrane, *J. Cell Physiol.* **68**, 269.

Waterson, A. P., 1962, Two kinds of myxovirus, *Nature (Lond.)* **193**, 1163.

Webster, R. G., 1970, Estimation of the molecular weights of the polypeptide chains from the isolated hemagglutinin and neuraminidase subunits of influenza viruses, *Virology* **40**, 643.

Webster, R. G., and Darlington, R. W., 1969, Disruption of myxoviruses with Tween 20 and isolation of biologically active hemagglutinin and neuraminidase subunits, *J. Virol.* **4**, 182.

Webster, R. G., and Laver, W. G., 1971, Antigenic variation in influenza virus, *Progr. Med. Virol.* **13**, 271.

Webster, R. G., Laver, W. G., Kilbourne, E. D., 1968, Reactions of antibodies with surface antigens of influenza virus, *J. Gen. Virol.* **3**, 315.

Webster, R. G., Campbell, C. H., and Granoff, A., 1973, The *in vivo* production of new influenza viruses. III. Isolation of recombinant influenza viruses under simulated conditions of natural transmission, *Virology* **51**, 149.

Wecker, E., 1957, Die Verteilung von ^{32}P im Virus der klassischen Geflügelpest bei verschiedenen Markierungsverfahren, *Z. Naturforsch.* **12b**, 208.

Weinstein, D. B., and Blough, H. A., 1972, Cited in Blough, H. A., and Tiffany, J. M., 1973, Lipids in viruses, *Adv. Lipid Res.* **11**, 267.

White, D. O., and Cheyne, I. M., 1965, Stimulation of Sendai virus multiplication by puromycin and actinomycin D, *Nature (Lond.)* **208**, 813.

White, D. O., Day, H. M., Batchelder, E. J., and Cheyne, I. M., and Wansbrough, A. J., 1965, Delay in the multiplication of influenza virus, *Virology* **25**, 289.

White, D. O., Taylor, J. M., Haslam, E. A., and Hampson, A. W., 1970, The polypeptides of influenza virus and their biosynthesis, *in* "The Biology of Large RNA Viruses" (R. D. Barry and B. W. J. Mahy, eds.), pp. 602–618, Academic Press, London.

Winzler, R. J., 1972, Glycoproteins of plasma membranes, *in* "Glycoproteins, Their Composition, Structure and Function," 2nd ed. (A. Gottschalk, ed.), p. 1268, Elsevier, Amsterdam.

Wrigley, N. G., Skehel, J. J., Charlwood, P. A., and Brand, C. M., 1973, The size and shape of influenza virus neuraminidase, *Virology* **51**, 525.

Young, R. J., and Content, J., 1971, 5´-terminus of influenza virus RNA, *Nat. New Biol.* **230**, 140.

Zimmermann, T., and Schäfer, W., 1960, Effect of p-fluorphenylalanine on fowl plaque virus multiplication, *Virology* **11**, 676.

CHAPTER 4

Reproduction of RNA Tumor Viruses

John P. Bader

Chemistry Branch
National Cancer Institute
National Institutes of Health
Bethesda, Maryland 20014

1. INTRODUCTION

The RNA-containing tumor viruses have been the objects of a surge of investigational activity during the past few years. This activity emanates from a conviction that cancer in man may be a direct consequence of infection by RNA tumor viruses, and it was prompted by the discovery of enzymes (reverse transcriptases) which have forced a conceptual change in notions about the transfer or exchange of genetic information among eukaryotic cells.

The RNA tumor viruses have been recognized for some time as the natural etiologic agents of leukemias of mice and fowl, and of mammary tumors among highly susceptible strains of mice. Investigations into other animal species have resulted in the isolation of many host-derivative (e.g., feline, cavian, hamster) strains of virus, resulting in the conclusion that leukemias caused by RNA tumor viruses are not restricted to a few vertebrate species. Similar viruses have been isolated from solid tumors of several species, and these viruses have tumorigenic potential. Nonetheless, the role of sarcoma-inducing viruses as tumor-inducing agents in natural disease has not been defined.

In contrast to most other types of animal viruses, infection by RNA tumor viruses rarely leads to destruction of the cell, and where cell death occurs as a result of infection it usually can be attributed to an increased selective sensitivity to an exogenous toxic agent. Cells infected with a sarcoma virus become transformed into malignant cells, and in a functional sense these cells are biologically useless. Nonetheless, such cells can propagate while producing large quantities of progeny virus. In cases of infection with leukosis or leukosislike viruses, there often may be no obvious deleterious effect on cellular physiologic properties. The implications of this become all the more interesting when we find that many animal cells which have never been deliberately infected, and which are apparently normal, can be induced to produce particles which resemble RNA tumor viruses in every physical and chemical respect (Aaronson *et al.*, 1969, 1971*b*; Lowy *et al.*, 1971; Weiss *et al.*, 1971).

In this review I have attempted to collate information on the structure of the virions of RNA tumor viruses, and to relate this to biological and biochemical observations made during the course of a reproductive cycle in infected cells. While many specific differences among different RNA tumor viruses are recognized, both in virion-specific molecules and in the consequence of infection, most general features are similar or identical, and these will often be treated without reference to the specific organism studied.

Some other types of viruses, not commonly recognized as tumorigenic, including visna virus, progressive pneumonia virus, and simian foamy virus, have properties similar to RNA tumor viruses (Lin and Thormar, 1970; Stone *et al.*, 1971). Also, several isolates of infectious virions with all the physical and chemical characteristics of RNA tumor viruses have not been shown to induce malignancies. These viruses will be included in this discussion. To avoid exciting those who may become annoyed at a restrictive nomenclature for a general group of viruses, I shall refer to all of the viruses containing general properties similar to RNA-containing tumor viruses simply as RTV,* giving deference to the title of this chapter.

I have taken the prerogative of speculating whenever information is incomplete. Many of the observations presented here can be considered phenomena, but to list those facts without relevance to their

---

* Editor's note: Oncornaviruses is one alternate name of this group of viruses preferred by many, and retraviruses (reverse transcriptase) may be the least controversial term. The author's use of the abbreviation RTV may be regarded as allowing for either terminology [H. F. -C.].

biological role relegates one's function to that of a taxonomist. The mysteries of reproduction of RTV, and of the role of these viruses in tumorigenesis, are too exciting to permit oneself to be cast in this sterile mold.

1.1. Production and Assay of RTV

Cell culture methods are almost exclusively the methods of choice for production or assay of RTV. Cultures once infected may be used continuously thereafter as a source of virus since such cells can simultaneously produce virus and function physiologically. Initial infections are most efficient when the receptive cells are actively dividing and the rate of DNA synthesis in the culture is high (Bader, 1967b; Weiss, 1971; Clark and Bader, 1974). Once infection is accomplished, however, virus production is no longer dependent on functions associated with cellular DNA synthesis or cell growth, and virus production proceeds given a reasonable rate of metabolic activity. Since infection by RTV usually does not lead to destruction of cells, collection of virions can often be made with a minimum of cellular materials in the virus-containing culture fluids. The advantages of such material become obvious when purification of virions is considered.

There are systems in which the intact animal can provide concentrations of virus unattainable by cell culture methods, e.g., the plasma of fowl infected with and producing avian myeloblastosis virus [see Beard *et al.* (1955)] and spleen homogenates or plasma of mice infected with murine leukemia viruses (Rauscher and Allen, 1964). While such systems may provide a valuable resource for an investigator interested in a large amount of a purifiable virus component (e.g., reverse transcriptase or a specific antigen), it is recognized that such preparations contain a high proportion of "old" virions with degraded molecular constituents, in addition to large amounts of contaminating cellular substances. These preparations are of little value in definitive studies on the structure of infectious virions or in the resolution of viral molecular constituents.

Cells of recent embryonic origin have been the cells of choice for production of RTV. Of particular advantage are virus-producing cells capable of growth in suspension. Cells transformed by sarcoma viruses acquire this property, and large amounts of virus can be obtained after growth and concentration of suspended virus-producing cells (Bader, 1968). This procedure only rarely has proven advantageous for the production of leukemia viruses, as in the production of avian myeloblastosis virus by myeloblasts (Beaudreau *et al.*, 1960), although non-virus-producing transformed cells should be expected in some instances to act as hosts for leukemia viruses. For undefined reasons serial cell lines have not been particularly useful for the production or assay of RTV.

Several quantitative or semiquantitative techniques have been developed for the assay of infectious RTV (Table 1). The focus-formation methods are based on the ability of transforming viruses to change the morphology and/or growth pattern of infected cells. A single infectious particle is sufficient to infect and transform a cell (Temin and Rubin, 1958). When more than one virion is required for recognizable transformation (Hartley and Rowe, 1966), the transforming virus may require simultaneous infection with a leuke-mialike virus to allow virus reproduction and secondary infection of adjacent cells. Although single transformed cells can be identified in cultures infected by Bryan "high-titer" strain of Rous sarcoma virus (Nakata and Bader, 1968a), quantitative recognition of infection by most strains of transforming viruses requires several cell divisions. Foci of transformed cells then are ascertained against a background of nontransformed cells.

Transforming viruses are able to alter the growth potential of cells, and such transformed cells are often able to grow in suspension, either in liquid or when relatively immobilized in a semisolid gel such as agar (Rubin, 1966; Bader, 1967a). Under similar conditions, many nontransformed cells, including cells infected by leukemia viruses, are

TABLE 1

Techniques for Assay or Detection of RTV

Infectivity	Particles	
Focus formation	Reverse transcriptase (a)	enzyme activity
Colonies in agar suspension	(b)	labeling of vRNA[a]
Syncytia formation	Radioactive labeling (a)	virions
Plaque formation	(b)	vRNA[a]
Interference	Electron microscopy	
Complement fixation	Rescue of defective viruses	
Fluorescent antibody		

[a] vRNA is the large-molecular-weight 60–70 S viral RNA.

unable to divide more than once or twice. Colonies of transformed cells appearing in agar gel suspension, therefore, can be easily recognized. This method is quantitatively less efficient than focus formation in assaying some transforming viruses, but it is valuable for selection of transformed clones where the growth of nontransformed cells is undesirable or where transformed foci in monolayer cultures cannot be easily distinguished from nontransformed cells.

Nontransforming viruses can, in some cases, be assayed quantitatively, although no general procedure applies to all types. Certain strains of avian leukosis virus, specifically subgroups B and D, can be assayed by plaque formation using chick embryo cells (Dougherty and Rasmussen, 1964; Graf, 1972). Plaque formation is dependent upon localized cytopathic changes, and one would not expect such drastic effects of leukosis viruses under physiological conditions. It seems that the artificial cell culture environment cannot sustain cell viability after infection by these strains of RTV. In one report, plaque formation did not occur unless the cells had been previously infected with a conditionally transforming mutant of Rous sarcoma virus (Kawai and Hanafusa, 1972a).

Murine leukemia viruses can be assayed by a variation of the plaque technique (Rowe et al., 1970). Mouse embryo cells, which can support full cycles of virus reproduction, are exposed to murine leukemia virus and are then mixed with rat XC cells (rat embryo cells which are infected and transformed by avian sarcoma virus, but are producing no virus). The murine leukemia virus causes coalescence of XC cell membranes resulting in multicellular syncytia (Johnson et al., 1971). As in the focus-formation and plaque methods, these syncytia can be identified and enumerated. Most infectious murine leukemia viruses can be assayed by this method, or by a variation employing an indicator a cell line other than XC (Bassin et al., 1971).

Since each focus, plaque, or syncytium is a consequence of infection with a single virus particle, the quantitative sensitivity is high. Less-sensitive methods utilize (1) homologous interference, where cells infected with a nontransforming virus are refractory to infection with transforming virus from the same subgroup (Rubin, 1960; Vogt and Ishizaki, 1966), (2) complement fixation, in which infected cells synthesize sufficient viral antigen to be detected by complement fixation (Huebner et al., 1964; Hartley et al., 1965), or (3) fluorescent antibody to viral antigens (Vogt and Rubin, 1962; Ubertini et al., 1971). These methods are most often used in the detection of generalized virus infection, or have specific application in experiments.

1.2. Detection of Virus Particles

A number of methods have been devised to detect virions of RTV (Table 1), and the current demand that viruses be identified as etiologic agents in human cancer requires methods other than those used in classical infectious-disease studies. For example, increasingly rigorous criteria have been developed by electron microscopists in the identification of particles as virions, including size, shape, display of internal structure, and the arrest of virions in the process of budding from the host cell membrane.

Radioactive labeling of virions after exposure of cells to radioactive precursors, with subsequent isopycnic banding in density gradients can be used to detect virions (Robinson *et al.*, 1965; Valentine and Bader, 1968). However, inadvertant lysis of cells can result in radioactive vesicles banding in the region of virions, thus resulting in an erroneous determination. Therefore, extraction and resolution of high-molecular-weight (60–70 S) RNA from suspected virions is particularly demonstrative.

Since it is likely that all infectious virions of RTV contain reverse transcriptase (viral RNA-dependent DNA polymerase), the detection of this enzyme in an unknown preparation would encourage one to inquire further into the possibility that virions are present. To increase the specificity for detection of viral transcriptase, specific polynucleotide templates have been recommended to distinguish the viral enzyme from cellular polymerases [see Temin and Baltimore (1972) and Baltimore *et al.* (1973)]. Also the incorporation of radioactive deoxyribonucleotides into DNA associated with 60–70 S RNA can be used to detect virions undetectable by other means. Spiegelman and his co-workers have used this method to identify mouse mammary tumor virus (Schlom and Spiegelman, 1971), and also in attempts to detect virions associated with human breast cancer (Schlom *et al.*, 1971; Axel *et al.*, 1972c).

The ability of one virus to complement functions defective in other viruses, either by forming phenotypic variants or by aiding in enzymatic requirements, has elicited hope for the use of known RTV in the "rescue" and identification of otherwise undetectable viruses. Few investigations of this type have been recorded thus far, and success has been limited to experimental systems. Cells transformed by murine sarcoma virus may produce no detectable virions, but after superinfection with murine leukemia virus complete infectious sarcoma virus can be found in the extracellular fluids (Aaronson and Rowe, 1970; Rowe,

1972*a*). Similarly, cells transformed by avian sarcoma virus may produce virions with limited host range; superinfection of these cells with a host range variant of avian leukosis virus can result in release of sarcoma virus with the host range of the superinfecting leukosis virus (Hanafusa, 1965). Complementation and rescue are restricted to related viruses, and the success of such methods in revealing unknown viruses will depend on the ability to predict relatedness between the rescuing and unknown viruses, or on luck.

Molecular hybridization techniques, employing DNA synthesized on a viral RNA template and RNA extracted from tumor cells, have been used in attempts to identify viral nucleotide sequences in tumor cells. The validity of such studies depends upon the absolute purity of the virions, or on the purity of the viral RNA template used in the synthesis of the putative viral DNA, since contamination with cellular DNA or RNA could result in synthesis of DNA which may recognize nucleotide sequences other than viral RNA sequences. On this basis it is difficult to be convinced of the validity of studies which purport the demonstration of RNA identical to murine leukemia viral RNA in a variety of human neoplasms (Hehlmann *et al.*, 1972*a,b*) and the demonstration of mouse mammary tumor virus RNA sequences in human breast tumors (Axel *et al.*, 1972*b,c*).

2. VIRION STRUCTURE

2.1. Purification and Physical Properties

A variety of experiments addressed to the elucidation of the structure of RTV, or particularly in the use of RTV or components of RTV as reagents, require some confidence in the relative purity of the RTV preparation. Although minor consistent differences between strains can be found, virions of RTV have a characteristic buoyant density, and centrifugation to equilibrium in density gradients is the preferred technique for purification of RTV. Virions band at a density of 1.18–1.16 g/ml in solutes of high osmotic pressure (e.g., sucrose or potassium tartrate) (Robinson *et al.*, 1965; Valentine and Bader, 1968). In Ficoll (polysucrose) or in Dextran 110 (polydextrose), which have minimal osmotic effects, the RTV band at 1.08 and 1.06 g/ml, respectively (J. P. Bader, unpublished). Unfortunately, cellular components also can be found banding at the density of the virus, especially the membraneous vesicles which may enclose other cellular constituents, including nucleic acids. Consideration must also be given to virions binding cellular molecules or organelles which might otherwise separate from virions during purification. No published technique has overcome these encumbrances to virus purification. In lieu of documentation to the contrary, one must assume that all preparations of virions contain contaminating cellular elements. In my experience, heavily contaminated virions can be purified to only a limited extent by density gradient centrifugation, and the best virion preparations are obtained by selection of virus-containing fluids in which contamination is precluded by careful treatment of the virus-producing cell cultures prior to banding of virions in a density gradient.

RTV are essentially spherical, and diameters ranging from 65 to 150 nm have been reported. Individual strains have a consistent average diameter which may be different from that of another strain. Nonspherical forms have been described and the possibility that virions of RTV might have tails analogous to those of certain bacteriophages has even been considered (Dalton *et al.*, 1964). These aberrant forms are almost certainly due to osmotic effects, introduced during preparation of the virions for electron microscopy, which result in dehydration of virions and collapse of the outer envelope (deHarven and Friend, 1964).

Particles resembling RTV, but which are rodlike, similar to the filamentous forms of myxoviruses, have been induced in cultures of liver cells by chemical carcinogens (Weinstein *et al.*, 1972). However, other criteria necessary for the identification of these particles as virus have not been satisfied, and whether such filamentous forms are ever found among RTV is an open question.

Electron microscopy of sectioned specimens has revealed a general morphological structure characteristic of RTV. The virion can be considered as three concentric spheres: (1) an outer lipoprotein envelope, similar in appearance to cell surface membrane, (2) an internal electron-dense layer, sometimes referred to as the intermediate layer, or intermediate membrane, and (3) a central nucleoid, which contains the RNA.

Morphological differences between virions occasionally can be used to distinguish RTV virions, especially when the viruses originate in hosts of heterologous species. Preparations of avian leuko-sarcoma viruses can easily be distinguished from their murine counterparts by the more prominent intermediate layer of the former [see Bader (1969)]. Differences between individual virions within an otherwise homologous preparation can usually be attributed to exposure of the virions to exogenous factors. For example, virions of murine leukemia virus more commonly contain nucleoids with electron-lucent centers when harvested and examined soon after being released from infected cells (deHarven, 1968). Extended exposure of virions to incubator temperatures results in a population of virions containing electron-dense nucleoids. This morphological change was the basis for the use of the terms "immature" and "mature" in describing virions of murine leukemia virus, as well as the morphological classification, Type A and Type C, respectively (Bernhard, 1960; deHarven, 1968), Type B being reserved for virions with eccentric electron-dense nucleoids, such as those of mouse mammary tumor virus. The terms "immature" and "mature" are perhaps inappropriate in a biological sense since it seems likely that fresh, "immature" virions are infectious, while "mature" virions may contain degraded constituents and be noninfectious. Nonetheless, no strict correlation between morphology and infectivity has been reported, and any generalization on this matter may be premature.

2.2. Chemical Composition

The exact chemical composition of RTV cannot be described since virions devoid of cellular constituents have rarely been realized. Nonetheless, the constancy of several components as revealed by radioactive labeling or antigenic analysis presents us with a reasonable chemical description of the RTV virion. In general, the virions are composed of approximately 30% lipid, 62% protein, 6% hexose, and less than 2% RNA (Bonar and Beard, 1959; Quigley *et al.*, 1971).

Several discoveries of intravirion DNA have been reported (Levinson *et al.*, 1970; Riman and Beaudreau, 1970; Biswal *et al.*, 1970, 1971). The cellular origin of the DNA was suggested by molecular hybridization experiments (Varmus *et al.*, 1971), and such DNA was almost certainly a contaminant since adequate criteria for virion purification were not presented. We have examined the nucleic acid species of scores of "purified" virion preparations by gel electrophoresis, and found DNA to be a variable component, many samples containing no detectable DNA (in some instances, less than 1/100 the content of viral RNA). Other laboratories (Robinson *et al.*, 1965), as well as mine, have failed to find DNA in virions after exposing virus productive cells to high levels of $^{32}PO_4$ or ^3H-thymidine.

Studies on the metabolic requirements for infection by RTV have shown that DNA synthesis is a requirement, but only during the first several hours after exposure of cells to virus (Bader, 1964a, 1965a,

1966*a*). Once this DNA requirement is fulfilled, DNA synthesis can be suppressed without affecting production of progeny virus. In one study (Bader, 1965*a*), DNA synthesis was continuously inhibited by maintenance of infected chick embryo cells in serum-free medium, yet Rous sarcoma virus was produced in large quantities for as long as 40 days. Furthermore, the virion enzyme which transcribes the viral RNA into DNA (reverse transcriptase) has no requirement for polydeoxyribonucleotides, either as template or as primer (Temin and Mizutani, 1970; Baltimore, 1970; Baltimore and Smoler, 1971). Since this enzyme can synthesize new DNA complementary to virtually the entire viral genome, one can construct a scheme for reproduction of RTV exclusive of a putative intravirion DNA. Intravirion DNA seems unlikely when (1) no virus-specific DNA has been identified within virions, (2) virus can be produced in the absence of DNA synthesis, and (3) there is no apparent functional basis for intravirion DNA and no reasonable role for intravirion DNA has been suggested.

2.3. Virion Lipids

Virion lipids are probably exclusively in the membraneous envelope, although the instability of virion cores after detergent treatment (Bader *et al.*, 1970; Duesberg, 1970) possibly can be attributed to internal lipids. Crawford (1960) found that Rous sarcoma virus presented a broad density distribution in RbCl gradients, but that density differences were maintained when heavy and light fractions were rebanded. Cells infected with these separated virion populations produced viral progeny, which in both cases banded heterologously and indistinguishibly. He concluded that the observed phenotypic differences were due to a variable content of lipid in the viral membrane. (At that time he could not have known that the strain of Rous sarcoma virus studied was in fact a mixture of two avian RTV, and that phenotypic mixing and masking occur regularly among avian RTV. The possibility that observed densities were due to such mixtures would have had to be considered).

Subsequent studies showed that the lipid composition of virions was qualitatively, and in some respects quantitatively, similar to the lipid composition of the host cell membrane (Rao *et al.*, 1966; Quigley *et al.*, 1971, 1972*b*). Rous sarcoma virus was grown in either chick embryo cells or Japanese quail cells, hosts of differing lipid constitution, and progeny virions contained lipid reflecting the composition of the host (Quigley *et al.*, 1972*b*). Also, other types of enveloped viruses, including Newcastle disease virus, Sendai virus, and Sindbis virus, when grown on the same host cells, contained similar phospholipids (Quigley *et al.*, 1971). An exception to these general observations are the observed increases in sphingomyelin and phosphatidylethanolamine, and lesser amounts of phosphatidylcholine, in virions compared to host cell membranes. Also, cholesterol compared to phospholipid, and cholesterol ester compared to total cholesterol, were higher in virions than in plasma membranes. Two interesting possibilities arise: (1) virion structural proteins may seek out specific areas on the membrane having the observed lipid proportions, or (2) viral envelopes are restricted in the amounts of specific lipids incorporated. A more trivial explanation is the possible selective contamination of host surface membranes with other cellular lipids, of virions preparations with host cell lipids, or both.

2.4. Viral Proteins

The similarity in gross structure among RTV is reflected in a general similarity in proteins extractable from the virions. Seven major structural proteins have been identified in avian RTV and six proteins in murine RTV using gel electrophoresis or gel filtration techniques. These structural proteins can be divided into two classes, glycosylated and nonglycosylated proteins. Furthermore, there is at least one other protein within virions, the reverse transcriptase, which is not easily identifiable by gross protein analysis. It would hardly be surprising if other unidentified proteins, present in small concentrations, constitute integral constitutents of RTV. There is no consistency in the nomenclature of resolved polypeptides among the published works. Therefore, after separating into glycosylated and nonglycosylated proteins, I have adopted a simple numbering system beginning with highest apparent molecular weight.

2.4.1. Glycoproteins

The two largest proteins regularly found in RTV are glycoproteins, with molecular weights approximately 80,000 and 40,000. These proteins contain the type-specific antigenic activity of the virions and are found exclusively in the virion envelope (Duesberg *et al.*, 1970; Bolognesi and Bauer, 1970; Bolognesi *et al.*, 1972a; Witte *et al.*, 1973). The specificity of the virions in initial virus–host interactions resides in these glycoproteins. While the specific amino acid sequence almost certainly is determined by the viral genome, and is different for different strains of RTV, at least some degree of glycosylation is specified by the cell.

The migration of viral glycoproteins during electrophoresis in polyacrylamide gels was found to be dependent not only upon the strain of virus examined, but on the physiological state of the cell as well. The large glycoprotein of Rous sarcoma virus was observed to move more slowly than that of a related avian leukosis virus, but when the leukosis virus was produced by Rous-transformed cells its glycoprotein could not be distinguished from that of Rous virions (Robinson *et al.*, 1970; Duesberg *et al.*, 1970). Lai and Duesberg (1972*b*) used a mutant of the Schmidt-Ruppin strain of Rous sarcoma virus to examine the nature of virion glycoproteins. Cells infected with this mutant were capable of producing virus at both a high (41°C) and low (36°C) temperature, but cells were morphologically transformed only at the lower temperature. The glycoproteins from virions produced by the transformed cells at 36°C had a lower electrophoretic mobility than glycoproteins from virions produced at 41°C. After digestion with protease, the slowly migrating glycoproteins released glycopeptides (molecular weight *ca.* 5100) which were larger than the glycopeptides (molecular weight *ca.* 3900) released from virions produced at the nontransforming temperature.

Certain strains of avian sarcoma virus have counterpart viruses which are nontransforming, although antigenically indistinguishable from the transforming viruses. In each of several cases, the glycoproteins of transforming virions produced by transformed cells were larger than the glycoproteins from the nontransforming virions produced by nontransformed cells, and derivative glycopeptides reflected this difference. It seems clear that the degree of glycosylation in itself is insuffient to confer viral antigenic specificity since there are no obvious antigenic differences between these related sarcoma and leukosis viruses.

Lest we become too enthusiastic about these noted glycoprotein and glycopeptide differences, it should be noted that the differences, while consistent, are not great, that there is considerable overlap in migration patterns of the glycoproteins, and that the separation of glycopeptides is incomplete. These experiments leave unresolved the possibilities that (1) several similar glycopeptides are present in virions grown in either type of cell, but the relative proportions are different, or (2) qualitative differences exist among the glycopeptides of homologous proteins or between glycopeptides of the two types of virions.

Different strains of avian sarcoma viruses are found to contain distinguishable large-molecular-weight glycoproteins (Duesberg *et al.*, 1970). Since transformation by one virus may alter glycosylation enzymes in a manner different from another virus, it is not possible to determine from the data whether the electrophoretic separation of virion glycoproteins is due to degrees of glycosylation of proteins, the amino acid substructure of the proteins, or both.

2.4.2. Nonglycosylated Proteins

Five nonglycosylated proteins have been identified in avian RTV and at least four in murine RTV. Several of these including P_1, P_2, P_4, and P_5 (Table 2) contain complement-fixing activity when mixed with appropriate antisera lacking infectivity-neutralizing activity (Hung *et al.*, 1971; Oroszlan *et al.*, 1971*b*). Immunological studies employing fluorescence techniques demonstrated that the complement-fixing antigens were unexposed in intact virions (Kelloff and Vogt, 1966);

TABLE 2

Proteins of RTV[a]

Protein	Approximate mol. wt., $\times 10^3$ daltons	Isoelectric point	Relative percentage	Antigenicity[b]
gp₁ (a) (b)	115–70	4.9–6.3	12	Type specific
Reverse transcriptase	110 and 70	—	Low	Interspecies specific
gp₂	37–50	6.3	6.0	?CF
(gp₃)	—	3.5	—	No CF
P₁	27–32	8.9	32	CF, species specific
P₂	19–21	6.3 / 9.9	13	CF / No CF
P₃	14–17	4.9	27	CF
P₄	12–13	7.4		CF, interspecies specific
P₅	10–11	3.5	—	No CF

[a] Summarization of data extracted from the following sources: Allen *et al.* (1970), Duesberg (1970), Hung *et al.* (1971), Oroszlan *et al.* (1970, 1971*b*, 1972), Robinson *et al.* (1970), Fleissner (1971), Rifkin and Compans (1971), Bolognesi *et al.* (1972*a, b*), Schäfer *et al.* (1972*a, b*), Witte *et al.* (1973).
[b] CF = complement fixing.

virions were impermeable to the antibody unless previously treated with acetone.

That at least some of these antigens are internal proteins was confirmed by the identification of complement-fixing antigen in isolated virion cores stripped of the external envelope by detergent (Bader *et al.*, 1970; Fleissner, 1971). Proteins P_1 (the dominant virion protein) and P_4 exhibit highest antigenic activity, and these have been extracted from virion cores (Allen *et al.*, 1970; Quigley *et al.*, 1972a; Oroszlan *et al.*, 1970, 1971b; Lange *et al.*, 1973).

The complement-fixing proteins of avian RTV cross-react with antibody to other avian strains. Oroszlan *et al.* (1971b, 1972) have shown that leukosis viruses from mouse, rat, and hamster have a distinguishable "species-specific" gs1 antigen, and an indistinguishable "interspecies-specific" gs3 antigen. The dominant protein, P_1, is antigenically specific for RTV produced by the particular animal species (has gs1 antigen), but also has determinants cross-reactive with other mammalian virus antigens (gs3) (Gilden and Oroszlan, 1972). Trypsinization of P_1 resulted in a polypeptide which had lost most of the species-specific antigenic activity, but retained interspecies-specific antigenicity (Davis *et al.*, 1973). Another protein, P_4, also may cross-react with RTV antigen originating in heterologous rodent hosts.

The demonstration that a virus of unknown origin contained an identifiable gs1 antigen and/or gs3 antigen would be a significant step toward resolving the history of origin and identification of the virus. On the other hand, the failure to find cross-reacting antigens, does not exclude the host of a tested virus as progenitor of the unknown virus. This should be clear when one notes that reticuloendotheliosis virus of fowl appears to have no antigens in common with the classsical avian leuko-sarcoma virsues (Maldonado and Bose, 1971), and that mouse mammary tumor virus probably is unrelated antigenically to the murine leukemia viruses. Many similar discrepancies are likely to surface in future investigations.

The lesson was dramatized during two recent publicity-laden incidents purporting the discovery of human tumor viruses. In the first, human lymphoid cells in culture were found to produce a virus, called ESP-1 which was morphologically in the RTV class (Priori *et al.*, 1971). Preliminary immunological examination of ESP-1 virus failed to reveal similarity to known viruses (Shigematsu *et al.*, 1971), but other studies demonstrated strong cross-reactions with antibody directed against murine RTV (Gilden *et al.*, 1971). Furthermore, the reverse transcriptase of ESP-1 virions was inhibited by antiserum elicited by murine leukemia virus (Gallo *et al.*, 1971) or by feline leukemia virus (Scolnick *et al.*, 1972*b*). While discussion on this matter continues, the conclusion that ESP-1 is a murine virus is inescapable.

In the second case, cells from a human rhabdomyosarcoma were transplanted into fetal cats. Cells later were removed, and after propagation in culture, electron microscopic examination revealed RTV-like particles (termed RD 114 virus) in the culture medium (McAllister *et al.*, 1971). Viral material in excess of that required to give complement-fixing reactivity failed to react with antibody directed against a variety of RTV, including various isolates of feline leukemia virus (McAllister *et al*, 1972). Nonetheless, molecular hybridization experiments suggested a greater relatedness of RD 114 to feline cells than to human cells (Gillespie *et al.*, 1973; Okabe *et al.*, 1973; Baluda and Roy-Burman, 1973; Neiman, 1973). Subsequent experimentation with cat cells resulted in the isolation independently by three laboratories of RTV different from feline leukemia virus, but similar to RD 114 virus (Livingston and Todaro, 1973; Fischinger *et al.*, 1973; Sarma *et al.*, 1973).

2.5. Viral RNA

Less than 2% of the total dry weight of virions is RNA (Bonar and Beard, 1959). Description of the molecules comprising this RNA range the gamut of biologically active RNAs, from 4 S tRNAs to the large 70 S RNA characteristic of RTV. Ribosomal RNAs have often been considered virus constitutents (Bonar *et al.*, 1967). While generally considered to be cellular contaminants of virions, some investigators have attempted to attribute a function to the presence of ribosomal RNAs, and estimates of one ribosome per virion have been made. When one considers the difficulties in purification of RTV, the variable amounts of cellular RNAs observed in virion preparations compared with viral 60–70 S RNA suggest that the cellular RNAs, when found, are contaminants. Virions from cultures exposed to high levels of ^{3}H-uridine for as long as 24 hours have been isolated and found devoid of 28 S or 18 S ribosomal RNAs. Preparations of Rauscher leukemia virus, and Rous sarcoma virus processed in my laboratory have contained no more than one ribosome for every hundred virions. Also, protein synthesis can be completely suppressed without effect on the early stages of infection with RTV. Without protein synthesis it is difficult to conceive of a role for intravirion ribosomes in virus reproduction.

Intravirion degradation of the large-molecular-weight RNA may be responsible for the appearance of a variety of species smaller than 60–70 S RNA, and, when these as well as associated cellular RNAs are found and given serious consideration, confusion reigns. A number of molecular sizes (McCain *et al.*, 1973) may emerge after mistreatment of virions, but these signal degradation and cannot be accepted as original virion species.

Some 15 to 20 different species of low-molecular-weight RNAs (4–7 S) are regularly found in virion preparations (Bishop *et al.*, 1970*a,b*; Sawyer and Dahlberg, 1973). The suspicion that at least some of this RNA originates in 60–70 S RNA is supported by quantitation of RNA classes of a number of preparations of avian myeloblastosis virus (Bonar *et al.*, 1967). Amounts of low-molecular-weight RNA in these studies increased in inverse proportion to 60 S RNA, while that of associated ribosomal RNAs did not change. We have found that extended incubation of virions at 37°C results in loss of 60–70 S RNA from virions of murine leukemia or avian leuko-sarcoma viruses, while amounts of low-molecular-weight RNAs progressively increase. Also, several low-molecular-weight species can be found after heating the 60–70 S RNA (Emanoil-Ravicovitch *et al.*, 1973).

Some 4 S RNA extracted from virion preparations is legitimate tRNA with amino acid-accepting activity (Beaudreau *et al.*, 1964; Carnegie *et al.*, 1969; Travnicek, 1968; Travnicek and Riman, 1970; Erikson and Erikson, 1970). Is it contaminant, or is it viral, and if viral, is it functional? The relative amino acid-accepting activities of the 4 S RNA from avian myeloblastosis virus were examined and certain activities were enhanced compared to those from host cells, while other activities were absent. These investigators suggested that virions selectively incorporated specific tRNAs. Other workers (Bishop *et al.*, 1970*b*; Randerath *et al.*, 1971) have attempted to draw conclusions about the origin of low-molecular-weight viral RNAs on base composition alone. In the absence of supportive data, such studies do not seem meaningful since contaminating cellular RNA, degraded 60–70 S RNA, and the possible intravirion tRNA may all be contributors.

Let us consider a role for intravirion tRNA in infection by RTV. It can be assumed that intravirion components are required only during the first few hours (i.e., the early stages) of infection. No new protein synthesis is required during this time (Bader, 1966*a*, 1972*a*); it thus seems unlikely that "intravirion tRNA" is involved in recognition of unusual viral RNA codons (e.g., suppression of terminator sequences), that this tRNA allows for a localized increase in availability of specific tRNAs, or that such tRNA is used in any other activity related to protein synthesis. This is the same argument advanced against the occurrence of ribosomal RNAs in virions.

Another possibility is that amino acid-accepting RNA is structurally associated with the 60–70 S RNA and functions to produce structural restraints in contributing to a specific secondary structure, or perhaps is used as the primer for initiation in the reverse transcriptase reaction. The isolated 60–70 S RNA of avian myeloblastosis virus was shown to contain 4 S RNA (Erikson and Erikson, 1971), which could be dissociated by heat, and contained amino acid-accepting activity (Rosenthal and Zamecnik, 1973). Various amino acid-acceptor species were found, and the latter authors reported an enrichment in lysyl-tRNA, perhaps a tenuous conclusion. It remains to be determined whether the released polynucleotides with amino acid-acceptor activity are identical with cellular tRNA.

2.5.1.   60–70 S RNA

Large-molecular-weight RNA was found originally by Robinson *et al.* (1967) to be characteristic of RTV of avian and murine origin, and these observations were eventually extended to all recognized RTV. Resolution of 60–70 S RNA has been the predominant identifying factor in analyses for RTV, and can be used to measure quantitatively the production of RTV which may be missing other components, e.g., reverse transcriptase (Hanafusa and Hanafusa, 1971), or may be otherwise defective (Bader and Bader, 1970).

The molecular weight of the viral RNA has been estimated by sedimentation relative to RNA markers of known molecular weight (Robinson *et al.*, 1965), by mobility after electrophoresis in polyacrylamide gels (Bader and Steck, 1969), or by sedimentation equilibrium analysis (Luborsky, 1971). These extrapolations agree on a common molecular weight of about $8-11 \times 10^6$ daltons for the RNA from avian leuko-sarcoma viruses. Murine leuko-sarcoma viruses are found to be slightly larger, about $10-13 \times 10^6$ daltons, perhaps in keeping with the slightly larger size of the murine virions.

Most strains of RTV have 60–70 S RNA with a characteristic apparent molecular weight, which may be distinguished from other strains in double-labeling experiments. This large-molecular-weight 60–70 S viral RNA will be referred to herein as "vRNA." Among avian leuko-sarcoma viruses, Bolognesi and Graf (1971) demonstrated a variety of vRNA molecular sizes, and no correlation could be drawn on the basis of (1) whether the viruses were transforming or nontransforming, (2) antigenic subgroup, or (3) the capacity of the virus to induce tumors in animals. Duesberg and Vogt (1970; 1973a) showed similar results, but suggested that transforming viruses may contain larger RNAs than similar nontransforming viruses.

2.5.2. Denatured Viral RNA

When vRNA in solution is boiled briefly, its sedimentation rate decreases and its electrophoretic mobility in polyacrylamide gels increases (Fig. 1), (Duesberg, 1968; Erikson, 1969; Bader and Steck, 1969). We shall refer to this form as vRNA'. For Rauscher murine leukemia virus the projected molecular weight of vRNA decreases from 12×10^6 to 4×10^6 daltons, and for Rous sarcoma virus (RAV1) the decrease is from about 9×10^6 to 3×10^6 daltons (J. P. Bader and D. A. Ray, unpublished). Duesberg (1968) first suggested that the vRNA was composed of several subunits, and the observed decreases in molecular weights indicated that vRNA contains 2–4 vRNA' subunits, if one ignores the contribution of the secondary structure of vRNA to molecular weight estimates.

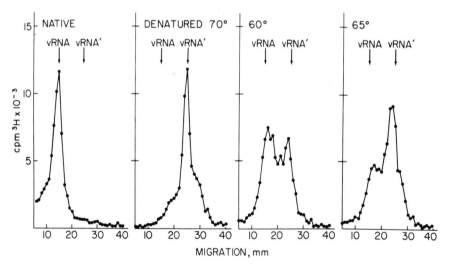

Fig. 1. Denaturation of RTV RNA. RNA extracted from Rous sarcoma virus (RSV-BH + RAV1) was suspended in buffer containing 0.13 M NaCl and heated for 3 minutes at 60°C, 65°C, or 70°C. Heating at 70°C denatured the vRNA, changing its electrophoretic mobility from a slowly moving peak (left panel), to a more rapidly moving one (vRNA', middle left panel). Incomplete denaturation was found after heating at 60°C or 65°C, with the appearance of forms intermediate to vRNA and vRNA (right panels).

While vRNA′ probably has the "random-coil" configuration, vRNA probably is different. Native vRNA extracted from virions has a linear extended configuration when viewed by electron microscopy, but after denaturation, vRNA′ is found in a collapsed form (Kakefuda and Bader, 1969). Secondary structure of vRNA′ seems to have no aberrant effect on molecular weight determinations; sedimentation in gradients containing dimethyl sulfoxide (Duesberg, 1968) or electrophoresis in formamide-containing gels (Duesberg and Vogt, 1973a), treatments designed to disengage base-paired regions, gave molecular weight values of vRNA′ similar to those estimated without such treatments. Scissions in the viral RNA chain(s) may not affect the characteristic slow electrophoretic mobility of native vRNA, but these chain interruptions are revealed when vRNA is denatured, and, instead of a sharp vRNA′ electrophoretic peak, a heterogenous distribution of rapidly migrating RNA is found (Bader and Steck, 1969).

Any of a number of treatments which dissociate hydrogen bonds will convert vRNA to vRNA′, including exposure to dimethyl sulfoxide, urea, or formadehyde (Duesberg, 1968; Bader and Steck, 1969). Other treatments which do not dissociate hydrogen bonds, including high salt concentrations, mercaptoethanol, protease, and DNase, fail to effect conversion. It seems, therefore, that maintenance of the vRNA configuration depends upon hydrogen bonds. Whether the hydrogen bonding occurs through specific nucleotide base pairing or some other manner has not been determined. Digestion with pancreatic RNase suggests that vRNA can be considered predominantly single-stranded, although Leis and Hurwitz (1972a) have shown that about 50% of vRNA is base paired. Also, denaturation of vRNA occurs over a wide range of temperatures (45–70°C), increasing with increasing salt concentration (Bader and Steck, 1969), while reovirus RNA, a completely double-stranded RNA, has a narrow range of denaturation (80–85°C) at similar salt concentrations. As shown in Fig. 1, when vRNA is incompletely denatured, forms migrating intermediate to vRNA and vRNA′ are observed (Bader and Steck, 1969). One may envision a vRNA molecule composed of subunits held together by short, perhaps nonidentical, lengths of nucleotide base pairs.

On the other hand, base pairing might be essential to the maintenance of a certain degree of secondary structure, but association of subunits may be due to the binding to RNA of molecules other than nucleic acids. Some secondary structure is required in order for viral RNA to act as specific template in a reverse-transcriptase reaction. Loss of template activity occurs upon denaturation by heating, and this loss of activity is thought to be due to the dissociation of a short strand of "primer" RNA which is bound through base pairing to the larger viral RNA. The loss of template activity is not due to the conversion of vRNA to vRNA´ however. When conversion of vRNA to vRNA´ was compared with template activity after exposure of vRNA to various temperatures, most of the template activity could be found still intact after conversion was complete, (Canaani and Duesberg, 1972). While one can easily imagine that retention of the vRNA structure requires less extensive base pairing than that involved in reverse-transcriptase activity, the possibility that other types of molecules may be involved in the binding together of subunits has not been excluded.

The molecular weight of intravirion RNA of any RTV probably cannot be stated with any degree of authority as of this writing. Let us consider for a moment how the figure "approximately 10^7 daltons" for the molecular weight of RTV RNA was derived. The first estimates of molecular weight for RTV RNA were based upon quantitative determinations of RNA per virion, after sedimentation of avian myeloblastosis virus (Bonar and Beard, 1959), and after isopycnic density banding of Rous sarcoma virus in RbCl gradients (Crawford, and Crawford, 1961). The estimated molecular weight for the viral RNAs of both preparations was approximately 9.5×10^6 daltons. Subsequent publications of Bonar and his co-workers showed considerable ribosomal and perhaps other cellular RNAs in their virion preparations. No similar manifestation of heterogeneity of RNA species is available for Crawford's preparations, but in the absence of any contradictory documentation, one can assume that such preparations likewise contained cellular RNA. Base ratios of the RNA from Crawford's Rous sarcoma virus preparation were quite different from the base ratios of purified 60–70 S vRNA determined later (Robinson et al., 1965; Bishop et al., 1970b). Since extraneous RNAs probably constituted a significant proportion of the RNA measured, the number 9.5×10^6 daltons for the intravirion molecular weight of avian myeloblastosis virus RNA, and Rous sarcoma virus RNA, probably is an overestimate.

Similar molecular weights extrapolated from the sedimentation rates and electrophoretic mobilities of the large viral RNAs from the same viruses seem too coincidental to be disregarded. However, as discussed earlier, the contribution of secondary structure to the hydrodynamic properties of vRNA cannot be predicted, and any estimate of molecular weight on the basis of the available data must be taken, at this time, as crude estimates indeed.

Subunits of reovirus RNA or influenza virus RNA are of several different sizes. Subunits of RTV are probably of identical size for any given strain; that is, denaturation of vRNA (Fig. 1) results in vRNA′ which migrates electrophoretically in a single sharp peak, (Bader and Steck, 1969, and unpublished observations). Duesberg and Vogt (1970) argued that sarcoma viruses contain two classes of subunits, one identical with the subunits of counterpart nontransforming viruses and another, larger, class. All of these transforming-virus preparations examined probably contained nontransforming viruses as well, and later analysis of virus from recently cloned sarcoma-producing cells showed that only the larger-sized RNA was present in virions (Duesberg and Vogt, 1973b). Therefore, the existence of two sizes of vRNA′ molecules within a single virion is suspect, except perhaps in cases such as heterozygosis (Weiss et al., 1973), where two or more similar genomic regions are found in the same virion. Scheele and Hanafusa (1972) were unable to detect differences between vRNA′ from several transforming and nontransforming avian RTV. Any generalization about sizes of subunits of transforming vs. nontransforming RTV probably should be withheld until more information is available.

As indicated above, the size of vRNA′ may not be identical among all strains of RTV. Comparative studies of murine and avian leuko-sarcoma viruses performed in my laboratory indicate that the size of vRNA′ is directly proportional to the estimated size of the native vRNA.

A somewhat puzzling phenomenon should be presented at this point. Virions of avian leuko-sarcoma viruses, when collected from cell cultures within a few minutes after completion, contain a high proportion of RNA in the vRNA′ form, or in forms intermediate between vRNA and vRNA′ (Cheung et al., 1972; Canaani et al., 1973). If these same preparations are incubated at 37–41°C for 1 hour before viral RNA is extracted, all of the RNA is found in the vRNA form. In a comparative study in which these results on avian viruses were confirmed, virions of Rauscher murine leukemia virus presented only the vRNA form in freshly collected samples (J. P. Bader and D. A. Ray, unpublished). The observations cannot be explained at this time. Suggestions that fresh virions are relatively noninfectious, or that they represent morphologically "immature" (Type A) virions cannot be taken seriously without supporting data.

The above data fail to exclude configurational changes in the RNA as the basis for changes in hydrodynamic properties. One such configuration which fits well with electron microscopic observations, and which could result in the observed sedimentation and electrophoretic properties of vRNA and vRNA′, is that of a tight, symmetrical coil, which after denaturation assumes a random-coil configuration. Resolution of the character of vRNA probably will require procedures which allow renaturation of vRNA from the vRNA′ form.

2.5.3. Polyadenylic Acid and Viral RNA

The role of polyadenylic acid (poly A) in the activity of mRNA has caught the attention of scientists interested in the biological transfer of information. Most mRNAs contain extended consecutive sequences of adenylic acid (Lee *et al.*, 1971; Darnell *et al.*, 1971; Edmonds *et al.*, 1971). This poly A may contain as many as 200 nucleotides, covalently attached to the 3′ OH end of the RNA molecules (Burr and Lingrel, 1971). Since the strand of RNA contained within the virion of RTV probably is identical to the strand translated intracellularly into virus-specific proteins, the presence or absence of poly A would bear on the activity of viral RNA as mRNA.

The RNAs of several RTV were found to contain poly A consisting of 100–200 nucleotides (Lai and Duesberg, 1972*a*, Gillespie *et al.*, 1972; Ross *et al.*, 1972; Green and Cartas, 1972). The poly A is found in the denatured as well as native forms of viral RNA. Unfortunately, the exact location of the poly A has not been determined, although it is presumed to be attached to the viral genome at the 3′ OH end. This attachment would be consistent with the finding of adenine at the 3′ terminus of virus (Stephenson *et al.*, 1972*b*). On the other hand, Maruyama *et al.* (1971) determined the 3′ end of the vRNAs from a variety of RTV to be uracil, and Erikson *et al.*, (1971) using avian myeloblastosis virus, showed uracil to be the terminus of the denatured form, vRNA′. It is possible that poly A is attached near the 3′ end of viral RNA, but the molecule is terminated by uracil.

In any case, the function of poly A in viral RNA is unknown. There is some question about its transcription into DNA, although Duesberg *et al.* (1971) observed synthesis of deoxythymidine-rich polynucleotide in a reverse-transcriptase reaction. Translation of poly A might result in polylysine, which has not been described in virions or infected cells. If the poly A is involved in maintaining secondary structure, sequences of uridylic acid might also be expected. Deliberate experiments failed to indicate the existence of polyuridylic acid in viral RNA (Marshall and Gillespie, 1972).

2.5.4. Irradiation Experiments

Irradiation experiments have been used in attempts to gain information on the nucleic acid substructure of RTV virions. Exposure to UV results in inactivation of infectivity following "single-hit" kinetics (Levinson and Rubin, 1966). Comparison of the UV-inactivation rates of the transforming ability of the Bryan strain of Rous sarcoma virus (RSV-BH) and the reproductive activity of a related leukosis virus, Rous-associated virus, revealed no differences (Levinson and Rubin, 1966). Nonetheless, rates of inactivation may be different for different RTV. Friis (1971) found that several other strains of avian sarcoma virus were inactivated at rates 50% or more greater than RSV-BH. The differences could not be related to host cell differences or envelope phenotype. Since minor, if any, differences in the sizes of the viral RNA are found between RSV-BH and the other sarcoma viruses, rates of inactivation cannot be attributed to size of viral RNA alone. In fact, Newcastle disease virus infectivity is inactivated by UV at a rate about 10 times that of RSV-BH, despite the vRNA of RSV-BH being larger than Newcastle disease viral RNA (Rubin and Temin, 1959; Levinson and Rubin, 1966). In contrast, X rays inactivated RSV-BH and Newcastle disease virus (NDV) at similar rates.

No easy explanation for these data is at hand, but one could imagine that (1) only a portion of the RTV RNA is involved in reproduction, (2) a different portion of the RNA is involved in transformation, (3) UV inactivation of one area of the genome may or may not prevent functioning of another portion of the genome, (4) the gene(s) responsible for transformation may be of different size in different strains of sarcoma virus, (5) secondary structure makes RTV RNA less sensitive than the RNA of NDV to the effects of UV, and/or (6) on the basis of secondary structure specific regions of the RTV genome are more or less sensitive to UV than other regions.

Studies of mutants of several avian sarcoma viruses have shown that the functioning of the genes responsible for transformation are not required for virus reproduction (Martin, 1970; Bader and Brown, 1971). These virus mutants have the capability of full cycles of reproduction at both 41°C and 37°C, but they transform cells only at the lower temperature. Also, differences in morphology of transformed cells after infection by different sarcoma viruses suggest that transformation by one virus may have a biochemically different basis, and therefore a genetically different basis, than transformation by another virus. It is not difficult to envision the "transformation gene" of one avian sarcoma virus being of different size or of different genomic location than the transformation gene of another avian sarcoma virus.

2.6. Reverse Transcriptase

Reverse transcriptase is the name commonly given to the viral RNA-dependent (RNA-specified, RNA-directed, or RNA-instructed) DNA polymerase found in all RTV, and also in several other viruses not usually considered in the tumor virus group (e.g., visna virus, simian foamy virus). An enzyme which synthesizes DNA using viral RNA as template was anticipated by studies demonstrating that no new protein synthesis was required for the synthesis of a presumptive viral DNA during the early stages of infection of cells by Rous sarcoma virus (Bader, 1966a). Temin and Mizutani (1970) and Baltimore (1970) simultaneously reported on the occurrence of reverse transcriptase in virions of avian leuko-sarcoma and murine leukemia viruses, and subsequent analysis of a number of RTV from a variety of hosts of origin showed that the enzyme was characteristic of RTV, but not of several other RNA-containing animal viruses which do not require DNA synthesis in their reproductive cycles.

Although the reverse transcriptase can often be demonstrated in virion preparations without any deliberate disruption of the virions, the enzyme is an internal component of the virion, and highest activity is found after exposure to small amounts of detergent. A core fraction of virions partially stripped of outer envelope was found to retain reverse-transcriptase activity (Coffin and Temin, 1971).

Enzyme activities in different RTV often can be distinguished with antiserum to a given reverse transcriptase (Oroszlan et al., 1971a; Parks et al., 1972). Antibody to the Schmidt-Ruppin strain of Rous sarcoma virus inhibits the activity of the avian sarcoma viral enzyme, but not that of Rauscher murine leukemia virus. Similarly, antibody to Rauscher murine leukemia virus enzyme fails to inhibit the activity of avian sarcoma virus or viper virus. Nonetheless, immunological cross-reactivity is found among the reverse transcriptases of murine, feline, rat, and hamster leukosarcoma viruses (Aaronson et al., 1971a). This cross-reactivity is also found with the viral interspecies-specific complement-fixing antigen (gs3), although the reverse transcriptase is a different protein. The molecular weight of murine leukemia virus reverse transcriptase is considerably larger than that of the gs3 antigens (Tronick et al., 1972), and antibody directed against purified enzyme from avian myeloblastosis virus in immunodiffusion studies failed to react with any of the major proteins of the virus (Watson et al., 1972).

On the other hand, antibody to reverse transcriptase from avian myeloblastosis virus did not inhibit the activity of avian reticuloendo- theliosis virus (Watson et al., 1972), and antiserum which inhibited the enzyme of a murine leukemia virus had little effect on the activity of murine mammary tumor virus. These results demonstrate that dif- ferent viruses from the same host of origin may have different forms of reverse transcriptase, and suggest that reverse transcriptase is specified by the viral genome.

The reverse transcriptase of avian myeloblastosis virus has a molecular weight of about 170,000 daltons and can be separated into two polypeptide subunits of 65,000 and 105,000 daltons (Kacian et al., 1971; Hurwitz and Leis, 1972; Grandgenett et al., 1973). The lower- molecular-weight subunit contains the DNA-polymerizing activity, as well as a ribonuclease specific for DNA–RNA hybrid polymers. The function of the larger polypeptide is unknown, but it possibly assists in the polymerization of DNA by denaturing the secondary structure of native viral RNA. Only one polypeptide, of about 70,000 daltons molecular weight, has been identified in the reverse transcriptase of murine leukemia virus (Tronick et al., 1972).

2.6.1.   Role of Reverse Transcriptase in Virus Infection

Enzymes similar to viral reverse transcriptase are found in noninfected cells. These enzymes either show different cofactor re- quirements or utilize synthetic polynucleotide templates with a dif- ferent efficiency than viral enzyme (Baltimore et al., 1973). The "R- DNA polymerase" of chick embryo cells described by Weissbach et al. (1972) can copy polyriboadenylic acid in a poly-rA/oligo-dT template, but cannot copy from poly-rC/oligo-dG or natural RNAs. A similar enzyme described by Kang and Temin (1972) synthesized DNA from an endogenous chick embryo RNA template, but could not use poly- rA/oligo-dT. Also, antisera against enzymes from avian or murine RTV failed to react with enzymes from uninfected avian and murine cells, respectively (Nowinski et al., 1971; Ross et al., 1971). While it has not been excluded that viral reverse transcriptases are cellular enzymes, the failure to find identical enzymes in uninfected, non-virus- producing cells supports the theory of a viral origin for these enzymes.

This belief is strengthened when certain defective RTV are considered. Certain chick embryo cells infected with RSV 0 produce virions which cannot infect any known cells, including certain cells which are responsive to the viral envelope involved in initial interactions. Examination of these virions showed them to be deficient in reverse-transcriptase activity (Hanafusa and Hanafusa, 1971; Robinson and Robinson, 1971) and in the protein with which enzymatic activity is associated (H. Hanafusa *et al.*, 1972). In addition, cells producing this defective virus contain no detectable viral reverse transcriptase (Weissbach *et al.*, 1972). Similar cases have been reported for cells transformed by murine sarcoma virus in which noninfectious virions without polymerase activity were produced (May *et al.*, 1972; Peebles *et al.*, 1972). One could argue that the viruses failed to induce the specific cellular enzyme identified as reverse transcriptase, which was to be incorporated into virions. A solution to this problem, it seems, would be to compare immunologically the enzyme from avian leuko-sarcoma viruses grown in avian cells with the same viruses grown in mammalian cells.

The deficiency of reverse transcriptase in defective virions is, in the absence of any other observable defect, evidence for a role for this enzyme in infection of cells by RTV. The demand for DNA synthesis early in the course of infection, which almost certainly represents synthesis of viral DNA, requires an enzyme capable of using viral RNA as a template for complementary DNA. The associated viral enzyme fulfills at least some of the requirements for synthesizing viral DNA.

2.6.2. Polynucleotide Requirements for Transcriptase Activity

Synthesis of DNA by reverse transcriptase requires two forms of polynucleotide, the template and a primer. The template is the RNA, specifically the viral RNA, which is transcribed into DNA. The natural primer is also an RNA polynucleotide, not necessarily long, which provides the new DNA a beginning point for elongation complementary to the template. The primer may be either a result of intramolecular base pairing, forming a "hairpin" structure with a free 3′ OH end, or an associated polynucleotide not covalently bound to the viral RNA. This latter possibility is favored by the observed priming activity of synthetic oligonucleotides: vRNA upon denaturation loses template activity which can be reconstituted by the addition of low-molecular-weight polynucleotides (Duesberg *et al.*, 1971; Canaani and Duesberg, 1972). No unequivocal statement can be made about the nature of the native primer molecule since the integrity of the native viral RNA in these studies was not discussed; partial degradation of the native viral RNA could result in loss of primer upon denaturation. Nonetheless, short polynucleotide chains may serve as primer. Bishop *et al.* (1973) found that the primer could be selectly separated from the template after initiating DNA synthesis, and they have tentatively identified the bases comprising the 3′-terminal fragment of the primer.

The primer probably is a dispensable segment of the virus genome, no matter what its association to the bulk of the viral RNA. Since the primer begins the DNA chain, it cannot be transcribed until the second strand of DNA is synthesized. In another sense, the primer may be redundant information since it probably is base paired to its complementary viral RNA.

2.6.3. The DNA Product

Using the endogenous viral RNA as template, the DNA product of the transcriptase reaction is initially associated with the viral RNA (Garapin *et al.*, 1970; Fujinaga *et al.*, 1970; Faras *et al.*, 1971; Manly *et al.*, 1971), and later is found as free DNA (Fanshier *et al.*, 1971). The initial association was found to be a covalent link between the 3′ OH of the ribonucleotide primer molecule through a phosphodiester bond to the 5′ OH end of the growing deoxyribonucleotide chain. The linked nucleotides of avian myeloblastosis virus have been identified by Verma *et al.*, (1971, 1972) and of murine leukemia by Okabe *et al.* (1972) as . . . rA3′-p-5′ dA. . . . Flugel and Wells (1972), using ether instead of detergent to permeate avian myeloblastosis virions, found the rA-p-dA linkage to constitute only about one-fifth of the linkage regions, and rU-p-dC to constitute the majority of linked ribo–deoxynucleotides. Perhaps this disagreement was not unexpected since the 3′ OH ends of avian myeloblastosis virus RNA (Erikson *et al.*, 1971), as well as murine, feline, and viper virus RNAs (Maruyama *et al.*, 1971), had been determined to be rU, while Stephenson *et al.* (1972b) found rA to be the predominant ribonucelotide at the 3′ terminus. In addition, however, the linkage rC-p-dC, as well as rA-p-dA, was found by Flugel *et al.* (1973) in the transcription products of both B77 virus (avian) and Rauscher leukemia virus (murine).

If the primer is simply a hairpin loop in the viral RNA, then one should expect one 3′ terminus per subunit in vRNA, and the same number after denaturation to vRNA′. Maruyama *et al.* (1971) found four 3′ termini in the vRNA of a murine sarcoma virus, but the integrity of the molecules was not assessed and no measurements on vRNA´ were done. If primer is a small polynucleotide attached by base pairing, then two or more 3´ termini with nonidentical bases could be found per subunit in vRNA. This number should be reduced after denaturation and loss of primer from vRNA´. In the latter case, the 3´ end of the vRNA´ could be different for the 3´ end of the primer, and one might come to a different conclusion about the nature of the 3´ end of vRNA´ compared with vRNA. Virus preparations used in analyses of these types often contain partially degraded RNA, despite retaining the high 60–70 S sedimentation rate. Even when fresh virion preparations are used in reverse-transcriptase reactions using the endogenous viral RNA scissions in the RNA are commonplace. Interruptions in the ribonucleotide chains might not only present an erroneous 3´ OH determination, but might also provide priming activity not available in an intact molecule. That this occurs is suggested by the favored synthesis of the linkage, rC-p-dC, over rA-p-dA in fresh virions, and the reverse in older, incubated virions, (Flugel *et al.*, 1973). Until guarantees about the integrity of the RNA template are presented, there seems to be no obligation to make a decision about either the base at the 3´ terminus or the nucleotide composition of the linkage region.

As stated before, the initial DNA product of an endogenous transcriptase reaction is associated with the RNA, and later appears as double-stranded DNA. There are two circumstances in which double-stranded DNA apparently does not appear. In the first case, purified enzyme from avian myeloblastosis virus is used to transcribe isolated viral RNA into DNA; only RNA–DNA hybrid results (Leis and Hurwitz, 1972*a*). This result demonstrates that intravirion factors other than the reverse transcriptase are required to obtain double-stranded DNA, suggesting that double-stranded DNA is (1) an artifact of synthesis induced by the degradative processes of the reaction system, (2) synthesized by additional DNA-polymerizing enzymes such as a separate DNA-dependent DNA polymerase and/or ligase, or (3) promoted by a protein factor which stimulates DNA synthesis (Leis and Hurwitz, 1972*b*).

The second case in which the synthesis of double-stranded DNA is inhibited occurs after the addition of actinomycin D to the reaction mixture. Synthesized DNA is found hybridized to the viral RNA (Garapin *et al.*, 1973). Since it is well known that actinomycin D binds selectively to double-stranded DNA, it is likely that this interaction impedes further synthesis. Still, this reaction has been useful since it allows practically the entire viral genome to be transcribed into DNA, whereas under the usual reaction conditions, only a small portion of the genome is selectively transcribed.

The fact that it is possible to obtain almost complete transcripts from viral RNA (Duesberg and Canaani, 1970) suggests that the natural mode of genomic reduplication involves transcription of the entire genome into viral DNA. Unfortunately, the largest DNAs obtained from *in vitro* transcription reactions have been about 100,000 daltons of single-stranded DNA. Each of these strands represent considerably less than $\frac{1}{20}$, perhaps as little as $\frac{1}{100}$, of the viral genome. In a reaction system in which the total viral RNA is represented in the transcription product, there must be 20–100 initiation sites. But we know from our earlier discussion that if subunits comprise the native viral RNA, there are probably four or less 3′ OH ends of template RNA in native vRNA. This suggests that there are more than 20 primer molecules attached intermittently along any single viral polynucleotide template, or that nicks are introduced into the template RNA which then allow the template to act as its own primer.

An alternative, which I have not seen previously considered, is that the initiating regions of the viral genomes are randomly permuted, i.e., any molecule in a population of viral RNAs may have initiating template region which is different from another molecule, and because of this, all regions of the genome are represented in the initiator regions of a population of viral RNAs. The plot thickens when one makes the extrapolation to a hypothetical circular form of the genome during some stage of reduplication, which is cleaved at random to a linear form.

2.7. Other Enzymes

Reverse transcriptase gave a biochemical validity to the notion that RNA could be transcribed into DNA, but the enzyme by itself is insufficent to complete an uninterrupted polydeoxyribonucleotide chain equivalent to vRNA′. However, almost any other enzyme which one might implicate in DNA synthesis has been discovered in preparations of RTV. The question which inexorably surfaces is which of these enzymes are virus specific and which contaminant? Even contamination need not be invoked if one considers the classical example of adenosine triphosphatase (ATPase) associated with avian myeloblastosis virus (de The, 1964; de-The *et al.*, 1964). This ATPase was considered so consistent a component of virions that their number was often determined by the relative activity of the enzyme. Examination of virus-producing cells revealed enzyme activity on the cell surfaces. However, virus-producing kidney tumors, and virions emanating from them, had virtually no ATPase activity, and the presence or absence of enzyme in virions was shown to depend upon cell-specific, not virus-specific, factors.

Besides reverse transcriptase, the only enzyme which seems unequivocally to be virus specific, is the virus-associated RNase H (Molling *et al.*, 1971). This enzyme, apparently a processive exonuclease which attacks both ends of the polynucleotide (Keller and Crouch, 1972; Leis *et al.*, 1973), digests only the RNA strand of a DNA–RNA hybrid, and was found in all RTVs examined by Grandgenett *et al.* (1972). Furthermore, RNase H activity may be associated with the same polypeptide (molecular weight of 70,000 daltons) as the reverse transcriptase (Grandgenett *et al.*, 1973), although the purified DNA polymerase from Kirsten murine sarcoma-leukemia virus had no RNase H activity (Wang and Duesberg, 1973). A biological function for the RNase H of RTV has yet to be described. One obvious possibility is the degradation of the viral RNA strand complementary to the newly synthesized viral DNA, which might render the DNA more accessible to complementary synthesis of the second DNA strand. The requirement for a free RNA end for RNase H activity would necessitate either completion of a DNA strand equivalent to the vRNA′ before the enzyme could act, or prior nicking of the RNA opposite a completed DNA sequence. For various reasons, neither of these possibilities readily acceptable, and it is possible that the nuclease is an extraordinary activity of the reverse transcriptase.

The synthesis of short segments of DNA *in vitro* suggests that a ligase is involved in the covalent attachment of 3′ to 5′ ends and the eventual attainment of a DNA-size equivalent to vRNA′. DNA-dependent DNA polymerase would be useful in synthesizing the second strand of DNA and/or perhaps in completing gaps in DNA left after reverse transcriptase. Both ligase and DNA-dependent DNA-polymerizing activities have been described in virion preparations (Spiegelman *et al.*, 1970; Mizutani *et al.*, 1970, 1971). However, if these enzymes are involved in the joining of DNA segments, they clearly do not do this in the *in vitro* reverse-transcriptase reaction, and other factors must be invoked. Also, since reverse transcriptase can use DNA as template, and a separate DNA polymerase has not been identified in virions, one need not describe a separate biological function for the observed DNA-dependent DNA polymerase.

Other enzyme activities associated with nucleic acid synthesis found in virion preparations include DNA endonuclease and exonuclease (Rosenbergová, 1965; Mizutani *et al.*, 1970, 1971; Quintrell *et al.*, 1971; Maly and Riman, 1971; Hung, 1973), RNA methylase (Gantt *et al.*, 1971), nucleoside triphosphate phosphotransferase (Roy and Bishop, 1971), nucleotide kinase (Mizutani and Temin, 1971), and tRNA synthetases (Erikson and Erikson, 1972). Hexokinase, lactic dehydrogenase, phosphatase (Mizutani and Temin, 1971), protein kinase (Strand and August, 1971; Hatanaka *et al.*, 1972), and ATPase (de-The *et al.*, 1964) are among other activities found in virus preparations. It is difficult to be convinced that these are anything but inadvertant associates of virions. Reasonable assessment of purity of the virions is lacking in all of these studies, and a specific role for any single enzyme in virus reproduction is not easily identifiable.

2.8. Organization of Virion Components

A diagrammatic model of a typical RTV virion is presented in Fig. 2.

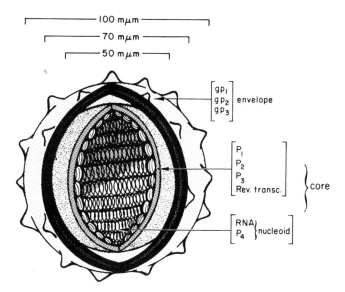

Fig. 2. Model of a virion of RTV. The virion is composed of an envelope and a core. The envelope contains lipid, glycoproteins, and perhaps other proteins. The core contains several nonglycosylated proteins, including the reverse transcriptase. The RNA-containing nucleoid constitutes the internal part of the core.

2.8.1. The Envelope

The viral envelope is composed of lipid and proteins, including the glycoproteins. Projections of the envelope, called "spicules" or "spikes," can be visualized microscopically and are removed by treatment of the virions with proteolytic enzymes (Bonar *et al.*, 1964; Rifkin and Compans, 1971). The envelope is responsible for the initial interaction of the virion with the cell, and host-range specificity is determined by the polypeptide portion of at least one glycoprotein (Scheele and Hanafusa, 1971; Duesberg *et al.*, 1970). The envelope appears microscopically as a typical "unit" membrane and is separate from the core. This membrane is semipermeable and virions typically respond to changes in osmotic pressure.

Dimethyl sulfoxide (less than 10%) protects RTV from inactivation by freezing and thawing, and brief exposure of virions to low concentrations (less than 0.001%) of the nonionic detergent, Triton X-100, inactivates infectivity (unpublished observations). Proteolytic enzymes which remove spike proteins, but which leave other proteins intact, also inactivate infectivity. These observations suggest that the integrity of the envelope is essential to the infectivity of the virion.

2.8.2. The Core

A virion core can be obtained by exposure of intact virions to detergents, or other treatments which strip off the outer envelope (de-The and O'Connor, 1966; Bader *et al.*, 1970; Stromberg, 1972). These cores are unstable in usual extraction media (Bader *et al.*, 1970; Duesberg, 1970), and neither these nor the nucleoids can be considered analogous to nucleocapsids of other types of virions. This instability perhaps is responsible for the discrepancies in certain parameters found during characterization. Buoyant densities of 1.23, (Coffin and Temin, 1971), 1.26–1.27 (de-The and O'Connor, 1966; Bader *et al.*, 1970), and 1.34 g/ml (Davis and Rueckert, 1972) have been reported for cores. Densities of 1.23–1.27 in sucrose are somewhat lower than that expected of only RNA and protein, suggesting that cores found in this range of densities still contain lipid.

Cores found at 1.34 g/ml may be substructures (nucleoids) of cores since the viral RNA is associated largely with a single protein (molecular weight, 14,000 daltons) different from the major internal proteins of the virion (molecular weights, 30,000 and 11,000) (Davis and Rueckert, 1972; Oroszlan *et al.*, 1971*b*). Quigley *et al.*, (1972*a*) also found a 14,000-dalton-molecular-weight protein predominating in cores banding at 1.26 g/ml. About 2300 molecules per virion were estimated, or about one polypeptide for every 15 nucleotides. A similar protein was shown by Fleissner and Tress (1973*b*) to contain a larger proportion of arginine residues than other viral proteins, perhaps aiding in the neutralization of the acidic groups of the RNA within the virion.

A core structure without RNA has not been isolated. In fact, exposure of cores to RNase released both protein and RNA (Duesberg, 1970), suggesting that the RNA participates in the binding of protein in the core.

Although core preparations have been observed to retain some infectivity (Shibley *et al.*, 1969; Bolognesi *et al.*, 1972*b*) cores have generally been found to be noninfectious. The lability of viral RNA upon dissociation of the envelope suggests that the retention of core infectivity would require special procedures to protect the RNA from degradation.

2.8.3. The Nucleoid

The nucleoid is the internal RNA-containing portion of the virion observed in thin sections by electron microscopy. Isolation of nucleoids has not been reported, unless the "cores" of Davis and Rueckert (1972) are, in fact, nucleoids. Nonetheless, no particles of defined structure having the morphology of nucleoids have been described.

Consideration of the electron-lucent centers of virions, and the location of the RNA in the nucleoid, led us to suggest that viral RNA is arranged in a ropelike coil, forming a hollow sphere within the virion (Kakefuda and Bader, 1969; Bader *et al.*, 1970). The thickness of the electron-dense RNA region within the nucleoid as observed in sectioned virions suggests also that the RNA is twisted in a secondary tight coil, similar to a spring, and it is this springlike molecule which is wound in larger turns within the nucleoid.

Isolated, native viral RNA occasionally exhibits a linear, twisted-coil structure which has not been noticed in other species of RNA (Kakefuda and Bader, 1969). Nonetheless, one must be cautious in accepting this as the native configuration, since disruption of the virion may confer a configuration which is merely a reflection of its form in the nucleoid. Electron micrographs from studies purporting to demonstrate a coiled-filament configuration within the virion unfortunately lack definition (Lacour *et al.*, 1970; Nowinski *et al.*, 1970;

Luftig and Kilham, 1971; Sarkar *et al.*, 1971). Viewing of the natural configuration probably will require methods allowing the removal of the obscuring outer envelope and intermediate layer without disturbing the nucleoid.

3. THE REPRODUCTIVE CYCLE

The reproductive cycle of RTV begins with the initial interactions of viral envelope and cellular membranes, and the unveiling of the viral RNA genome, proceeds through the synthesis of viral DNA, transcription of viral DNA into RNA, translation of viral RNA into proteins, the association of viral proteins and viral RNA in the developing virion, and ends as the virion buds from the cell surface membrane. The entire procedure requires a minimum of 8 hours. While the time course of some of the intracellular stages have been described, the molecular events are not nearly so well defined.

3.1.   Initial Interactions

The infection of cells by RTV requires interaction between a specific component of the viral envelope and a specific component of the cell. The cell component has been presumed to be located on or in the cell surface membrane, although direct evidence for this is lacking.

Avian leuko-sarcoma viruses have been classified into subgroups on the basis of antigenicity and homologous interference reactions, and these subgroups are maintained when susceptibility to given chick embryo cells are examined. Chick embryo cells resistant to subgroup A viruses, C/A cells, are susceptible to subgroup B viruses; C/B cells are resistant to subgroup B viruses but not to subgroup A (Vogt and Ishizaki, 1965). Susceptibility to both A and B subgroups has been found dominant to resistance in genetic crossover experiments in chickens, and the A and B genes are nonallelic (Payne and Pani, 1971). Cells susceptible to both A and B viruses presumably are dominant at both A and B loci (called *tva* and *tvb*, respectively), while C/AB, which are resistant to both A and B, probably are homozygous recessive in both loci.

Another type of control has been found in susceptibility to subgroup E viruses (Payne *et al.*, 1971). As with A and B subgroups, a dominant autosomal gene (e^s) controls susceptibility to RSV (RAV 0), a subgroup E virus. In addition, a second unlinked epistatic gene (I^e) inhibits the action of e^s. The I^e gene is dominant to i^e for inhibition;

therefore, cells with $e^s I^e$ are resistant to infection by RSV (RAV 0), $e^s i^e$ are susceptible, and $e^r I^e$ and $e^r i^e$ are resistant. These observations may explain why resistance to some tumor viruses is inherited as a dominant trait (Dhaliwal, 1963; Waters and Burmester, 1963).

Genetic experiments have also been used to analyze suceptibility and resistance to murine leukemia viruses. With these viruses, however, no correlation could be made between host range and serotype. Murine leukemia viruses can be separated into three host-range categories, N-tropic, B-tropic, and NB-tropic. This nomenclature is used to indicate relative ability to infect cells from NIH-Swiss mice or BALB/c mice, or both, respectively (Hartley *et al.*, 1970; Ware and Axelrod, 1972). A single gene (*Fv-1*), dominant for susceptibility to Friend leukemia virus, was shown to control the susceptibility of the cell (Odaka, 1969).

In some cases, the efficiency of infection of cells can be improved by treating the cells with DEAE-dextran (Vogt, 1967*b*), or with other substances which can alter the charge of the cell surface. In this way, one can effect a hundredfold increase in the number of chick embryo cells infected with Schmidt-Ruppin Rous sarcoma virus, subgroup D, or rat embryo cells infected with murine sarcoma virus (Ting, 1966). Possibly a similar change in relative charge is responsible for the increased susceptibility to superinfection noted in certain infected cells. Rous sarcoma virus-RAV2 infects chick embryo cells more efficiently if the cells are previously infected with and producing the Rous-associated virus, RAV1 (Hanafusa, 1964; Hanafusa and Hanafusa, 1968).

Mere attachment of a virion to the cell is insufficient for infection, since subgroup A and B avian leuko-sarcoma viruses adsorb equally well to susceptible or resistant cells (Steck and Rubin, 1966; Piraino, 1967; Crittenden, 1968). It is possible, however, that a different type of binding occurs between the cell surface membrane and viral envelope at compatible sites.

Host-range specificity can be extended for some viruses by incorporating envelope proteins from another virus in a phenotypic mixture. In this way the Bryan strain of Rous sarcoma virus has been made infectious for several genetic types of chick embryo cells which it could not otherwise infect. By growing Bryan virus in a mixed infection with RAV1 (subgroup A), normally resistant C/B cells can now be infected by the sarcoma virus containing envelope components of the leukemia virus. Likewise, Bryan virus grown with RAV2 (subgroup B) are capable of infecting normally resistant C/A cells (Vogt and Ishizaki, 1965).

   Interspecies barriers can be broken also, as Hanafusa and Hanafusa (1966) showed with a nontransforming derivative (RAV50) of an
avian sarcoma virus capable of infecting hamster cells. Bryan Rous
sarcoma virus was grown in cells mixedly infected with RAV50. Normally resistant hamster cells became transformed after exposure to this
virus, and tumors could be induced in hamsters. The same phenomena
are noted among murine leukemia and sarcoma viruses. As in the case
of some avian sarcoma viruses, murine sarcoma viruses depend upon
the envelope of an accompanying leukemia virus for transmissibility.
   The processes leading to disclosure of the viral RNA for DNA
synthesis are unknown. Several possibilities can be considered: (1) coalescence of viral and cellular membranes at the cell surface allowing
the viral core access to the cytoplasm, (2) penetration of the complete
virion into the cytoplasm, and later digestion of the envelope, and (3)
engulfment of the virion within a membranous vesicle, followed by
membrane coalescence, penetration, or combining of vesicles with
lysosomes. In electron microscopy studies Miyamoto and Gilden
(1971) found evidence for all three possibilities, but none were excluded. Virions were found coalescing with cell surface membranes,
intact within the cytoplasm, and contained within phagocytic vesicles.
However, the process involved in infection could not be distinguished
from processes which lead to destruction of the virion. Whatever the
mechanism, the penetration and uncoating process is rapid. The next
step, DNA synthesis, begins within the first hour after exposure of cells
to RTV (Bader, 1972a).
   Two stages in the initiation process after attachment could be resolved by Steck and Rubin (1966). In the first, addition of neutralizing
antibody immediately after adsorption prevented infection by Rous
sarcoma virus. After incubating a few minutes at 37°C antibody was
no longer effective. Brief exposure of cell–virus complexes to pH 2.2
also inactivated the virus, and susceptibility to low-pH inactivation was
lost rapidly. By varying the temperature, the rates of inactivation by
antibody and low pH could be differentiated, and resistance to antibody was found to proceed at a faster rate than resistance to pH 2.2.
   In studies involving electron microscopy and radioactive labeling,
Dales and Hanafusa (1972) concluded that virions migrated directly to
the nucleus, where the RNA was uncoated. Within an hour after addition of virus to cells, Rous sarcoma virions were observed in vesicles
adjacent to the nucleus, and radioactive viral RNA could be extracted
from fractionated nuclei. These enticing experiments would have
benefited from additional controls, such as using virus to which the

cells were resistant, and a monitor for cytoplasmic contamination of nuclear fractions.

Hatanaka *et al.* (1971) came to a different conclusion, using autoradiography to reveal the location of newly synthesized intracellular viral DNA, and thereby the viral RNA genome. Addition of ^{3}H-thymidine to cells recently infected with murine sarcoma or leukemia virus resulted in a large number of autoradiographic grains occurring in the cytoplasm. Curiously, cytoplasmic grains were found when labeling was delayed as long as 30–50 hours after infection. This could occur only if the viral DNA were replicating within the cytoplasm. The efficiency of infection in this system seems disproportionately low in comparison with the numbers of grains observed, and, without further supporting data, these results must be regarded as tentative.

3.2. Synthesis of Viral DNA

3.2.1. Physiological Requirements

Cellular factors involved in the early stages of the reproductive cycle of RTV, or of transforming by RTV, can generally be related to the synthesis of cellular DNA. This is not to say that cellular DNA itself must be synthesized, since such synthesis probably is unnecessary. Temin (1967) has reported that cells in the G2 phase of the mitotic cycle, which have completed their synthesis of DNA for that round, can be infected by Rous sarcoma virus. There is some doubt, however, about the ability of cells in G2 to be distinguished from those in S in the synchronization system employed in these experiments. More likely than a specific requirement for cellular DNA synthesis in RTV reproduction is the increased availability of enzymes synthesizing DNA precursors, and perhaps even DNA-polymerizing enzymes, at the time when cellular DNA is being synthesized. In semisynchronized cell populations, successful infection of cells by Rous sarcoma virus varied during the cell cycle (Bader, 1967*b*). The efficiency of infection was highest during the S phase, and fell off during and immediately after mitosis. In contrast, the efficiency of infection by Newcastle disease virus remained constant throughout the cell cycle (Bader, 1967*b*; Hobom-Schnegg *et al.*, 1970).

When virus reproduction was analyzed, infection immediately prior to, or during early S was found to produce the largest amounts of virus, and virus yield diminished in cultures infected at subsequent progressive stages through S and G2. Hobom-Schnegg *et al.*, (1970) observed no variation in the efficiency of infection for transformation during the cell cycle, but they found that cells infected in G1 required longer to yield the equivalent amount of Rous sarcoma virus than cells infected during S. A similar result was reported by Temin (1967) and by Yoshikura (1970) using murine sarcoma virus. These authors suggested that the S phase and mitosis had to be traversed in order for virus to be produced. Considering this requirement and their observed invariability of the efficiency of infection, one might expect that a given time after the first mitosis virus production would be the same regardless of the stage of the cell cycle at the time of infection; this is consistent with their observations. An alternative explanation is that cells infected during S are capable of reduplicating viral DNA to a greater extent than at any other time, and in turn the greater number of replicative genomes lessens the "latent" stage of virus reproduction, and results in greater yields of virus per unit time.

Cultures which have attained a high cell density, and in which cell growth and DNA synthesis has decreased to low levels, are resistant to infection by RTV (Temin and Rubin, 1958, 1959; Nakata and Bader, 1968*b*; Baker and Simons, 1971; Golde and Villaudy, 1971; Weiss, 1971). If such confluent cells are dispersed with trypsin within a few hours after exposure to virus, thus inducing DNA synthesis and cellular divisions, or if the cells are stimulated to induce DNA synthesis by replenishing depleted nutrients, infection is "established;" otherwise, infections may be aborted, and if cells are dispersed a day or more later, few infected cells can be found (Nakata and Bader, 1968*b*).

A similar phenomenon can be seen in cells suspended in growth medium. Chick embryo cells proceed through only one or two divisions after suspension in spinner cultures. After this time, the suspended cells cannot be infected by Rous sarcoma virus, but if allowed to settle onto a substratum, cell growth is renewed and cells again are susceptible to infection (Bader, 1967*a*).

Cultures exposed to serumless medium stop synthesizing DNA within a few days, although RNA synthesis continues (Bader, 1966*a*). Such cells are resistant to infection by Rous sarcoma virus, although even a brief exposure to serum allows infection to occur, and cells become transformed and produce virus. Cells infected prior to serum depletion have been observed to produce high levels of virus for over a month in the absence of serum.

A related phenomenon is the observed failure to infect X-irradiated cells if virus is added to cells after irradiation, when DNA synthesis has decreased to low levels (Rubin, 1960; Nakata and Bader,

1968*a*). However, if virus is added before irradiation, cells become infected and can release virus for several days.

In all of the above observations, a strict correlation can be drawn between successful infection and cellular DNA synthesis, while susceptibility changes in virus adsorption or penetration are not implicated. Also, such conditions which fail to allow for infection by RTV have little effect on other viruses, such as NDV or vesicular stomatitis (VS) virus, which require no DNA synthesis for reproduction. Nonetheless, a role for cellular DNA synthesis has never been defined experimentally. Some viral DNA undoubtedly becomes integrated into chromosomal DNA in the course of propagation of infected cells, and perhaps such integration involves synthesis of cellular DNA. However, an obligate integrative step has never been demonstrated, and in its absence it is difficult to envision a role for cellular DNA synthesis in infection by RTV. Cells grown in the presence of 5-bromodeoxyuridine, and in which the DNA contains large numbers of bromodeoxyuridine residues, are fully responsive to infection by Rous sarcoma virus if the bromodeoxyuridine is removed (Bader, 1964*a*). This suggests that even if cellular DNA synthesis is involved in RTV reproduction, the faithful complementation of specific nucleotide sequences may not be.

Implicit in the above observations is the failure of RTV to induce cellular DNA synthesis in inhibited cells. This suggested an important difference between RTV and DNA-containing tumor viruses, which had been reported to induce DNA synthesis in newly infected dormant cells. Deliberate experiments to examine this point failed to show any increase in DNA synthesis in confluent cells exposed to high multiplicities of murine leukemia virus or avian leuko-sarcoma viruses (Nakata and Bader, 1970), while under similar cell culture conditions polyoma virus induced DNA synthesis to three times the level of noninfected cells. Baker *et al.* (1972) obtained more than a tenfold increase in murine sarcoma virus if DNA synthesis of mouse embryo cells was stimulated by simultaneous infection with the papovavirus SV40. Other reports suggested that RTV, like DNA tumor viruses, could induce DNA synthesis (Macieira-Coelho and Ponten, 1967; Kara, 1968), but these results were probably due to other substances in the viral inoculum (Macieira-Coelho *et al.*, 1969).

3.2.2. Evidence for a DNA Replicative Genome

The first clear indication that DNA is involved in the reproduction of RTV came from the observed decrease in virus production of cells exposed to actinomycin D, an inhibitor of DNA transcription (Temin, 1963; Bader, 1964a; Vigier and Golde, 1964). Several other cytolytic RNA viruses had previously been shown to be unaffected by actinomycin D and could replicate independently of the participation of DNA (Reich et al., 1961).

A requirement for new DNA synthesis in the reproduction of RTV was demonstrated using 5-bromodeoxyuridine (Bader, 1964a,b) or 5-iododeoxyuridine (Bader, 1964b, 1965a). These nucleoside analogues substitute for thymidine during synthesis of DNA, thereby making a defective DNA. The reproduction of infectious Rous sarcoma virus was inhibited 10- to 1000-fold when either drug was added within the first few hours after infection.

Inhibition of DNA synthesis by cytosine arabinoside during the first 8–12 hours after infection gave a similar result; virus reproduction was almost completely inhibited (Bader, 1964a, 1965b). Other investigators (Temin, 1964a; Knudson et al., 1967) observed inhibitory effects of amethopterin and 5-fluorodeoxyuridine on the reproduction of avian leuko-sarcoma viruses, but the efficacy of these compounds in inhibiting DNA synthesis in chick embryo cells was not examined. Nonetheless, many subsequent studies established that any interference with DNA synthesis early in the course of RTV infection resulted in inhibition of virus reproduction. Inhibition of DNA synthesis also resulted in the failure of cells to become transformed after infection with Rous sarcoma virus (Bader, 1965b) or murine sarcoma virus (Nakata and Bader, 1968b). The requirement for DNA synthesis in the reproduction of RTV, or in transformation, was restricted to the first 8–12 hours after infection (Bader, 1965a,b, 1966a; Nakata and Bader, 1968b). Addition of cytosine arabinoside or 5-iododeoxyuridine after this time had no effect on virus production, although actinomycin D was still inhibitory.

Several RNA viruses which reproduce directly through an RNA replicative form, without the participation of DNA, induce RNA-dependent RNA polymerase in infected cells. Extensive experimentation failed to reveal RNA-dependent RNA polymerase in avian leukosis or sarcoma virus-infected cells (Wilson and Bader, 1965; J. P. Bader, unpublished).

On the basis of such studies, a DNA intermediate in the reproduction of RTV was proposed (Temin, 1963, 1964b; Bader, 1964a,b). These and all subsequent studies, were consistent with a new viral DNA being synthesized using the viral RNA as template. Theoretical objections to transcription of RNA into DNA, based upon notions of the unidirectional flow of biological information, were overcome with the discovery of the viral reverse transcriptases (Temin and Mizutani, 1970; Baltimore, 1970). Induction of mutations in Rous sarcoma virus by 5-bromodeoxyuridine demonstrated that the viral DNA functioned as the intracellular viral genome (Bader and Bader, 1970; Bader and Brown, 1971). Although viral DNA has not been isolated from infected cells in a form which can be characterized, the following are the studies which have helped to establish that the intracellular replicative genome of RTV is DNA.

3.2.3. Molecular Hybridization Studies

One might expect that a new intracellular DNA could be revealed through molecular hybridization experiments involving radioactive viral RNA and DNA extracted from infected and noninfected cells. Such experiments were hampered by (1) the inability to obtain viral RNA of high specific radioactivity, and (2) the existence in host cells of DNA regions homologous with viral RNA. Temin (1964b,c) first reported an increased binding capacity of infected-cell DNA for viral RNA, but the data were based upon levels of radioactivity too low to be convincing.

In my laboratory, no differences were found between infected and noninfected chick embryo cells in the binding of Rous sarcoma virus RNA and cellular DNA. However, the high natural background of homology found in chick embryo cells was absent in hamster cell DNA, and an increase in the binding capacity for Rous sarcoma virus RNA was revealed in DNA from hamster cells transformed by this virus (Bader, 1967c). Other unpublished studies showed that this increased binding capacity was specific when DNA from cells transformed by polyoma or murine sarcoma virus were compared with Rous sarcoma cells. Measuring RNA–DNA association rates, Varmus et al. (1973) confirmed that hamster cells transformed by Rous sarcoma virus contained DNA with a greater affinity for viral RNA than nontransformed hamster cells, and calculated that each cell contained two genome equivalents of viral DNA. Similar results were found using rat cells transformed with Rous sarcoma virus.

Baluda and Nayak (1970) found that the high natural affinity of chick embryo cell DNA for avian myeloblastosis virus RNA could be reduced by adding large amounts of cellular RNA to the system, thereby revealing increased homology in the DNA from infected cells. Using a similar system, Rosenthal et al. (1971) found DNAs in infected chick embryo cells homologous to several other avian leuko-sarcoma viruses. Similar studies using murine leukemia virus and mammalian cells also have shown an increase in hybridizable DNA in infected cells (Gelb *et al.*, 1971).

3.2.4. Specificity of DNA Synthesis

Experiments in which cells were grown in 5-bromodeoxyuridine, and the drug removed at the time of infection, suggested that alterations in cellular DNA were not responsible for inhibition of reproduction of RTV (Bader, 1964*a*). Duesberg and Vogt (1969) and Vigier (1970) infected chick embryo cells with one avian leuko-sarcoma virus and found that a second infection with another avian virus still required DNA synthesis.

These observations minimized the possibility that virus reproduction depended upon a cellular substance inducible during the S phase. Viruses in the process of production were unable to provide the necessary function demanded by the second virus during DNA synthesis, despite the fact that these strains of virus can complement each other in other functions. The DNA, therefore, is specific for each strain of virus.

3.2.5. The DNA Replicative Genome

Genetic evidence for a DNA replicative genome was provided by experiments involving 5-bromodeoxyuridine. This antimetabolite can be incorporated into DNA, resulting in the aberrant functioning of the DNA. Such DNA may make mistakes in base pairing during DNA replications or during transcription into RNA. It was reasoned that a defective viral DNA might produce defective viral RNA progeny, while specific cistrons on the same viral RNA used as message might retain the ability to be translated into functional proteins. Thereby, intracellular complementarity could occur; i.e., all essential viral proteins would be functionally represented if (1) the defective DNA only occasionally made mistakes in any single cistron, (2) during the reduplication of viral genomes, different mistakes were introduced into different DNA molecules, or (3) under conditions of high multiplicity DNA transcripts received defects in different cistrons.

First, 5-bromodeoxyuridine was shown to be ineffective as an inhibitor of Rous sarcoma virus production if the DNA synthesis phase had been completed. Also, the drug had no effect on any phase of the reproduction of NDV. Cellular macromolecular synthesis was quantitatively unaffected during the first 24 hours after exposure of cells to the drug, and cells proceeded as normal cells through mitoses. Also, radioactive 5-bromodeoxyuridine was not incorporated into cellular RNA. These observations established that 5-bromodeoxyuridine had little effect on cellular or viral RNA synthesis or on several cellular processes essential to viability.

The addition of 5-bromodeoxyuridine to cells newly infected with Rous sarcoma virus resulted in a substantial decrease in the *infectivity* of virions produced by treated cultures compared to nontreated cultures, but the *number* of virions produced was unaffected. Virus particles were determined by the relative incorporation of radioactive uridine into particles banding about 1.16 g/ml in sucrose gradients, by incorporation of radioactive uridine into viral RNA resolved by gel electrophoresis, and by direct counting by electron microscopy. In addition, the production of virus-specific complement-fixing antigen was undiminished in cultures receiving 5-bromodeoxyuridine, and transformation occurred to a similar extent in treated and nontreated cultures. Only viral infectivity was affected.

These noninfectious virions could be considered defective mutants, thus raising the possibility that conditionally active mutants could be isolated. The demonstrations by Toyoshima and Vogt (1969) and by Martin (1970) that virions temperature sensitive for transformation could be found led us to the isolation of similar mutants after treatment of newly infected cells with 5-bromodeoxyuridine (Bader and Brown, 1971). These studies demonstrated unequivocally that at least part of the intracellular viral replicative genome of avian leuko-sarcoma viruses was constituted of DNA.

Another type of experiment involving 5-bromodeoxyuridine was performed by Boettiger and Temin (1970) and Balducci and Morgan (1970). Chick embryo cells were exposed to serum-deficient medium for a few days until cellular DNA synthesis reached low levels. Avian sarcoma viruses were then added along with 5-bromodeoxyuridine, and, after a reasonable interval, serum-containing medium was added to allow resumption of cell growth. Exposure to light then resulted in a decrease in the number of developing foci of transformed cells, supposedly by selectively inactivating the hypersensitive 5-bromodeoxyuridine-containing viral genome. These authors tendered the results as evidence for the intracellular synthesis of viral DNA. However, the data are compromised by the considerations that the cells most likely to be successfully infected in these experiments are those in which DNA synthesis is in progress, in which 5-bromodeoxyuridine would be incorporated, and which would be most sensitive to the DNA-inactivating action of UV-irradiation. Thus, infected cells would be among the most likely to be killed by irradiation.

3.2.6. Infectious DNA

Hill and Hillova (1972a) recently announced that DNA extracted from cells transformed by Rous sarcoma virus was infectious for chick embryo cells. Using a temperature-sensitive virus they found that the infected-cell DNA could transmit the infection, and the resulting progeny were temperature sensitive (Hill and Hillova, 1972b). Similar results on transfection with DNA isolated from rat cells transformed by Rous sarcoma virus were reported by Svoboda et al. (1972). These are exciting results, unfortunately tempered by the inefficiencies of the systems employed and certain experimental inconsistencies. Resolution of an efficient transfection system certainly would be a tremendous advance in defining the intracellular replicative intermediate of RTV.

3.2.7. Kinetics and Integration

Studies involving the inhibition of protein synthesis demonstrated that the viral DNA is synthesized by virion enzymes existing before infection. Addition of puromycin (Bader, 1966b) or cycloheximide (Bader, 1972a) for a few hours after infection had little effect on the efficiency of infection of Rous sarcoma virus, as measured by eventual transformation or on reproduction of infectious virus. The DNA-synthetic phase was not merely delayed in these experiments since DNA synthesis could be specifically inhibited immediately after removal of the protein-inhibiting drugs without affecting virus infection. Therefore, the viral DNA was synthesized without a requirement for new protein synthesis. A corollary is that the incoming viral RNA acts only as a template for transcription and not as a messenger RNA.

Not only are DNA-synthesizing enzymes pre-existing, but any other enzymes which may be required in steps prior to or accompanying DNA synthesis are also pre-existing. Inhibition of protein synthesis can be initiated prior to exposure of cells to virus, and infections still proceed.

Viral DNA synthesis begins within the first hour after exposure of suceptible cells to virus, and continues for 6–8 hours, (Bader, 1972a). Pulse-temporal additions of 5-iododeoxyuridine produce the greatest inhibition of infectious progeny when the drug is added during the first hour after exposure of cells to Rous sarcoma virus. The effect diminishes thereafter, until about 8 hours has elapsed since infection, when addition of 5-iododeoxyuridine no longer has an effect on virus production. These results suggest that either viral DNA molecules transcribed from viral RNA have a random completion time up to 8 hours, with more than 50% requiring longer than 5 hours, or that viral DNAs are reduplicated. A plot of the degree of inhibition as a function of time of addition of 5-iododeoxyuridine shows that inhibition decreases logarithmically after the first hour. The many factors involved in virus reproduction caution one not to be too enthusiastic about an interpretation for this result, but superficially it fits a pattern for logarithmic reduplication of DNA genomes. A rate of reduplication can be calculated and from it one can conclude that about 50–100 viral DNAs emanate from each infectious viral RNA. The prospect of reduplication of DNAs is contradictory to the "provirus" concept as developed by Temin (1970).

An interesting matter to consider is the termination of the synthesis of viral DNA. If only one DNA molecule is made per viral RNA, there is no problem. On the other hand, the duration of viral DNA synthesis is close to that of a complete S phase. It would not be unreasonable to suppose that *all* DNA synthesis in the cell terminates at a given time, perhaps by a critical reduction in the precursor pool or inactivation of polymerases, or that the completion of cellular DNA synthesis signals a reduction in the DNA-synthesizing machine. In any case, it is unlikely that viral DNA synthesis continues through mitosis.

Another consideration is the integration of viral DNA into the chromosome. Again, a single replicative genome poses no problem since thoughts of integration of a single DNA molecule into chromosomal DNA are hardly flabbergasting. In AKR mice, which congenitally acquire the murine leukemia virus genome, genetic crossover experiments have revealed two separated loci which contain the genes for virus production (Rowe *et al.*, 1972). At least in this case, it seems that integration has occurred twice. But supposing 50–100 reduplicated DNAs exist in each cell 8 hours after infection, or even that one cell is multiply infected by 10 or 20 virions to give multiple intracellular viral DNAs, must we expect each DNA molecule to be integrated in order to function? I think not. More likely is the possibility that multiple viral DNAs can exist extrachromosomally, in the manner of episomes, and that they function in transcription into viral RNA for the synthesis of viral proteins and progeny. Integration is not precluded and probably would occur; viral DNA would then be replicated coordinately with the chromosome. Extrachromosomal DNAs might be replicated with each ensuing S phase and/or discarded or segregated during cellular divisions.

It is unlikely that a single viral DNA molecule is synthesized from one viral RNA since most cells infected even with a single virion produce two infected daughter cells at the first division (Nakata and Bader, 1968a). Reinfection by progeny virus can hardly be blamed for this result since cellular divisions occurred probably before any viral progeny had formed, and viral RNA by itself is undoubtedly noninfectious. The hypothesis of a single viral DNA molecule would require that the viral DNA be integrated, and then that the chromosome be duplicated by synthesis of DNA, before the strands of DNA are separated for distribution into daughter cells.

The location of the synthesis of the viral DNA has not been established. There is disagreement about the site of early interactions (Hatanaka et al., 1971; Dales and Hanafusa, 1972), and definitive experiments to resolve this have not been presented.

3.3. Mitosis and the Reproductive Cycle

A possible requirement for cellular mitosis in the reproductive cycle of Rous sarcoma virus was examined by Temin (1967). Using colchicine to prevent cellular divisions, he found that virus reproduction was prevented. This result probably was due to an unfortunate choice in the strain (Schmidt-Ruppin) of sarcoma virus, or was possibly due to the accumulation of treated cells in the state of mitosis, a state which does not allow for production of virus even in cells in which infection is fully established (unpublished observations).

Chick embryo cells exposed to vinblastine sulfate cannot divide, but not all cells reach the rounded mitotic stage commonly recognized as the stage inhibited by vinblastine. About one-third of the cells remain flattened on the culture substratum, and these cells can support full cycles of reproduction of the Bryan strain of Rous sarcoma virus and Rous-associated virus, (Bader, 1972b). Furthermore, infected cells become morphologically transformed, and metabolic changes associated with malignant transformation occur in these cells which have not divided after exposure to virus and vinblastine (J. P. Bader, 1972b, 1973). These studies demonstrated that cellular divisions *per se* were not an obligate step in virus reproduction, and that the role of mitosis could be removed from further consideration.

3.4. Synthesis of Viral RNA

The continuous production of virus by infected virus-producing cells, and the synthesis of viral RNA in these cells, is rigorously dependent upon transcription of DNA. Actinomycin D stops further virus synthesis within an hour after its addition (Temin, 1963; Bader, 1964a, 1970; Bases and King, 1967). The RNAs of several other RNA viruses can be synthesized in the presence of actinomycin D (Reich et al., 1961; Bader, 1967b), and the intracellular synthesis of these viral RNAs can be revealed by using this drug to suppress synthesis of cellular RNA. After many unsuccessful attempts to find the intracellular RNA of RTV using actinomycin D (unpublished observations), we concluded that the inhibition of virus production by actinomycin D was due to an inhibition of viral RNA synthesis, and that viral RNA synthesis was dependent upon transcription of DNA. Duesberg and Robinson (1967) came to a similar conclusion after some hesitation (Robinson, 1966).

A complicating feature to this dependence is the possible role of cellular DNA in the production of virus. Exposure of Rous sarcoma virus-producing chick embryo cells to UV irradiation prevents the further production of virus (Rubin and Temin, 1959; Bader, 1966b). Doses of UV irradiation far less than those affecting the infectivity of free virus produce this effect, and the required dose level is similar whether the cells are irradiated prior to infection or at any time after infection (Bader, 1966b). Equivalent irradiation has no effect on the capacity of cells to support the reproduction of NDV or VS virus.

Sensitization of cellular DNA to UV irradiation by growing cells in 5-bromodeoxyuridine before infection demonstrated that it was cellular DNA which was being affected (Bader, 1966b). Yoshikura (1970, 1972) obtained different results, finding increased resistance of the virus-producing capacity of cells to UV irradiation with time after infection. However, he failed to take into account the radiation resistance of virus already completed in the culture at the time of irradiation.

Whether cellular DNA is responsible for a protein involved in virus synthesis, or is more directly involved in viral RNA synthesis, has not been determined. The intracellular synthesis of viral RNA in irradiated cells has not been examined, and the kinetics of decreased production are not definitive enough to provide a rational explanation.

3.4.1. Detection of Intracellular Viral RNA

Viral RNA is not easily detected in virus-producing cells after labeling with radioactive uridine. Biswal et al. (1968) and Watson (1971) have reported the direct resolution of intracellular viral RNA from cellular RNAs, but completed, cell-associated virus could account for these observations. In a large number of experiments, involving separation of cytoplasm from nuclei, and including isolation of polysomes and separation and denaturation of RNA fractions, we (J. P. Bader and E. J. Matthews, unpublished) were unable to find evidence of 60–70 S viral RNA within cells producing murine leukemia virus or avian leuko-sarcoma viruses. These experiments were restricted to the first hour after addition of radioactive uridine, before completed virions could contaminate the cellular extracts, and the techniques were sufficiently sensitive to easily identify viral RNA which was labeled during this period and eventually appeared in virions. We concluded that the intracellular viral RNA was in the vRNA′ (35–45 S), a size which may have been obscured by cellular RNA species.

Viral DNA synthesized by the reverse-transcriptase reactions has been used as a probe for intracellular viral RNA in molecular hybridization experiments. Green et al. (1971) detected viral RNA in both nuclei and cytoplasm of rat cells transformed by murine sarcoma virus. They estimated that about 1% of the total cellular RNA was viral RNA. This is more than tenfold the amount of radioactive uridine appearing in viral RNA of virions compared with the total cellular RNA (Bader, 1970; Watson, 1971; A. V. Bader, 1973), suggesting, if the systems are comparable, that only a small proportion of intracellular viral RNA ever appears in virions.

Virus-specific RNA has also been detected in tissues producing murine leukemia virus (Hehlmann et al., 1972a) and mouse mammary tumor virus (Axel et al., 1972a; Gulati et al., 1972). Avian and mammalian cells infected with Rous sarcoma virus contain RNA hybridization to virus DNA (Coffin and Temin, 1970; Garapin et al., 1971), but sedimentation studies showed the RNA to be heterogeneous in size, all the RNA being smaller than native vRNA (Leong et al., 1972a).

There seems to be no question that intracellular viral RNA can be detected in infected virus-producing cells where reasonably large quantities of viral RNA are expected. Whether or not the molecular hybridization techniques as presently employed can distinguish a small amount of viral RNA against a background of potentially hybridizable cellular RNA is another matter. Purified viral RNA is not usually separated from cellular RNAs or DNAs in the endogenous reaction used for the generation of labeled virus-specific DNA, and such contaminating nucleic acids may be transcribed in addition to the viral RNA. The DNA, in turn, might hybridize with nucleic acids extracted from infected, or questionably infected, cells, although a viral DNA generated in a heterologous system may not hybridize, calling attention to the "specificity" of the system. Reports of human tumor cells having nucleic acid sequences identical to those of murine viral RNAs (Hehlmann et al., 1972a,b; Axel et al., 1972b) must be considered with this reservation.

Another obstacle to the detection of intracellular viral RNA is the acknowledged homology of viral RNA to noninfected cellular DNA, and the likelihood that this cellular DNA is transcribed into hybridizable cellular RNA. While one might attribute this RNA to the presence of virus genes residing in the cell, another could point to the transposition of cellular genes to viral RNA.

3.4.2. The Viral mRNA

The RNA used as the message for viral proteins has almost certainly the same polarity as that found in the virion, and is perhaps identical to intravirion RNA. Hybridization experiments involving viral RNA and cellular RNA have not revealed the complementary negative strand of RNA (J. P. Bader, unpublished), and it is possible that negative strands of viral RNA are never synthesized.

It would be desirable to have information on viral RNA attached to ribosomes, that is, the mRNA at its functional site. RNA hybridizable to mouse mammary tumor virus DNA has been found in a sedimentable fraction from murine mammary carcinoma (Axel et al., 1972a). Although called "polysomal," the fractionation procedure would result in a wide range of rapidly sedimenting organelles, including free viral RNA and even virions.

The interval between completion of synthesis of viral RNA and its appearance in extracellular virions was determined to be about 75 minutes for murine leukemia virus (Bader, 1970). This was shown by adding ^{3}H-uridine to virus-producing cells and then examining cell culture fluids at 10- or 15-minute intervals for the appearance of radioactivity in extracted vRNA resolved by gel electrophoresis. Samples taken at hourly intervals gave similar, albeit less precise, results for chick embryo cells producing avian leuko-sarcoma viruses (Bader, 1970) and for myeloblasts producing avian myeloblastosis virus (Baluda and Nayack, 1969). Using autoradiography to detect radioactivity in virions, Okano and Rich (1969) found labeled virions after 2 hours in murine leukemia virus-producing cultures, and labeled Rous sarcoma virus was found in chick embryo cells after 3 hours (Rabotti et al., 1969).

The rate of increase in labeled vRNA within virions becomes linear within 10 minutes of its initial appearance, suggesting that viral

RNA is synthesized at a constant rate, and that synthesis of each molecule requires less than 10 minutes. The delay between viral RNA synthesis and its appearance in virions is also shown by delayed addition of actinomycin D after exposure of cells to ^{3}H-uridine. Labeled viral RNA eventually appears in virions even though further RNA synthesis is inhibited within 15 minutes after addition of ^{3}H-uridine. Most of the required 75 minutes between labeling of viral RNA and its appearance in virions, therefore, is used in the formation of the virion. This may include synthesis of viral RNA-associated protein or a metabolically labile protein, as well as the association of molecules at the cell surface for structural completion of the virion. Synthesis of viral RNA apparently does not involve ribosomal RNA synthesis, since the latter can be prevented by 5-fluorouridine without an immediate adverse effect on the labeling of virion RNA (Brdar et al., 1972).

Leong et al. (1972b) have reported that the rate of synthesis of Rous sarcoma viral RNA is highest in early S, while virus production is greatest in G1. According to this interpretation of their data, it would require 8–10 hours for viral RNA to reach its maximal rate of release in virions after synthesis. Direct labeling data do not support this (Bader, 1970), and their data need not be interpreted in terms of the cell cycle. Synchronization in their system was done by sequential serum depletion and serum addition. In cells synchronized using high levels of thymidine, I found the rate of virus production to be uniform throughout the cell cycle. Only if mitotic cells were separated from the rest of the population could differences be shown; cells maintained in mitosis by treatment with vinblastine sulfate produce practically no virus.

3.4.3. The Character of New Viral RNA

One might expect progeny viral RNAs to have the same gene content, the same base ratios, and indeed the same base sequences as the infecting parent, and this may be the case. Nonetheless, aside from low-level mutations, we can consider two possible exceptions which might result in progeny RTV containing different RNA than the parent.

First, if the cellular low-molecular-weight RNAs found in virion preparations are in fact within virions, then these RNAs might be expected to differ when the virus is grown in heterologous host cells. Strictly speaking, these would not be progeny viral RNAs, but nonetheless may constitute an indispensable function to the reproduction of the viral genome.

A second case might be found after integration of viral DNA into chromosomal DNA. If the viral has lost a significant portion of the infecting genome, either by cleavage or by failure to be synthesized, then integration of this DNA and subsequent transcription may result in a viral RNA extended by cellular RNA transcribed from adjacent regions. We are aware already of regions in the viral RNA genome which are nonfunctional with respect to virus reproduction (Martin, 1970; Bader and Brown, 1971), and as long as all of the cistrons required for virus reproduction are intact, this possibility is not unreasonable. Another related mechanism involves the hypothetical situation involving integration of the entire infecting genome, but during transcription adjacent cellular RNA is selected while at the other end dispensable viral RNA is removed.

3.5. Synthesis of Viral Proteins

It is a curious fact that little attention has been given to the synthesis of RTV proteins, although the tumorigenic potential of the virion almost certainly resides in protein translated from the viral RNA. No new protein synthesis is required in the synthesis of viral DNA, but the same cannot be said about the transcription of viral DNA into new viral RNA. After inhibition of protein synthesis by cycloheximide or inhibition of RNA synthesis by actinomycin D, virus production decreases at about the same rate (Bader, 1970). However, no choice can be made among several possibilities: (1) inhibition of protein synthesis also inhibits viral RNA synthesis, (2) inhibition of RNA synthesis reduces the synthesis of essential virus proteins, or (3) there is a coincidental synthesis of essential protein and viral RNA.

Virus-specific proteins can be recognized in infected cells by immunological methods using antisera reacting with viral structural proteins. Methods for the detection and assay of viruses (the CoFAL and CoMuLV tests) have been developed in which intracellular complement-fixing antigens react with virus-specific antigens (Huebner *et al.*, 1964; Hartley *et al.*, 1965). Studies with labeled antibody demonstrated that internal virion antigens are found generally within the cytoplasm (Kelloff and Vogt, 1966; Dougherty *et al.*, 1972), suggesting that synthesis of viral proteins is not localized at the cell surface, where virion assembly takes place.

The overwhelming amount and number of species of cellular proteins, whose synthesis cannot be selectively inhibited, has made the identification of specific intracellular viral proteins difficult. Fleissner and Tress (1973*a*) used antibody to precipitate viral protein aggregates away from bulk cellular proteins, and also to identify reactive proteins separated by gel chromatography or electrophoresis. Three internal virion proteins were identified in hamster cells, and two in chicken cells, which were transformed by Bryan Rous sarcoma virus. Viral antigens were found aggregated with cellular proteins, augmenting the difficulties already inherent in the system.

Shanmugam *et al*. (1972) added ^{14}C-labeled amino acids to virus-producing cells and found radioactivity in virus-specific proteins of extracellular virions within 40 minutes. This is at least 30 minutes earlier than the earliest time that new RNA was found in virions.

3.6. Assembly of the Virion

Once the virion constituents are synthesized, virion completion can occur without simultaneous RNA or protein synthesis. This is based upon studies which show the continuous release of ^{3}H-uridine-labeled murine leukemia virus, or infectious Rous sarcoma virus, from infected cells treated with actinomycin D or cycloheximide (Bader, 1970; A. V. Bader, 1973). However, information on assembly of viral RNA, proteins, and cellular lipids into completed virions is mainly restricted to electron microscopic observations.

No virus components can be visualized other than at the cell surface, and the observed stages of the budding process indicate that assembly occurs at the cell membrane. The consistent occurrence of intracytoplasmic A particles in mammary tumor cells of mice infected with the mammary tumor virus led to the conclusion that these A particles were viral cores which eventually became enveloped to become completed virions. Such a process would constitute an important deviation from the mechanism of formation of cores and virions of other RTV and is difficult to accept. It is more likely that A particles are aberrant condensations of viral macromolecules, are cores of reingested virions, or are particles unrelated to the mammary tumor virus. The nonidentity of proteins purified from A particles and mammary tumor virions (Smith and Wivel, 1972, 1973) suggests that the last possibility is the most probable.

The virion does not simply condense at the cell surface, but rather it appears to grow by accretion as the virion bud protrudes from the cell surface (Fig. 3). Let me offer a possible, rather general, mechanism for which there is no good supportive evidence: Mutually attractive viral proteins (glycoproteins) accumulate among cellular lipids in the cell surface membrane; core proteins recognize the viral glycoproteins,

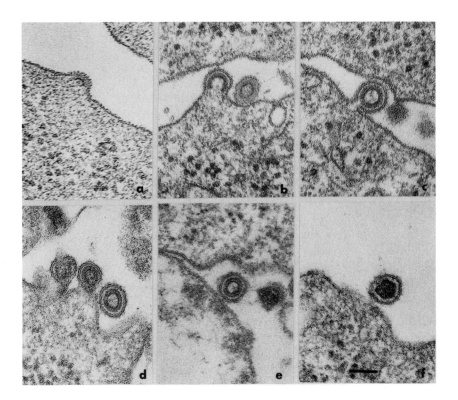

Fig. 3. Completion of RTV at the cell surface membrane. A series of electron micrographs depict the "budding" of virions of murine leukemia virus from the cell surface: (a) Early protrusion with faint outline of beginning core. (b) Budding virion with incomplete envelope and core. (c) Budding virion with completed core but incomplete membrane. (d) Virion at right and in (e) completed virions with electron-lucent centers (Type A). (f) Virion with electron-dense center (Type C). Marker = 0.1 μm Electron micrographs by A. V. Bader.

become aligned, and begin to form the intermediate layer; viral RNA, perhaps in association with the internal protein, recognizes the protein of the intermediate layer and begins to coil; the RNA–protein associations, while coiling, pull the emerging particle into a spherical configuration, which eventually is displaced from the cell surface by the mutual repulsion of cellular surface proteins and viral envelope proteins.

3.7. The Role of Mitochondria

Increased glycolysis has long been considered a characteristic of tumor cells, and Warburg (1956) advanced a theory of tumorigenesis based upon defects in aerobic metabolism. Since mitochondria are the organelles mainly associated with energy production through aerobic oxidation, the possibility that tumorigenic viruses might disrupt mitochondrial function is of reasonable concern. Particles thought to be virion precursors of Rous sarcoma virus were viewed in the electron microscope (Gazzolo *et al.*, 1969) in association with mitochondria, and infectious particles of Rous sarcoma virus were found in preparations of isolated mitochondria (Mach and Kara, 1971; Kara *et al.*, 1971). Localization of virus reproduction in mitochondria was suggested, with implications regarding the oncogenic potential of RTV. The association of intracytoplasmic virions or cores with mitochondria would be unusual since cores and virions of Rous sarcoma virus are constructed at the cell surface membrane. Nonetheless, one might imagine viral DNA residing in mitochondria, transcribing viral RNA, which eventually becomes incorporated into virions.

Ethidium bromide was used by my favorite electron microscopist to induce degenerative effects in mitochondria for the examination of the role of mitochondria in virus reproduction (A. V. Bader, 1973). She found that mouse cells continued to produce murine leukemia virus when practically all cellular mitochondria had degenerated. ^{3}H-uridine was incorporated into the vRNA of virions, and particles were observed budding from the surface of cells containing no intact mitochondria. Also, complete reproductive cycles of Rous sarcoma virus occurred in chick embryo cells containing aberrant mitochondria. In the face of these observations, it is difficult to find a role for mitochondria in reproduction of RTV. If mitochondria are affected at all by virus infection, one must look to the effects of virus gene products, or to secondary effects of cellular transformation.

4. GENETICS OF RNA TUMOR VIRUSES

4.1. Phenotypic Mixing

Phenotypic mixing is a common occurrence among related strains of RTV, and is often responsible for the infectivity of particles for a specific host. Virions produced from a cell infected with two or more viruses may contain envelope components of both viruses, and such phenotypically mixed virions may be neutralized by antiserum to either virus (Vogt, 1967*a*). Virions containing only envelope constituents of the opposite genotype are considered genotypically "masked" and are also common. Since phenotypic mixing and masking are basically the same phenomenon, they will not be further differentiated.

A historic example of the consequences of phenotypic mixing in RTV studies is described in the following sequence. The Bryan strain of Rous sarcoma virus (RSV-BH) was found to contain a nontransforming virus, RAV1, which was responsible for the type-specific antigenicity and host range of RSV-BH. Culture fluids from RSV-BH-transformed clones devoid of RAV1, could not reinfect the chick embryo cells commonly used at that time, and RSV-BH was deemed defective (Hanafusa, 1964). However, electron microscopic examination (Dougherty and DiStefano, 1965) and radioactive labeling (Robinson, 1967) of the transformed cells showed that virions were produced, and a survey of other avian cells showed that these particles were infectious, but with a more limited host range (Weiss, 1967; Vogt, 1967c; H. Hanafusa and Hanafusa, 1968). Extending these investigations revealed that a naturally occurring avian leukosis virus, RAV60, accompanied the sarcoma virus and was responsible for even this limited infectivity of RSV-BH (Hanafusa et al., 1970). Particles emanating from transformed cells without any identifiable leukosis virus indeed were defective, unable to infect any known cells, and defectiveness could be attributed to 2 factors: (1) a deficiency in the large virion glycoprotein (Scheele and Hanafusa, 1971), and (2) a deficiency in reverse transcriptase (Hanafusa and Hanafusa, 1971; H. Hanafusa et al., 1972).

The host range of RTV can be deliberately extended by mixedly infecting cells and producing virions of a different phenotype. In this way, Hanafusa and Hanafusa (1966) were able to transform hamster cells with a Rous sarcoma strain which normally could not do so. Extending the range of infectivity by phenotypic mixing has been invaluable to many investigations on RTV.

4.2. Genetic Recombination

Avian RTV of different subgroups can form stable recombinants after mixed infection of cells. Thus far, these recombinants have been limited to the regions responsible for transformation and for antigenic subgroup. Vogt (1971b) mixedly infected cells with the Prague strain of Rous sarcoma virus (subgroup A) and nontransforming avian viruses representative of subgroups B, C, or D. In each case, transforming viruses of subgroup B, C, or D, respectively, were obtained, which were stable upon passage. In a similar experiment, the Schmidt-Ruppin strain of Rous sarcoma virus (subgroup A) mixed with RAV2, a subgroup B leukosis virus, produced a recombinant transforming virus with subgroup B phenotype (Kawai and Hanafusa, 1972b). The extent of genetic transfer could not be determined for any of these recombinants; i.e., whether the sarcoma virus genome replaced only the region determining antigenicity, or whether the intact leukosis virus genome acquired transforming capacity. Reciprocal exchange, i.e., acquisition of the transforming subgroup determinant by the nontransforming particle, could not be shown by these experiments. Another unresolved question is whether different antigenic subgroups are allelic, and the possibility remains that several viral genes may be involved in the synthesis of antigenic determinants. The resolution of unstable heterozygotes of avian RTV (Weiss *et al.*, 1973) might be explained on this basis.

High rates of recombination were found in the studies discussed above, suggesting to these investigators a reassortment of genomic subunits as a mechanism of recombination, in contrast to molecular breakage and rejoining. This in turn favors the hypothesis of vRNA being composed of molecular subunits, and furthermore that the transformation gene is on a different subunit than the gene(s) determining antigenicity. However, an examination of vRNA′ after a recombinational event involving genomes of different sized vRNAs, indicated that crossing over had occurred. Vogt and Duesberg (1973) found only the larger-sized vRNA′ in a recombinant containing RAV3 (smaller vRNA′) antigen and the transforming potential of Prague sarcoma virus (larger vRNA′). Until other physiological or molecular markers are available, and recombination rates can be measured accurately, a firm decision about these matters cannot be made.

Recombination is not always the outcome of mixed infection with two genotypes. Recombinants of avian leukosis viruses and RSV-BH have not been found. Also, RAV7, a subgroup C leukosis virus, could not recombine with Prague Rous sarcoma virus under conditions where several other leukosis viruses recombined. Possibly the genes responsible for transformation in the Bryan sarcoma virus, or antigenicity in RAV7, are situated in regions unfavorable for the recombinants as selected, or are displaced during recombination. Another possibility, the obvious one, is that these viral genomes do not recombine at all with the related viruses examined.

4.3. Mutants of RTV

Genetic relatedness of RTV may be assumed only for those parameters which have been determined experimentally, and assumptions based on the original source of the virus are often invalid. A common misunderstanding which exemplifies this point concerns the group of viruses called Rous sarcoma virus. Although originating with the agent produced by Rous tumor No. 1 (Rous, 1911), the passage of the virus in laboratories around the world has resulted in a series of "strains" which can be distinguished by the morphology of cells transformed, as well as by other criteria (Dougherty *et al.*, 1963; Morgan, 1964). The isolation of antigenic variants might be attributed to recombination with naturally occurring leukosis viruses. However, such coincidences of infection with two transforming viruses are unlikely, and the differences in morphological transformation have been discussed in terms of mutations in the transformation gene (Temin, 1960; Yoshii and Yogt, 1970). A more likely explanation is that different transformation-causing genes have been selected during passage and the products of these genes are different in different strains. Temperature-sensitive mutants of Rous strains show that the product of the transformation gene is not essential for virus production, abrogating any reproductive requirement for retention of the original transformation gene. Also, often more similarity exists between a separate isolate of avian sarcoma virus and a strain of Rous sarcoma virus than between strains of Rous sarcoma virus. These considerations suggest that different strains of Rous sarcoma virus may be different avian sarcoma viruses with respect to malignant transformation.

True mutants of RTV have only recently arrived on the investigative scene. Mutants defective in reproductive capacity, but still capable of transformation, were isolated by Golde (1970) after exposure of Schmidt-Ruppin Rous sarcoma virus to γ irradiation. Similar mutants were detected by Toyoshima *et al.* (1970) after UV irradiation. Viruses capable of reproduction, but which had lost the property of transformation, were also isolated, and Vogt (1971*a*) later found that nontransforming viruses were regularly segregated from clones of antigenically identical transforming viruses. Isolation of such defective mutants demonstrated that, among transforming viruses at least, some of the processes required for virus production were not required for transformation, and that transformation was not required for virus reproduction.

This latter point was more firmly established with the isolation and characterization of temperature-sensitive mutants of avian sarcoma viruses. Several isolates were capable of complete cycles of reproduction at both high (41°C) and low (36°C) temperatures, but infected cells only became transformed at the lower temperature (Martin, 1970; Bader and Brown, 1971; Kawai and Hanafusa, 1971; Bader, 1972*c*; Biquard and Vigier, 1972), thus demonstrating that a sarcoma virus could be produced even though the product of the transformation gene was not functioning. Mutants temperature-sensitive for transformation may provide the experimental mechanism for the identification of the gene product directly responsible for malignant transformation.

A series of mutants temperature sensitive for virus reproduction and/or transformation have been induced in avian sarcoma viruses and partially characterized (Toyoshima and Vogt, 1969; Friis *et al.*, 1971; Wyke and Lineal, 1973). Six general categories dealing with transformation and early or late defects are recognized. Two of these isolates defective in early functions were shown to contain temperature-sensitive DNA polymerase (Lineal and Mason, 1973). Rigorous complementation or genetic recombination data have not yet been presented, but these mutants offer the anticipation of elucidating the entire reproductive cycle of avian tumor viruses.

The value of such mutants is becoming generally recognized and isolation of temperature-sensitive mutants of other RTV have been reported (Stephenson *et al.*, 1972a; Scolnick *et al.*, 1972a; Wong and McCarter, 1973), including a cold-sensitive mutant of murine sarcoma virus (Somers and Kit, 1973).

5. VIRUS GENES AND CELLULAR GENES

Several observations over the years have suggested that RTV, at least nontransforming types, could be inherited. The transmission of avian lymphomatosis virus through the female line in fowls was shown by Rubin *et al.* (1961), and the AKR inbred mouse line was recognized as a population in which virtually all mice harbored leukemia virus, an unusual occurrence for a contagious disease. Cross-breeding, foster-nursing, and ova-transfer experiments suggested that in some circumstances murine leukemia virus was transferred chromosomally, although leukemias induced by injection of virus followed an extrachromosomal pattern [see Gross (1970)].

Genetic analysis of AKR mice showed that transmission of the murine leukemia virus indeed followed Mendelian segregation patterns and that AKR mice contained two unlinked chromosomal loci capable of inducing leukemia virus (Rowe, 1972b; Rowe and Hartley, 1972; Rowe *et al.*, 1972).

Leukemia virus antigens have been detected in mouse fetuses (Huebner *et al.*, 1970; Abelev and Elgort, 1970), and cell cultures of mouse embryos were found to produce virus. Examination of individual embryonic cells by fluorescent antibody suggested to Aaronson *et al.* (1969) that virus was not being produced at early times after dispersal, but that virus production was spontaneously activated as the cells propagated. Possible objections to this interpretation on the basis of failure to detect a low initial level of infection were disseminated with the discovery that 5-iododeoxyuridine or 5-bromodeoxyuridine could increase the rate of activation of murine leukemia virus in several cloned lines of AKR cells in which no evidence of virus production had been apparent (Lowy *et al.*, 1971). This experiment was repeated in BALB/c mouse cells (Aaronson *et al.*, 1971*b*), and in the observation that a defective murine sarcoma virus was rescued from rat cells after inducing a presumptive rat leukemia virus by 5-bromodeoxyuridine (Klement *et al.*, 1971). Nonetheless, induction of RTV in cells, either spontaneously or with the help of deoxynucleoside analogues, is not a universal phenomenon, and the hope of some that all vertebrate cells would yield virus by these procedures has not been realized.

The heritable nature of an avian leukosis virus also has been analyzed in cross-breeding experiments and found to segregate as a dominant autosomal allele (Weiss and Payne, 1971). Virus can be recovered from otherwise nonproducing cells by superinfection with a defective sarcoma virus (Hanafusa *et al.*, 1970; Vogt and Friis, 1971; T. Hanafusa *et al.*, 1972) or after exposure to irradiation or chemical carcinogens (Weiss *et al.*, 1971).

5.1. Virogenes and Oncogenes

Noticing the apparent ubiquity of RNA tumor viruses, and the heritable nature of some leukemia viruses, Huebner and Todaro (1969) formulated a general theory of carcinogenesis. Briefly stated, all cells contain virus genomes (virogenes), usually in a repressed state, which with a proper stimulus can be activated to produce virus. The virogene contains at least one cistron (the oncogene) whose expression converts the normal cell into a tumor cell; activation of the oncogene is by itself sufficient to convert the cell to a tumor cell, even if other parts of the virogene remain repressed.

The main difficulty with the theory lies in its inability to be tested. The failure to detect viruses or virogenes in most cells can be taken as technical inadequacy, while virus-induced cells can be heralded as supportive evidence. Most tumors probably have a genetic basis, but to determine whether or not this is part of a virogene seems, at present, an impossible task.

A mechanism whereby a cell would have a section of its genome set aside for production of a substance which inactivates the physiological function of the cell, and which allows for the transfer of this tumorigenic potential to another cell, does not seem reasonable to me. Also, the theory implies a very limited number of genes responsible for tumorigenesis within a given organism. A more likely situation is that gene defects for any one of a number of regulatory processes could result in a tumor. The failure of leukemogenic viruses to induce sarcomalike transformation and the apparent differences in cells transformed by different tumor viruses point to a multiplicity of tumorigenic factors. Such consideration can also be given to the multiplicity of antigenic types found in murine tumors induced by a single chemical carcinogen (Klein and Klein, 1962).

5.2. Proviruses and Protoviruses

The intracellular replicative genome of RTV was termed "provirus" by Temin (1964b) to suggest that there were only one or two heritable structures per cell, integrated with and replicating coordinately with the chromosome. This is in distinction to many viral genomic intermediates replicating outside the chromosome and being transmitted more or less at random to daughter cells during mitosis. The provirus is a genetic concept (Temin, 1970) which has its proof in the heritable transmission of murine and avian leukosis viruses as described above. Nonetheless, reproduction of RTV has not been shown to reproduce exclusively though a provirus mechanism, and data favoring a large early pool of viral replicative genomes in some circumstances has been presented (Bader, 1972a).

The "protovirus" hypothesis is more general and encompasses proviruses. In light of the demonstration that RNA could be enzymatically transcribed into DNA, Temin (1971) has proposed protoviruses as a mechanism for gene transfer between somatic cells, with viruses acting as specialized agents in this transfer. In this scheme, RNA from one cell passes to a second cell, is transcribed into DNA, and the DNA is incorporated into the chromosome. Such transfer would provide for variability in the genome of somatic cells since genetic information could be amplified or placed under a different regulatory program. Occasionally germ cells would receive and integrate such information, which would then become a hereditable trait for subsequent generations. Cancer might result from a mutation in the protovirus eliminating or altering a cell function, or from integration of the protovirus at a site disruptive to another gene.

The major premise of the protovirus hypothesis is that RNA-to-DNA information transfer is a general biological phenomenon and is not restricted to RTV. Protoviruses could play an important role in differentiation, in antibody formation, and in evolution by the acquisition of new genetic materials. Such exciting possibilities cannot be peremptorily dismissed. Nonetheless, evidence in support of protoviruses is meager, and a suitable experimental test of the hypothesis is currently unavailable.

6. A MODEL FOR VIRUS REPRODUCTION AND VIRAL TRANSFORMATION

Information on the reproduction of RTV, as described in this chapter, can be summarized and, after applying some general knowledge of the molecular biology of other systems, a tentative model for virus reproduction and viral transformation can be drawn (Fig. 4). Cell surface membrane and viral envelope interact specifically, and, after coalescence of membranes at the surface, or after transport to some internal site, the viral core is exposed to the intracellular milieu. Transcription of the viral RNA into DNA via the reverse-transcriptase reaction proceeds immediately, provided that DNA precursors are available. Cellular DNA-synthesizing enzymes may participate in the synthesis of viral DNA by completing regions left vacant after reverse-transcriptase activity, by covalently linking adjacent unbound chains through a ligase, or by aiding in the synthesis of the second strand of viral DNA or the reduplication of DNA. Circularization of the DNA occurs at some stage prior to reduplication, perhaps as the RNA–DNA hybrid, or after synthesis of the complementary strand of DNA. Viral DNA reduplication proceeds until cellular physiological mechanisms prior to mitosis restrict further synthesis.

One or more viral genomes may be integrated into the chromosome at this time or in later cell cycles, and integrated viral DNA now in linear form would reduplicate coordinately with the chromosomal DNA. The transcription of integrated viral DNA would be sensitive to the regulatory controls for that chromosome or for the specific region of integration. Transcription may encompass the length of viral DNA, but regions of cellular DNA adjacent to viral DNA might also be transcribed and become a permanent part of the genome in viral progeny. In this manner the genome of a nontransforming leukemia virus DNA could be extended to include a cellular gene. The gene may come under less stringent regulatory controls in a future infection, driving the infected cell to malignancy; thus, the origin of a

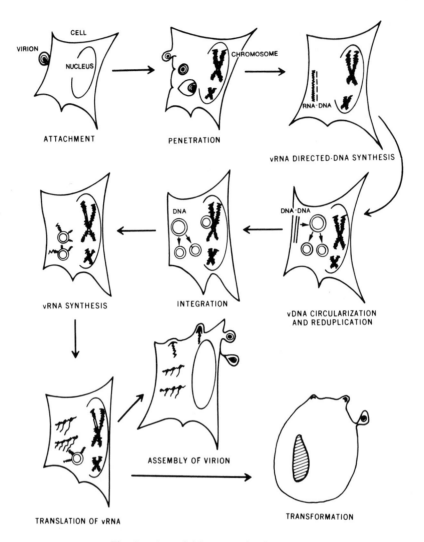

Fig. 4.   A model for reproduction of RTV.

transforming virus. Addition of cellular genes incapable of converting a newly infected cell to a malignant form, nonetheless, might provide for the transfer of other genetic information, as in transduction.

Nonintegrated DNA genomes might be incapable of reduplication after the first cycle, or subsequent replication might be coordinated with chromosomal doubling. These extrachromosomal DNAs could become segregated during cellular divisions, some cells completely losing the nonintegrated viral DNA. Transcription of nonintegrated DNA might be less rigorously controlled than that of integrated DNA, and virus production by cells containing both nonintegrated and integrated DNA might decrease or disappear when nonintegrated DNA is lost.

The translation of viral RNA into proteins, and the construction of an infectious agent as outlined above, are processes common to many viruses and will benefit from information derived more readily with other systems.

New transforming viruses probably are restricted to the animals of origin since the animal either dies of cancer or immunologically disposes of the tumor and the virus. Under rare circumstances, the virus might be rescued by chance infection of another animal or by the excision and extraction of the tumor by an alert scientist. In nature, however, it is unlikely that transforming RTV play a significant role as contagions in the induction of solid tumors.

Nontransforming RTV can be transmitted by contact, and if infection occurs at an early age or survives the immunological response of the animal, virus could be produced for long periods without killing the host. While the somatic cells might be most susceptible to infection, germ cells occasionally might also become infected, and integration of the viral DNA into a germ cell chromosome would insure transmission of the infection to the host's progeny.

7. REFERENCES

Aaronson, S. A., and Rowe, W. P., 1970, Nonproducer clones of murine sarcoma virus-transformed BALB/3T3 cells, *Virology* **42**, 9.

Aaronson, S. A., Hartley, J. W., and Todaro, G. J., 1969, Mouse leukemia virus: "Spontaneous" release by mouse embryo cells after long-term *in vitro* cultivation, *Proc. Natl. Acad. Sci. USA* **64**, 87.

Aaronson, S. A., Parks, W. P., Scolnick, E. M., and Todaro, G. J., 1971a, Antibody to the RNA-dependent DNA polymerase of mammalian C-type RNA tumor viruses, *Proc. Natl. Acad. Sci. USA* **68**, 920.

Aaronson, S. A., Todaro, G. J., and Scolnick, E. M., 1971b, Induction of murine C-type viruses from clonal lines of virus-free BALB/3T cells, *Science (Wash., D.C.)* **174**, 157.

Abelev, G. I., and Elgort, D. A., 1970, Group-specific antigen of murine leukemia viruses in mice of low leukemic strains, *Intl. J. Cancer* **6**, 145.

Allen, D. W., Sarma, P. S., Niall, H. D., and Saver, R., 1970, Isolation of a second avian leukosis group-specific antigen (gs-b) from myeloblastosis virus, *Proc. Natl. Acad. Sci. USA* **67**, 837.

Axel, R., Scholm, J., and Spiegelman, S., 1972a, Evidence for translation of viral-specific RNA in cells of a mouse mammary carcinoma, *Proc. Natl. Acad. Sci. USA* **69**, 535.

Axel, R., Scholm, J., and Spiegelman, S., 1972*b*, Presence in human breast cancer of RNA homologous to mouse mammary tumor virus RNA, *Nature (Lond.)* **235**, 32.

Axel, R., Gulati, S. C., and Spiegelman, S., 1972*c*, Particles containing RNA-instructed DNA polymerase and virus-related RNA in human breast cancers, *Proc. Natl. Acad. Sci. USA* **69**, 3133.

Bader, A. V., 1973, Role of mitochondria in the production of RNA-containing tumor viruses, *J. Virol.* **11**, 314.

Bader, J. P., 1964*a*, The role of deoxyribonucleic acid in the synthesis of Rous sarcoma virus, *Virology* **22**, 462.

Bader, J. P., 1964*b*, Nucleic acids of Rous sarcoma virus and infected cells, *Natl. Cancer Inst. Monograph* **17**, 781.

Bader, J. P., 1965*a*, The requirement for DNA synthesis in the growth of Rous sarcoma and Rous-associated viruses, *Virology* **26**, 253.

Bader, J. P., 1965*b*, Transformation by Rous sarcoma virus: A requirement for DNA synthesis, *Science (Wash., D.C.)* **149**, 757.

Bader, J. P., 1966*a*, Metabolic requirements for infection by Rous sarcoma virus. I. The transient requirement for DNA synthesis, *Virology* **29**, 444.

Bader, J. P., 1966*b*, Metabolic requirements for infection by Rous sarcoma virus. II. The participation of cellular DNA, *Virology* **29**, 452.

Bader, J. P., 1967*a*, A change in growth potential of cells after conversion by Rous sarcoma virus, *J. Cell. Physiol.* **70**, 301.

Bader, J. P., 1967*b*, Metabolic requirements in Rous sarcoma virus replication, *in* "The Molecular Biology of Viruses" (S. J. Colter and W. Parenchych, eds.), p. 697, Academic Press, New York.

Bader, J. P., 1967*c*, Metabolic requirements for infection by Rous sarcoma virus, *in* "Subviral Carcinogenesis" (Y. Ito, ed.), p. 144, Aichi Cancer Center, Nagoya, Japan.

Bader, J. P., 1968, A method for the propagation of large amounts of Rous sarcoma virus, *Virology* **36**, 140.

Bader, J. P., 1969, RNA tumor viruses, *in* "The Biochemistry of Viruses" (H. B. Levy, ed.), p. 293, Marcel Dekker, New York.

Bader, J. P., 1970, Synthesis of the RNA of RNA-containing tumor viruses. I. The interval between synthesis and environment, *Virology* **40**, 494.

Bader, J. P., 1972*a*, Metabolic requirements for infection by Rous sarcoma virus. III. The synthesis of viral DNA, *Virology* **48**, 485.

Bader, J. P., 1972*b*, Metabolic requirements for infection by Rous sarcoma virus. IV. Virus reproduction and transformation without cellular division, *Virology* **48**, 494.

Bader, J. P., 1972*c*, Temperature-dependent transformation of cells infected with a mutant of Bryan Rous sarcoma virus, *J. Virol.* **10**, 267.

Bader, J. P., 1973, Virus-induced transformation without cellular division, *Science (Wash., D.C.)* **180**, 1069.

Bader, J. P., and Bader, A. V., 1970, Evidence for a DNA replicative genome for RNA-containing tumor viruses, *Proc. Natl. Acad. Sci. USA* **67**, 843.

Bader, J. P., and Brown, N. R., 1971, Induction of mutations in an RNA tumor virus by an analogue of a DNA precursor, *Nat. New Biol.* **234**, 11.

Bader, J. P., and Steck, T. L., 1969, Analysis of the ribonucleic acid of murine leukemia virus, *J. Virol.* **4**, 454.

Bader, J. P., Brown, N., and Bader, A. V., 1970, Characteristics of cores of avian leuko-sarcoma viruses, *Virology* **41**, 718.

Baker, R. S. V., and Simons, P. J., 1971, Alterations in the susceptibility of cultured mouse cells to transformation by murine sarcoma virus (Harvey), *J. Gen. Virol.* **12,** 95.

Baker, R. S. V., Simons, P. J., and Rankin, B. J., 1972, Stimulation of DNA synthesis of DNA synthesis and enhancement of murine sarcoma virus replication in mouse embryo cells by SV40, *J. Gen. Virol.* **14,** 115.

Balducci, P., and Morgan, H. R., 1970, Mechanism of oncogenic transformation by Rous sarcoma virus. I. Intracellular inactivation of cell-transforming ability of Rous sarcoma virus by 5-bromodeoxyuridine and light, *J. Virol.* **5,** 470.

Baltimore, D., 1970, Viral RNA-dependent DNA polymerase, *Nature (Lond.)* **226,** 1209.

Baltimore, D., and Smoler, D., 1971, Primer requirement and template specificity of the DNA polymerase of RNA tumor viruses, *Proc. Natl. Acad. Sci. USA* **68,** 1507.

Baltimore, D., McCaffrey, R., and Smoler, D. F., 1973, Properties of reverse transcriptases, *in* "Second ICN-UCLA Symposium on Molecular Biology" (C. F. Fox and W. S. Robinson, eds.), p. 51, Academic Press, New York.

Baluda, M. A., and Nayak, D. P., 1969, Incorporation of precursors into RNA, protein, glycoprotein, and lipoprotein of avian myeloblastosis virus, *J. Virol.* **4,** 554.

Baluda, M. A., and Nayak, D. P., 1970, DNA complementary to viral RNA in leukemic cells induced by avian myeloblastosis virus, *Proc. Natl. Acad. Sci. USA* **66,** 329.

Baluda, M., and Roy-Burman, R., 1973, Partial characterization of RD114 virus by DNA–RNA hybridization studies, *Nat. New Biol.* **244,** 59.

Bases, R. E., and King, A. S., 1967, Inhibition of Rauscher murine leukemia virus growth *in vitro* by actinomycin D, *Virology* **32,** 175.

Bassin, R. H., Tuttle, N., and Fischinger, P. J., 1971, Rapid cell culture assay technique for murine leukaemia viruses, *Nature (Lond.)* **229,** 564.

Beard, J. W., Sharp, D. G., and Eckert, E. A., 1955, Tumor Viruses, *Adv. Virus Res.* **3,** 149.

Beaudreau, G. S., Becker, C., Stim, T., Wallbank, A. M., and Beard, J. W., 1960, Virus of avian myeloblastosis. XVI. Kinetics of cell growth and liberation of virus in cultures of myeloblasts, *Natl. Cancer Inst. Monograph* **4,** 167.

Beaudreau, G. S., Sverak, L., Zischka, R., and Beard, J. W., 1964, Attachment of C¹⁴-amino acids to BAI strain A (myeloblastosis) avian tumor virus RNA, *Natl. Cancer Inst. Monograph* **17,** 791.

Bernhard, W., 1960, The detection and study of tumor viruses with the electron microscope, *Cancer Res.* **20,** 712.

Biquard, J. M., and Vigier, P., 1972, Characteristics of a conditional mutant of Rous sarcoma virus defective in ability to transform cells at high temperature, *Virology* **47,** 444.

Bishop, J. M., Levinson, W. E., Quintrell, N., Sullivan, D., Fanshier, L., and Jackson, J., 1970a, The low-molecular-weight RNAs of Rous sarcoma virus. I. The 4S RNA, *Virology* **42,** 182.

Bishop, J. M., Levinson, W. E., Sullivan, D., Fanshier, L., Quintrell, N., and Jackson, J., 1970b, The low-molecular-weight RNAs of Rous sarcoma virus. II. 7S RNA, *Virology* **42,** 927.

Bishop, J. M., Tsan-Dung, C., Faras, A. J., Goodman, H. M., Levinson, W. E., Taylor, J. M., and Varmus, H. E., 1973, Transcription of the Rous sarcoma virus genome by RNA-directed DNA polymerase, *in* "Second ICN-UCLA Symposium on Molecular Biology" (C. F. Fox and W. S. Robinson, eds.), p. 15, Academic Press, New York.

Biswal, N., Grizzard, M. B., McCombs, R. M., and Benyesh-Melnick, M., 1968, Characterization of intracellular ribonucleic acid specific for the murine sarcoma-leukemia complex, *J. Virol.* **2**, 1346.

Biswal, N., McCain, B., and Benyesh-Melnick, M., 1970, Viral DNA dependent DNA polymerase and the properties of thymidine-labelled material in virions of an oncogenic RNA virus, *Nature (Lond.)* **228**, 427.

Biswal, N., McCain, B., and Benyesh-Melnick, M., 1971, The DNA of murine sarcoma-leukemia virus, *Virology* **45**, 697.

Boettiger, D., and Temin, H. M., 1970, Light inactivation of focus formation by chicken embryo fibroblasts infected with avian sarcoma virus in the presence of 5-bromodeoxyuridine, *Nature (Lond.)* **228**, 621.

Bolognesi, D. P., and Bauer, H., 1970, Polypeptides of avian RNA tumor viruses. I. Isolation and physical and chemical analysis, *Virology* **42**, 1097.

Bolognesi, D. P., and Graf, T., 1971, Size differences among the high-molecular-weight RNA's of avian tumor viruses, *Virology* **43**, 214.

Bolognesi, D. P., Bauer, H., Gelderblom, H., and Huper, G., 1972a, Polypeptides of avian RNA tumor viruses. IV. Components of the viral envelope, *Virology* **47**, 551.

Bolognesi, D. P., Gelderblom, H., Bauer, H., Mölling, F., and Huper, G., 1972b, Polypeptides of avian RNA tumor viruses. V. Analysis of the virus core, *Virology* **47**, 567.

Bonar, R. A., and Beard, J. W., 1959, Virus of avian myeloblastosis. XII. Chemical constitution, *J. Natl. Cancer Inst.* **23**, 183.

Bonar, R. A., Heine, U., and Beard, J. W., 1964, Structure of BAI strain A (myeloblastosis) avian tumor virus, *Natl. Cancer Inst. Monograph* **17**, 589.

Bonar, R. A., Sverak, L., Bolognesi, D. P., Langlois, A. S., Beard, D., and Beard, J. W., 1967, Ribonucleic acid components of BAI strain A (myeloblastosis) avian tumor virus, *Cancer Res.* **27**, 1138.

Brdar, B., Rifkin, D. B., and Reich, E., 1972, Specificity of Rous sarcoma virus synthesis, *FEBS (Fed. Evr. Biochem. Soc.) Lett.* **24**, 347.

Burr, H., and Lingrel, J. B., 1971, Poly A sequences at the 3′-termini of rabbit globin mRNAs, *Nat. New Biol.* **233**, 41.

Canaani, E., and Duesberg, P., 1972, Role of subunits of 60 to 70S avian tumor virus ribonucleic acid in its template activity for the viral deoxyribonucleic acid polymerase, *J. Virol.* **10**, 23.

Canaani, E., Helm, K. V. D., and Duesberg, P. H., 1973, Evidence for 30–40S RNA as precursor of the 60–70S RNA of Rous sarcoma virus, *Proc. Natl. Acad. Sci. USA* **72**, 401.

Carnegie, J. W., Deeney, A. O. C., Olson, K. C., and Beaudreau, G. S., 1969, An RNA fraction from myeloblastosis virus having properties similar to transfer RNA, *Biochim. Biophys. Acta* **190**, 274.

Cheung, K., Smith, R. E., Stone, M. P., and Joklik, W. K., 1972, Comparison of immature (rapid harvest) and mature Rous sarcoma virus particles, *Virology* **50**, 851.

Clark, J. M., and Bader, J. P., 1974, Inhibition of development of transformation by Rous sarcoma virus in cultures of high cell density, *J. Cell. Physiol.*, **83**, 203.

Coffin, J. M., and Temin, H. M., 1970, Hybridization of Rous sarcoma virus deoxyribonucleic acid polymerase product and ribonucleic acids from chicken and rat cells infected with Rous sarcoma virus, *J. Virol.* **9**, 766.

Coffin, J. M., and Temin, H. M., 1971, Comparison of Rous sarcoma virus-specific deoxyribonucleic acid polymerases in virions of Rous sarcoma virus and in Rous sarcoma virus-infected chicken cells, *J. Virol.* **7**, 625.

Crawford, L. V., 1960, A study of the Rous sarcoma virus by density gradient centrifugation, *Virology* **12,** 143.

Crawford, L. V., and Crawford, E. M., 1961, The properties of Rous sarcoma virus purified by density gradient centrifugation, *Virology* **13,** 227.

Crittenden, L. B., 1968, Observations on the nature of a genetic cellular resistance to avian tumor viruses, *J. Natl. Cancer. Inst.* **41,** 145.

Dales, S., and Hanafusa, H., 1972, Penetration and intracellular release of the genomes of avian RNA tumor viruses, *Virology* **50,** 440.

Dalton, A. J., Haguenau, F., and Moloney, J. B., 1964, Further electron microscopic studies on the morphology of the Moloney agent, *J. Natl. Cancer Inst.* **33,** 255.

Darnell, J. E., Wall, R., and Tushinski, R. J., 1971, An adenylic acid-rich sequence in messenger RNA of HeLa cells and its possible relationship to reiterated sites on DNA, *Proc. Natl. Acad. Sci. USA* **68,** 1321.

Davis, J., Gilden, R. V., and Oroszlan, S., 1973, Isolation of an immunogenic polypeptide after limited trypsin hydrolysis of murine leukemia virus group-specific antigen, *Virology* **56,** 411.

Davis, N. L., and Rueckert, R. R., 1972, Properties of a ribonucleoprotein particle isolated from Nonidet P-40-treated Rous sarcoma virus, *J. Virol.* **10,** 1010.

deHarven, E., 1968, Morphology of murine leukemia viruses, *in* "Experimental Leukemia" (M. A. Rich, ed.), p. 101, Appleton-Century-Crofts, New York.

deHarven, E., and Friend, C., 1964, Structure of virus particles partially purified from the blood of leukemic mice, *Virology* **23,** 119.

de-The, G., 1964, Localization and origin of the adenosine-triphosphatase activity of avian myeloblastosis virus. A review, *Natl. Cancer Inst. Monograph* **17,** 651.

de-The, G., and O'Connor, T. E., 1966, Structure of a murine leukemia virus after disruption with Tween ether, *Virology* **28,** 713.

de-The, G., Becker, C., and Beard, J. W., 1964, Virus of avian myeloblastosis (BAI strain A). XXV. Ultracytochemical study of virus and myeloblast phosphatase activity, *J. Natl. Cancer Inst.* **32,** 201.

Dhaliwal, S. S., 1963, Resistance of the chorioallantoic membrane of chick embryos to Rous sarcoma and MH2 reticuloendothelioma viruses, *J. Natl. Cancer Inst.* **30,** 323.

Dougherty, R. M., and DiStefano, H. S., 1965, Virus particles associated with "nonproducer" Rous sarcoma cells, *Virology* **27,** 351.

Dougherty, R. M., and Rasmussen, R., 1964, Properties of a strain of Rous sarcoma virus that infects mammals, *Natl. Cancer Inst. Monograph* **17,** 337.

Dougherty, R. M., Simons, P. J., and Chesterman, F. C., 1963, Biological properties of three variants of Rous sarcoma virus, *J. Natl. Cancer Inst.* **31,** 1285.

Dougherty, R. M., Marucci, A. A., and DiStefano, H. S., 1972, Application of immunohistochemistry to study of avian leukosis virus, *J. Gen. Virol.* **15,** 149.

Duesberg, P. H., 1968, Physical properties of Rous sarcoma virus RNA, *Proc. Natl. Acad. Sci. USA* **59,** 930.

Duesberg, P. H., 1970, On the structure of RNA tumor viruses, *Curr. Top. Microbiol. Immunol.* **51,** 79.

Duesberg, P. H., and Canaani, E., 1970, Complementarity between Rous sarcoma virus (RSV) RNA and the *in vitro*-synthesized DNA of the virus-associated DNA polymerase, *Virology* **42,** 783.

Duesberg, P. H., and Robinson, W. S., 1967, Inhibition of mouse leukemia virus (MLV) replication by actinomycin D, *Virology* **31,** 742.

Duesberg, P. H., and Vogt, P. K., 1969, On the role of DNA synthesis in avian tumor virus infection, *Proc. Natl. Acad. Sci. USA* **64,** 939.

Duesberg, P. H., and Vogt, P. K., 1970, Differences between the ribonucleic acids of transforming and nontransforming avian tumor viruses, *Proc. Natl. Acad. Sci. USA* **67**, 1673.

Duesberg, P. H., and Vogt, P. K., 1973*a*, Gel electrophoresis of avian leukosis and sarcoma viral RNA in formamide: Comparison with other viral and cellular RNA species, *J. Virol.* **12**, 594.

Duesberg, P. H., and Vogt, P. K., 1973*b*, RNA species obtained from clonal lines of avian sarcoma and from avian leukosis virus, *Virology* **54**, 207.

Duesberg, P. H., Martin, G. S., and Vogt, P. K., 1970, Glycoprotein components of avian and murine RNA tumor viruses, *Virology* **41**, 631.

Duesberg, P., Helm, K. V. D., and Canaani, E., 1971, Comparative properties of RNA and DNA templates for the DNA polymerase of Rous sarcoma virus, *Proc. Natl. Acad. Sci. USA* **68**, 2505.

Duesberg, P. H., Vogt, P. K., Maisel, J., Lai, M. M. C., and Canaani, E., 1973, Tracking defective tumor virus RNA, *in* "Second ICN-UCLA Symposium on Molecular Biology" (C. F. Fox and W. S. Robinson, eds.), p. 327, Academic Press, New York.

Edmonds, M., Vaughn, M. H., Jr., and Nakazato, H., 1971, Polyadenylic acid sequences in the heterogeneous nuclear RNA and rapidly-labeled polysomal RNA of HeLa cells: Possible evidence for a precursor relationship, *Proc. Natl. Acad. Sci. USA* **68**, 1336.

Emanoil-Ravicovitch, E., Larsen, C. J., Bazilier, M., Robin, J., Peries, J., and Boiron, M., 1973, Low-molecular-weight RNAs of murine sarcoma virus: Comparative studies of free and 70S RNA-associated components, *J. Virol.* **12**, 1625.

Erikson, E., and Erikson, R. L., 1970, Isolation of amino acid acceptor RNA from purified avian myeloblastosis virus, *J. Mol. Biol.* **52**, 387.

Erikson, E., and Erikson, R. L., 1971, Association of 4S ribonucleic acid with oncornavirus ribonucleic acids, *J. Virol.* **8**, 254.

Erikson, E., and Erikson, R. L., 1972, Transfer ribonucleic acid synthetase activity associated with avian myeloblastosis virus, *J. Virol.* **9**, 231.

Erikson, R. L., 1969, Studies on the RNA from avian myeloblastosis virus, *Virology* **37**, 124.

Erikson, R. L., Erikson, E., and Walker, T. A., 1971, The identification of the 3′-hydroxyl nucleoside terminus of avian myeloblastosis virus RNA, *Virology* **45**, 527.

Fanshier, L., Garapin, A., McDonnell, J., Faras, A., Levinson, W., and Bishop, J. M., 1971, DNA polymerase associated with avian tumor viruses: Secondary structure of the deoxyribonucleic acid product, *J. Virol.* **7**, 77.

Faras, A., Fanshier, L., Garapin, A., Levinson, W., and Bishop, J. M., 1971, Deoxyribonucleic acid polymerase of Rous sarcoma virus: Studies on the mechanism of double-stranded deoxyribonucleic acid synthesis, *J. Virol.* **7**, 539.

Fischinger, P. J., Peebles, P. T., Nomura, S., and Haapala, D. K., 1973, Isolation of an RD-114-like oncornavirus from a cat cell line, *J. Virol.* **11**, 978.

Fleissner, E., 1971, Chromatographic separation and antigenic analysis of proteins of the oncornaviruses. I. Avian leukemia-sarcoma viruses, *J. Virol.* **8**, 778.

Fleissner, E., and Tress, E., 1973*a*, Chromatographic and electrophoretic analysis of viral proteins from hamster and chicken cells transformed by Rous sarcoma virus, *J. Virol.* **11**, 250.

Fleissner, E., and Tress, E., 1973*b*, Isolation of a ribonucleoprotein structure from oncornaviruses, *J. Virol.* **12**, 1612.

Flugel, R. M., and Wells, R. D., 1972, Nucleotides at the RNA-DNA covalent bonds formed in the endogenous reaction by the avian myeloblastosis virus DNA polymerase, *Virology* **48**, 394.

Flugel, R. M., Rapp, U., and Wells, R. D., 1973, RNA-DNA covalent bonds between the RNA primers and the DNA products formed by RNA tumor virus DNA polymerase, *J. Virol.* **12**, 1491.

Friis, R. R., 1971, Inactivation of avian sarcoma viruses with UV light: A difference between helper-dependent and helper-independent strains, *Virology* **43**, 521.

Friis, R. R., Toyoshima, K., and Vogt, P. K., 1971, Conditional lethal mutants of avian sarcoma viruses. I. Physiology of *ts* 75 and *ts* 149, *Virology* **43**, 375.

Fujinaga, K., Parsons, J. T., Beard, J. W., Beard, D., and Green, M., 1970, Mechanism of carcinogenesis by RNA tumor viruses. III. Formation of carcinogenesis by RNA tumor viruses. III. Formation of RNA–DNA complex and duplex DNA molecules by the DNA polymerase(s) of avian myeloblastosis virus, *Proc. Natl. Acad. Sci. USA* **67**, 1432.

Gallo, R. C., Savin, P. S., Allen, P. T., Newton, W. A., Priori, E. S., Bower, J. M., and Dmochowski, L., 1971, Reverse transcriptase in type C virus particles of human origin, *Nat. New Biol.* **232**, 140.

Gantt, R. R., Stromberg, K. J., and Montes de Oca, F., 1971, Specific RNA methylase associated with avian myeloblastosis virus, *Nature (Lond.)* **234**, 35.

Garapin, A., McDonnell, J. P., Levinson, W., Quintrell, N., Fanshier, L., and Bishop, J. M., 1970, Deoxyribonucleic acid polymerase associated with Rous sarcoma virus and avian myeloblastosis virus: Properties of the enzyme and its product, *J. Virol.* **6**, 589.

Garapin, A. C., Leong, J., Fanshier, L., Levinson, W. E., and Bishop, J. M., 1971, Identification of virus-specific RNA in cells infected with Rous sarcoma virus, *Biochem. Biophys. Res. Commun.* **42**, 919.

Garapin, A. C., Varmus, H. E., Faras, A. J., Levinson, W. E., and Bishop, J. M., 1973, RNA-directed DNA synthesis by virions of Rous sarcoma virus: Further characterization of the templates and the extent of their transcription, *Virology* **52**, 264.

Gazzolo, L., de-The, G., Vigier, P., and Sarma, P. S., 1969, Presence de particules a l'aspect de nucleo-capsides associces aur mitochondries dans cellules de hamster transformees par le virus de Rous, *C. R. Hebd. Seances Acad. Sci. Ser. D Sci. Nat.* **268**, 1668.

Gelb, L. D., Aaronson, S. A., and Martin, M. A., 1971, Heterogeneity of murine leukemia virus *in vitro* DNA; Detection of viral DNA in mammalian cells, *Science (Wash., D.C.)* **172**, 1353.

Gilden, R. V., and Oroszlan, S., 1972, Group-specific antigens of RNA tumor viruses as markers for subinfectious expression of the RNA virus genome, *Proc. Natl. Acad. Sci. USA* **69**, 1021.

Gilden, R. V., Parks, W. P., Huebner, R. J., and Todaro, G. J., 1971, Murine leukemia virus group-specific antigen in the C-type virus-containing human cell line, ESP-1, *Nature (Lond.)* **233**, 102.

Gillespie, D., Marshall, S., and Gallo, R. C., 1972, RNA of RNA tumor viruses contains poly A, *Nat. New Biol.* **236**, 227.

Gillespie, D., Gillespie, S., Gallo, R. C., East, J. L., and Dmochowski, L., 1973, Genetic origin of RD 114 and other RNA tumor viruses assayed by molecular hybridization, *Nat. New Biol.* **244**, 51.

Golde, A., 1970, Radio-induced mutants of the Schmidt-Ruppin strain of Rous sarcoma virus, *Virology* **40**, 1022.

Goldé, A., and Laterjet, R., 1966, Dissociation, par irradiation, des fonctions oncogene et infectieuse du virus de Rous, souche de Schmidt-Ruppin, *C. R. Hebd. Seances Acad. Sci. Ser D Sci. Nat.* **262**, 420.

Goldé, A., and Villaudy, J., 1971, The effect of ageing and cell density on the infection and the morphological conversion *in vitro* by Rous sarcoma virus of chick embryo fibroblasts *in* "The Biology of Oncogenic Viruses Lepetit Colloquia on Biology and Medicine," Vol. 2, p. 124. American Elsevier Publishing Co., New York.

Graf, T., 1972, A plaque assay for avian tumor viruses, *Virology* **50**, 567.

Grandgenett, D. P., Gerard, G. F., and Green, M., 1972, Ribonuclease H: A ubiquitous activity in virions of ribonucleic acid tumor viruses, *J. Gen. Virol.* **10**, 1136.

Grandgenett, D. P., Gerard, G. F., and Green, M., 1973, A single subunit from avian myeloblastosis virus with both RNA-directed DNA polymerase and ribonuclease H activity, *Proc. Natl. Acad. Sci. USA* **70**, 230.

Green, M., and Cartas, M., 1972, The genome of RNA tumor viruses contains polyadenylic acid sequences, *Proc. Natl. Acad. Sci. USA* **69**, 791.

Green, M., Rokutanda, H., and Rokutanda, M., 1971, Virus-specific RNA in cells transformed by RNA tumour viruses, *Nat. New Biol.* **230**, 229.

Gross, L., 1970, "Oncogenic Viruses," p. 424, Pergamon Press, New York.

Gulati, S. C., Axel, R., and Spiegelman, S., 1972, Detection of RNA-instructed DNA polymerase and high-molecular-weight RNA in malignant tissue, *Proc. Natl. Acad. Sci. USA* **69**, 2020.

Hanafusa, H. 1964, Nature of the defectiveness of Rous sarcoma virus, *Natl. Cancer Inst. Monograph* **17**, 523.

Hanafusa, H., 1965, Analysis of the defectiveness of Rous sarcoma virus. 3. Determining influence of a new helper virus on the host range and susceptibility to interference of RSV, *Virology* **25**, 248.

Hanafusa, H., and Hanafusa, T., 1966, Determining factor in the capacity of Rous sarcoma virus to induce tumors in mammals, *Proc. Natl. Acad. Sci. USA* **55**, 532.

Hanafusa, H., and Hanafusa, T., 1968, Further studies on RSV production from transformed cells, *Virology* **34**, 630.

Hanafusa, H., and Hanafusa, T., 1971, Noninfectious RSV deficient in DNA polymerase, *Virology* **43**, 313.

Hanafusa, H., Miyamoto, T., and Hanafusa, T., 1970, Recovery of a new virus from apparently normal chick cells by infection with avian tumor viruses, *Proc. Natl. Acad. Sci. USA* **67**, 1797.

Hanafusa, H., Baltimore, D., Smoler, D., Watson, K. F., Yaniv, A., and Spiegelman, S., 1972, Absence of polymerase protein in virions of alpha-type Rous sarcoma virus, *Science (Wash., D.C.)* **177**, 1188.

Hanafusa, T., and Hanafusa, H., 1968, Interaction among avian tumor viruses giving enhanced infectivity, *Proc. Natl. Acad. Sci. USA* **58**, 818.

Hanafusa, T., and Hanafusa, H., 1973, Isolation of leukosis-type virus from pheasant embryo cells: Possible presence of viral genes in cells, *Virology* **51**, 247.

Hanafusa, T., Hanafusa, H., Miyamoto, T., and Fleissner, E., 1972, Existence and expression of tumor virus genes in chick embryo cells, *Virology* **47**, 475.

Hartley, J. W., and Rowe, W. P., 1966, Production of altered cell foci in tissue culture by defective Moloney sarcoma virus particles, *Proc. Natl. Acad. Sci. USA* **55**, 780.

Hartley, J. W., Rowe, W. P., Capps, W. I., and Huebner, R. J., 1965, Complement fixation and tissue culture assays for mouse leukemia viruses, *Proc. Natl. Acad. Sci. USA* **53**, 931.

Hartley, J. W., Rowe, W. P., and Huebner, R. J., 1970, Host-range restrictions of murine leukemia viruses in mouse embryo cell cultures, *J. Virol.* **5,** 221.

Hatanaka, M., Kakefuda, T., Gilden, R. V., and Callan, E. A. O., 1971, Cytoplasmic DNA synthesis induced by RNA tumor viruses, *Proc. Natl. Acad. Sci. USA* **68,** 1844.

Hatanaka, M., Twiddy, E., and Gilden, R. V., 1972, Protein kinase associated with RNA tumor viruses and other budding RNA viruses, *Virology* **47,** 536.

Hehlmann, R., Kufe, D., and Spiegelman, S., 1972a, RNA in human leukemic cells related to the RNA of a mouse leukemia virus, *Proc. Natl. Acad. Sci. USA* **69,** 435.

Hehlmann, R., Kufe, D., and Spiegelman, S., 1972b, Viral-related RNA in Hodgkins' disease and other human lymphomas, *Proc. Natl. Acad. Sci. USA* **69,** 1727.

Hill, M., and Hillova, J., 1972a, Virus recovery in chicken cells tested with Rous sarcoma cell DNA, *Nat. New Biol.* **237,** 35.

Hill, M., and Hillova, J., 1972b, Recovery of the temperature-sensitive mutant of Rous sarcoma virus from chicken cells exposed to DNA extracted from hamster cells transformed by the mutant, *Virology* **49,** 309.

Hobom-Schnegg, B., Robinson, H. L., and Robinson, W. S., 1970, Replication of Rous sarcoma virus in synchronized cells, *J. Gen. Virol.* **4,** 85.

Huebner, R. J., and Todaro, G. J., 1969, Oncogenes of RNA tumor viruses as determinants of cancer, *Proc. Natl. Acad. Sci. USA* **64,** 1087.

Huebner, R. J., Armstrong, D., Okuyan, M., Sarma, P. S., and Turner, H. C., 1964, Specific complement-fixing viral antigens in hamster and guinea pig tumors induced by the Schmidt-Ruppin strain of avian sarcoma, *Proc. Natl. Acad. Sci. USA* **51,** 742.

Huebner, R. J., Felloff, G. J., Sarma, P. S., Lane, W. T., Turner, H. C., Gilden, R. V., Oroszlan, S., Meier, H., Myers, D. D., and Peters, R. L., 1970, Group-specific antigen expression during embryogenesis of the genome of the C-type RNA tumor virus: Implications for ontogenesis and oncogenesis, *Proc. Natl. Acad. Sci. USA* **67,** 366.

Hung, P. P., 1973, Ribonucleases of Rous sarcoma virus, *Virology* **51,** 287.

Hung, P. P., Robinson, H. L., and Robinson, W. S., 1971, Isolation and characterization of proteins from Rous sarcoma virus, *Virology* **43,** 251.

Hurwitz, J., and Leis, J. P., 1972, RNA-dependent DNA polymerase activity of RNA tumor viruses. I. Directing influence of DNA in the reaction, *J. Virol.* **9,** 116.

Johnson, G. S., Friedman, R. M., and Pastan, I., 1971, Analysis of the fusion of XC cells induced by homogenates of murine leukemia virus-infected cells and by purified murine leukemia virus, *J. Virol.* **7,** 753.

Kacian, D. C., Watson, K. F., Burny, A., and Spiegelman, S., 1971, Purification of the DNA polymerase of avian myeloblastosis virus, *Biochim. Biophys. Acta* **246,** 365.

Kakefuda, T., and Bader, J. P., 1969, Electron microscopic observations on the ribonucleic acid of murine leukemia virus, *J. Virol.* **4,** 460.

Kang, C., and Temin, H. M., 1972, Endogenous RNA-directed DNA polymerase activity in uninfected chicken embryos, *Proc. Natl. Acad. Sci. USA* **69,** 1550.

Kara, J., 1968, Induction of cellular DNA synthesis in chick embryo fibroblasts infected with Rous sarcoma virus in culture, *Biochem. Biophys. Res. Commun.* **32,** 817.

Kara, J., Mach, O., and Cerna, H., 1971, Replication of Rous sarcoma virus and the biosynthesis of the oncogenic subviral ribonucleoprotein particles ("virosomes") in the mitochondria, *Biochem. Biophys. Res. Commun.* **44,** 162.

Kawai, S., and Hanafusa, H., 1971, The effects of reciprocal changes in temperature on the transformed state of cells infected with a Rous sarcoma mutant, *Virology* **46**, 470.

Kawai, S., and Hanafusa, H., 1972a, Plaque assay for some strains of avian leukosis virus, *Virology* **48**, 126.

Kawai, S., and Hanafusa, H., 1972b, Genetic recombination with avian tumor virus, *Virology* **49**, 37.

Keller, W., and Crouch, R., 1972, Degradation of DNA–RNA hybrids by ribonuclease H and DNA polymerases of cellular and viral origin, *Proc. Natl. Acad. Sci. USA* **11**, 3360.

Kelloff, G., and Vogt, P. K., 1966, Localization of avian tumor virus group-specific antigen in cell and virus, *Virology* **29**, 377.

Klein, G., and Klein, E., 1962, Antigenic properties of other experimental tumors, *Cold Spring Harbor Symp. Quant. Biol.* **27**, 463.

Klement, V., Nicholson, M. D., and Huebner, R. J., 1971, Rescue of the genome of focus forming virus from rat non-productive lines by 5′-bromodeoxyuridine, *Nat. New Biol.* **234**, 12.

Knudson, A. G., Brodetsky, A. M., and Baluda, M. A., 1967, Transient inhibition of avian myeloblastosis virus reproduction by amethopterin and fluorodeoxyuridine, *J. Virol.* **1**, 1150.

Lacour, F., Foureade, A., Verger, C., and Delain, F., 1970, Coiled structure of the nucleocapsid of avian myeloblastosis virus, *J. Gen. Virol.* **9**, 89.

Lai, M. M. C., and Duesberg, P. H., 1972a, Adenylic acid-rich sequence in RNAs of Rous sarcoma virus and Rauscher mouse leukemia virus, *Nature (Lond.)* **235**, 383.

Lai, M. M. C., and Duesberg, P. H., 1972b, Differences between the envelope glyco-proteins and glycopeptides of avian tumor viruses released from transformed and from nontransformed cells, *Virology* **50**, 359.

Lange, J., Frank, H., Hunsman, G., Moenning, V., Wollman, R., and Schafer, W., 1973, Properties of mouse leukemia viruses. VI. The core of Friend virus isolation and constituents, *Virology* **53**, 457.

Lee, S. Y., Mendecki, J., and Brawerman, G., 1971, A polynucleotide segment rich in adenylic acid in the rapidly-labeled polyribosomal RNA component of mouse sarcoma 180 ascites cells, *Proc. Natl. Acad. Sci. USA* **68**, 1331.

Leis, J. P., and Hurwitz, J., 1972a, RNA-dependent DNA pplymerase activity of RNA tumor viruses. II. Directing influence of RNA in the reaction, *J. Virol.* **9**, 130.

Leis, J. P., and Hurwitz, J., 1972b, Isolation and characterization of a protein that stimulates DNA synthesis from avian myeloblastosis virus, *Proc. Natl. Acad. Sci. USA* **69**, 2331.

Leis, J. P., Berkower, I., and Hurwitz, J., 1973, Mechanism of action of ribonuclease H isolated from avian myeloblastosis virus and *Escherichia coli, Proc. Natl. Acad. Sci. USA* **70**, 466.

Leong, J., Garapin, A., Jackson, N., Fanshier, L., Levinson, W., and Bishop, J. M., 1972a, Virus-specific ribonucleic acid in cells producing Rous sarcoma virus: Detection and characterization, *J. Virol.* **9**, 891.

Leong, J. A., Levinson, W., and Bishop, J. M., 1972b, Synchronization of Rous sarcoma virus production in chick embryo cells, *Virology* **47**, 133.

Levinson, W., and Rubin, H., 1966, Radiation studies of avian tumor viruses and of Newcastle disease virus, *Virology* **28**, 533.

Levinson, W., Bishop, J. M., Quintrell, N., and Jackson, J., 1970, Presence of DNA in Rous sarcoma virus, *Nature (Lond.)* **227**, 1023.

Lin, F. H., and Thormar, H., 1970, On visna virus: Purification and nucleic acid content, *Virology* **42**, 1140.

Linial, M., and Mason, W. S., 1973, Characterization of two conditional early mutants of Rous sarcoma virus, *Virology* **53**, 258.

Livingston, D., and Todaro, G. J., 1973, Endogenous type C virus from a cat cell clone with properties distinct from previously described feline type C virus, *Virology* **53**, 142.

Lowy, D. R., Rowe, W. P., Teich, N., and Hartley, J. W., 1971, Murine leukemia virus high-frequency activation *in vitro* by 5-iododeoxyuridine and 5-bromodeoxyuridine, *Science (Wash., D.C.)* **174**, 155.

Luborsky, S. W., 1971, Sedimentation equilibrium analysis of the molecular weight of a tumor virus RNA, *Virology* **45**, 782.

Luftig, R. B., and Kilham, S. S., 1971, An electron microscope study of Rauscher leukemia virus, *Virology* **46**, 277.

McAllister, R. M., Nelson-Rees, W. A., Johnson, E. Y., Rongey, R. W., and Gardner, M. B., 1971, Disseminated rhabdomyosarcomas formed in kittens by cultured human rhabdomyosarcoma cells, *J. Natl. Cancer Inst.* **47**, 603.

McAllister, R. M., Nicholson, M., Gardner, M. B., Rongey, R. W., Rasheed, S., Sarma, P. S., Huebner, R. J., Hatanaka, M., Oroszlan, S., Gilden, R. V., Kabigting, A., and Vernon, L., 1972, C-type virus released from cultured human rhabdomyosarcoma cells, *Nat. New Biol.* **235**, 3.

McCain, B., Biswal, N., and Benyesh-Melnick, M., 1973, The subunits of murine sarcoma-leukemia virus RNA, *J. Gen. Virol.* **18**, 69.

Mach, O., and Kara, J., 1971, Presence of Rous sarcoma virus inside the mitochondria isolated by zonal and differential centrifugation from Rous sarcoma cells, *Folia Biol. (Prague)* **17**, 65.

Macieira-Coelho, A., and Ponten, J., 1967, Induction of the division cycle in resting stage human fibroblasts after RSV infection, *Biochem. Biophys. Res. Commun.* **29**, 316.

Macieira-Coelho, A., Hiu, I. J., and Garcia-Giralt, E., 1969, Stimulation of DNA synthesis in resting stage human fibroblasts after infection with Rous sarcoma virus, *Nature (Lond.)* **222**, 1172.

Maldonado, R. L., and Bose, H. R., 1971, Separation of reticuloendotheliosis virus from avian tumor viruses, *J. Virol.* **8**, 813.

Maly, A., and Riman, J., 1971, Presence and origin of DNA endonuclease activities in oncogenic DNA virus preparations, *Neoplasma* **18**, 575.

Manly, K., Smoler, D. F., Bromfeld, E., and Baltimore, D., 1971, Forms of deoxyribonucleic acid produced by virions of the ribonucleic acid tumor viruses, *J. Virol.* **7**, 106.

Marshall, S., and Gillespie, D., 1972, Poly U tracts absent from viral RNA, *Nat. New Biol.* **240**, 43.

Martin, G. S., 1970, Rous sarcoma virus: A function required for maintenance of the transformed state, *Nature (Lond.)* **227**, 1021.

Maruyama, H. B., Hatanaka, M., and Gilden, R. V., 1971, The 3′-terminal nucleosides of the high-molecular-weight RNA of C-type viruses, *Proc. Natl. Acad. Sci. USA* **68**, 1999.

May, J. T., Somers, K. D., and Kit, S., 1972, Defective mouse sarcoma virus deficient in DNA polymerase activity, *J. Gen. Virol.* **16**, 223.

Miyamoto, K., and Gilden, R. V., 1971, Electron microscopic studies of tumor viruses. I. Entry of murine leukemia virus into mouse embryo fibroblasts, *J. Virol.* **7**, 395.

Mizutani, S., and Temin, H. M., 1971, Enzymes and nucleotides in virions of Rous sarcoma virus, *J. Virol.* **8**, 409.

Mizutani, S., Boettiger, D., and Temin, H., 1970, A DNA-dependent DNA polymerase and a DNA endonuclease in virions of Rous sarcoma virus, *Nature (Lond.)* **228**, 424.

Mizutani, S., Temin, H. M., Kodama, M., and Wells, R. O., 1971, DNA ligase and exonuclease activities in virions of Rous sarcoma virus, *Nat. New Biol.* **230**, 232.

Molling, F., Bolognesi, D. P., Bauer, H., Busen, W., Plassman, H. W., and Hansen, P., 1971, Association of viral reverse transcriptase with an enzyme degrading the RNA moiety of RNA–DNA hybrids, *Nat. New Biol.* **234**, 240.

Morgan, H. R., 1964, The biologic properties of cells infected with Rous sarcoma virus *in vitro, Natl. Cancer Inst. Monograph* **17**, 395.

Nakata, Y., and Bader, J. P., 1968*a*, Studies on the fixation and development of cellular transformation by Rous sarcoma virus, *Virology* **36**, 401.

Nakata, Y., and Bader, J. P., 1968*b*, Transformation by murine sarcoma virus: Fixation (deoxyribonucleic and synthesis) and development, *J. Virol.* **2**, 1255.

Nakata, Y., and Bader, J. P., 1970, *Abstr. Tenth Intl Cancer Congr.* (*Houston*) p. 234.

Neiman, P., 1973, Measurement of RD114 virus nucleotide sequences in feline cellular DNA, *Nat. New Biol.* **244**, 62.

Nowinski, R. C., Old, L. J., Sarkar, N. H., and Moore, D. H., 1970, Common properties of the oncogenic RNA viruses (oncornaviruses), *Virology* **42**, 1152.

Nowinski, R. C., Sarkar, N. H., Old, L. J., Moore, D. H., Scheer, D. I., and Hilgers, J., 1971, Viral proteins and antigens, *Virology* **46**, 21.

Odaka, T., 1969, Inheritance of susceptibility to Friend mouse leukemia virus. V. Introduction of a gene responsible for susceptibility in the genetic complement of resistant mice, *J. Virol.* **3**, 543.

Okabe, H., Loringer, G., G., Gilden, R. V., and Hatanaka, M., 1972, The nucleotides at the RNA–DNA joint formed by the DNA polymerase of Rauscher leukemia virus, *Virology* **50**, 935.

Okabe, H., Gilden, R. V., and Hatanaka, M., 1973, Extensive homology of RD114 virus DNA with RNA of of feline cell origin, *Nat. New Biol.* **244**, 54.

Okano, H., and Rich, M. A., 1969, Time cycle for intracellular synthesis of murine leukemia virus, *Nature (Lond.)* **224**, 77.

Oroszlan, S., Fisher, C. L., Stanley, T. B., and Gilden, R. V., 1970, Proteins of the murine C-type RNA tumor viruses: Isolation of a group-specific antigen by isoelectric focusing, *J. Gen. Virol.* **8**, 1.

Oroszlan, S., Hatanaka, M., Gilden, R. V., and Huebner, R. J., 1971*a*, Specific inhibition of mammalian ribonucleic acid C-type virus deoxyribonucleic acid polymerases by rat antisera, *J. Virol.* **8**, 816.

Oroszlan, S., Foreman, C., Kelloff, G., and Gilden, R. V., 1971*b*, The group-specific antigen and other structural proteins of hamster and mouse C-type viruses, *Virology* **43**, 665.

Oroszlan, S., Bova, D., Huebner, R. J., and Gilden, R. V., 1972, Major group-specific protein of rat type C viruses, *J. Virol.* **10**, 746.

Parks, W. P., Scolnick, E. M., Ross, J., Todaro, G. J., and Aaronson, S. A., 1972, Immunological relationships of reverse transcriptases from ribonucleic acid tumor viruses, *J. Virol.* **9**, 110.

Payne, L. N., and Pani, P. K., 1971, Evidence for linkage between genetic loci controlling response of fowl to subgroup A and subgroup C sarcoma viruses, *J. Gen. Virol.* **13**, 253.

Payne, L. N., Pani, P. K., and Weiss, R. A., 1971, A dominant epistatic gene which inhibits cellular susceptibility to RSV (RAV-o), *J. Gen. Virol.* **13**, 455.

Peebles, P. T., Haapala, D. K., and Gazdar, A. F., 1972, Deficiency of viral ribonucleic acid-dependent deoxyribonucleic acid polymerase in noninfectious virus-like particles released from murine sarcoma virus-transformed hamster cells, *J. Virol.* **9**, 488.

Piraino, F., 1967, The mechanism of genetic resistance of chick embryo cells to infection by Rous sarcoma virus-Bryan strain (BS-RSV), *Virology* **32**, 700.

Priori, E. S., Dmochowski, I., Myers, B., and Wilbur, J. R., 1971, Constant production of type C virus particles in a continuous tissue culture derived from pleural effusion cells of a lymphoma patient, *Nat. New Biol.* **232**, 61.

Quigley, J. P., Rifkin, D. B., and Reich, E., 1971, Phospholipid composition of Rous sarcoma virus, host cell membranes and other enveloped RNA viruses, *Virology* **46**, 106.

Quigley, J. P., Rifkin, D. B., and Compans, R. W., 1972*a*, Isolation and characterization of ribonucleoprotein substructures from Rous sarcoma virus, *Virology* **50**, 65.

Quigley, J. P., Rifkin, D. B., and Reich, E., 1972*b*, Lipid studies of Rous sarcoma virus and host cell membranes, *Virology* **50**, 550.

Quintrell, N., Fanshier, L., Evans, B., Levinson, W., and Bishop, J. M., 1971, Deoxyribonucleic acid polymerase(s) of Rous sarcoma virus: Effects of virion-associated endonuclease on the enzymatic product, *J. Virol.* **8**, 17.

Rabotti, G. F., Michelson-Fiske, and Haguenau, F., 1969, Cinetique du developpement du virus du sarcome de Rous (souche Schmidt-Ruppin). Estimation du temps de synthese de l'ARN. Etude par autoradiographie au microscope e'lectronique, *C. R. Hebd. Seances Acad. Sci. Ser. D Sci. Nat.* **269**, 2291.

Randerath, K., Rosenthal, L. J., and Zamecnik, P. C., 1971, Base composition differences between avian myeloblastosis virus transfer RNA and transfer RNA isolated from host cells, *Proc. Natl. Acad. Sci. USA* **68**, 3233.

Rao, P. R., Bonar, R. A., and Beard, J. W., 1966, Lipids of the BAI strain A avian tumor virus and of the myeloblast host cell, *Exp. Mol. Pathol.* **5**, 374.

Rauscher, F. J., and Allen, B. V., 1964, Growth curve of a murine leukemia virus in mice, *J. Natl. Cancer Inst.* **32**, 269.

Reich, E., Franklin, R. M., Shatkin, A. J., and Tatum, E. L., 1961, The effect of actinomycin D on cellular nucleic acid synthesis and virus production, *Science (Wash., D.C.)* **134**, 556.

Rifkin, D. B., and Compans, R. W., 1971, Identification of the spike proteins of Rous sarcoma virus, *Virology* **46**, 485.

Riman, J., and Beaudreau, G. S., 1970, Viral DNA-dependent DNA polymerase and the properties of thymidine-labelled material in virions of an oncogenic virus, *Nature (Lond.)* **228**, 427.

Robinson, H. L., 1967, Isolation of noninfectious particles containing Rous sarcoma virus RNA from the medium of Rous sarcoma virus-transformed nonproducer cells, *Proc. Natl. Acad. Sci. USA* **57**, 1655.

Robinson, W. S., 1966, The nucleic acid of Rous sarcoma virus, *in* "Viruses Inducing Cancer" (W. J. Burdette, ed.), p. 107, University of Utah Press, Salt Lake City, Utah.

Robinson, W. S., and Robinson, H. L., 1971, DNA polymerase in defective Rous sarcoma virus, *Virology* **44**, 457.

Robinson, W. S., Pitkanen, A., and Rubin, H., 1965, The nucleic acid of the Bryan strain of Rous sarcoma virus: Purification of the virus and isolation of the nucleic acid, *Proc. Natl. Acad. Sci. USA* **54**, 137.

Robinson, W. S., Robinson, H. L., and Duesberg, P. H., 1967, Tumor virus RNAs, *Proc. Natl. Acad. Sci. USA* **58**, 825.

Robinson, W. S., Hung, P., Robinson, H. L., and Ralph, D. D., 1970, Proteins of avian tumor viruses with different coat antigens, *J. Virol.* **6**, 695.

Rosenbergová, M., Lacour, F., and Huppert, J., 1965, Misc en endeuce d'une activite nucleasique associee en virus de la myeloblastose aviare, lors de tentatives de purification de ce virus et de son acid ribonucleique, *C. R. Hebd. Seances Acad. Sci. Ser. D Sci. Nat.* **260**, 5145.

Rosenthal, L. J., and Zamecnik, P. C., 1973, Amino-acid acceptor activity of the 70S-associate 4S RNA from avian myeloblastosis virus, *Proc. Natl. Acad. Sci. USA* **70**, 1184.

Rosenthal, P. M., Robinson, H. L., Robinson, W. S., Hanafusa, T., and Hanafusa, H., 1971, DNA in uninfected and virus-infected cells complementary to avian tumor virus RNA, *Proc. Natl. Acad. Sci. USA* **68**, 2336.

Ross, J., Scolnick, E. M., Todaro, G. J., and Aaronson, S. A., 1971, Separation of murine cellular and murine leukemia virus DNA polymerases, *Nat. New Biol.* **231**, 163.

Ross, J., Tronick, S. R., and Scolnick, E. M., 1972, Polyadenylate-rich RNA in the 70S RNA of murine leukemia-sarcoma virus, *Virology* **49**, 230.

Rous, P., 1911, A sarcoma of the fowl transmissible by an agent from the tumor cells, *J. Exp. Med.* **13**, 397.

Rowe, W. P., 1972a, The kinetics of rescue of the murine sarcoma virus genome from a nonproducer line of transformed mouse cells, *Virology* **46**, 369.

Rowe, W. P., 1972b, Studies of genetic transmission of murine leukemia virus by AKR mice. I. Crosses with FV-1[n] strains of mice, *J. Exp. Med.* **136**, 1272.

Rowe, W. P., and Hartley, J. W., 1972, Studies of genetic transmission of murine leukemia virus by AKR mice. II. Crosses with Fv-1[b] strains of mice, *J. Exp. Med.* **136**, 1286.

Rowe, W. R., Pugh, W. E., and Hartley, J. W., 1970, Plaque assay techniques for murine leukemia viruses, *Virology* **46**, 1136.

Rowe, W. P., Hartley, J. W., and Brenner, T., 1972, Genetic mapping of a murine leukemia virus-inducing locus of AKR mice, *Science (Wash., D.C.)* **178**, 860.

Roy, P., and Bishop, D. H. L., 1971, Nucleoside triphosphate phosphotransferase. A new enzyme activity of oncogenic and non-oncogenic "budding" viruses, *Biochim. Biophys. Acta* **235**, 191.

Rubin, H., 1960, A virus in chick embryos which induces resistance *in vitro* to infection with Rous sarcoma virus, *Proc. Natl. Acad. Sci. USA* **46**, 1105.

Rubin, H., 1966, The inhibition of chick embryo cell growth by medium obtained from cultures of Rous sarcoma cells, *Exp. Cell Res.* **41**, 149.

Rubin, H., and Temin, H. M., 1959, A radiological study of cell virus interaction in the Rous sarcoma, *Virology* **7**, 75.

Rubin, H., Cornelius, A., Fanshier, L., 1961, The pattern of congenital transmission of an avian leukosis virus, *Proc. Natl. Acad. Sci. USA* **47**, 1058.

Sarma, P. S., Tseng, J., Lee, Y. K., and Gilden, R. V., 1973, Virus similar to RD114 virus in cat cells, *Nat. New Biol.* **244**, 56.

Sarkar, N. H., Nowinski, R. C., and Moore, D. H., 1971, Helical nucleocapsid structure of the oncogenic ribonucleic acid viruses (oncornaviruses), *J. Virol.* **8**, 564.

Sawyer, R. C., and Dahlberg, J. E., 1973, Small RNAs of Rous sarcoma virus: Characterization by two-dimensional polyacrylamide gel electrophoresis and fingerprint analysis, *J. Virol.* **12**, 1226.

Schäfer, W., Fischinger, P. J., Lange, J., and Pister, L., 1972a, Properties of mouse leukemia viruses: 1. Characterization of various antisera and serological identification of viral components, *Virology* **47**, 197.

Schäfer, W., Lange, J., Fischinger, P. J., Frank, H., Bolognesi, D. P., and Pister, L., 1972b, Isolation of viral components, *Virology* **47**, 210.

Scheele, C. M., and Hanafusa, H., 1971, Proteins of helper-dependent RSV, *Virology* **45**, 401.

Scheele, C. M., and Hanafusa, H., 1972, Electrophoretic analysis of the RNA of avian tumor viruses, *Virology* **50**, 753.

Schlom, J., and Spiegelman, S., 1971, Simultaneous detection of reverse transcriptase and high-molecular-weight RNA unique to oncogenic RNA viruses, *Science (Wash., D.C.)* **174**, 840.

Schlom, J., Spiegelman, S., and Moore, D., 1971, RNA-dependent DNA polymerase activity in virus-like particles isolated from human milk, *Nature (Lond.)* **235**, 35.

Schlom, J., Spiegelman, S., and Moore, D. H., 1972, Detection of high-molecular-weight RNA in particles from human milk, *Science (Wash., D.C.)* **175**, 542.

Scolnick, E. M., Stephenson, J. R., and Aaronson, S. A., 1972a, Isolation of temperature-sensitive mutants of murine sarcoma virus, *J. Virol.* **10**, 653.

Scolnick, E. M., Parks, W. P., Todaro, G., and Aaronson, S. A., 1972b, Immunological characterization of primate C-type virus reverse transcriptase, *Nat. New Biol.* **235**, 35.

Shanmugam, G., Vecchio, G., Ahardi, D., and Green, M., 1972, Immunological studies on viral polypeptide synthesis in cells replicating murine sarcoma-leukemia virus, *J. Virol.* **10**, 447.

Shibley, G. P., Carleton, F. J., and Wright, B. S., 1969, Comparison of the biologic and biophysical properties of the progeny of intact and ether-extracted Rauscher leukemia viruses, *Cancer Res.* **29**, 905.

Shigematsu, T., Priori, E. S., Dmochowski, L., and Wilbur, J. R., 1971, Immunoelectron microscopic studies of type C virus particles in ESP-1 and HEK-1-HRLV cell lines, *Nature (Lond.)* **234**, 412.

Smith, G. H., and Wivel, N. A., 1972, Isolation and partial characterization of intracytoplasmic A particles, *Virology* **48**, 270.

Smith, G. H., and Wivel, N. A., 1973, Intracytoplasmic particles: Mouse mammary tumor virus nucleoprotein cores, *J. Virol.* **11**, 575.

Somers, K., and Kit, S., 1973, Temperature-dependent expression of transformation by a cold-sensitive mutant of murine sarcoma virus, *Proc. Natl. Acad. Sci. USA* **70**, 2206.

Spiegelman, S., Burry, A., Das, M. R., Keydar, J., Schlom, J., Travnicek, N., and Watson, K., 1970, DNA-directed DNA polymerase activity in oncogenic RNA viruses, *Nature (Lond.)* **227**, 1029.

Steck, T. F., and Rubin, H., 1966, The mechanism of interference between an avian leukosis virus and Rous sarcoma virus. II. Early steps of infection by RSV of cells under conditions of interference, *Virology* **29**, 642.

Stephenson, J. R., Reynolds, R. K., and Aaronson, S. A., 1972a, Isolation of temperature-sensitive mutants of murine leukemia virus, *Virology* **48**, 749.

Stephenson, M. L., Wirthlin, L. R. S., Scott, J. F., and Zamecnik, P. C., 1972b, The 3′-terminal nucleosides of the high-molecular-weight RNA of avian myeloblastosis virus, *Proc. Natl. Acad. Sci. USA* **69**, 1176.

Stone, L. B., Takemoto, K. K., and Martin, M. A., 1971, Physical and biochemical properties of progressive pneumonia virus, *J. Virol.* **8**, 573.

Strand, M., and August, J. T. 1971, Protein kinase and phosphate acceptor proteins in Rauscher murine leukemia virus, *Nat. New Biol.* **233**, 137.

Stromberg, K., 1972, Surface-active agents for isolation the core component of avian myeloblastosis virus, *J. Virol.* **9**, 684.

Svoboda, J., Hlozanek, I., and Mach, O., 1972, Detection of chicken sarcoma virus after transfection of chicken fibroblasts with DNA isolated from mammalian cells transformed with Rous virus, *Folia Biol. (Prague)* **18**, 149.

Temin, H. M., 1960, The control of cellular morphology in embryonic cells infected with Rous sarcoma virus *in vitro, Virology* **10**, 182.

Temin, H. M., 1963, The effects of actinomycin D on growth of Rous sarcoma virus *in vitro, Virology* **20**, 557.

Temin, H. M., 1964*a*, The participation of DNA in Rous sarcoma virus production, *Virology* **23**, 486.

Temin, H. M., 1964*b*, The nature of the provirus of Rous sarcoma, *Natl. Cancer Inst. Monograph* **17**, 557.

Temin, H. M., 1964*c*, Homology between RNA from Rous sarcoma virus and DNA from Rous sarcoma virus-infected cells, *Proc. Natl. Acad. Sci. USA* **52**, 323.

Temin, H. M., 1967, Studies on carcinogenesis by avian sarcoma viruses. V. Requirement for new DNA synthesis and for cell division, *J. Cell. Physiol.* **69**, 53.

Temin, H. M., 1970, Formation and activation of the provirus of RNA sarcoma viruses, *in* "The Biology of Large RNA Viruses" (R. D. Barry and B. J. W. Mahy, eds.) p. 233, Academic Press, New York.

Temin, H. M., 1971, The protovirus hypothesis: Speculations on the significance of RNA-directed DNA synthesis for normal development and for carcinogenesis, *J. Natl. Cancer Inst.* **46** III–VII.

Temin, H. M., and Baltimore, D., 1972, RNA-directed DNA synthesis and RNA tumor viruses, *Adv. Virus Res.* **17**, 129.

Temin, H., and Mizutani, S., 1970, RNA-dependent DNA polymerase in virions of Rous sarcoma virus, *Nature (Lond.)* **226**, 1211.

Temin, H. M., and Rubin, H., 1958, Characteristics of an assay for Rous sarcoma virus and Rous sarcoma cells in tissue culture, *Virology* **6**, 669.

Temin, H. M., and Rubin, H., 1959, A kinetic study of infection of chick embryo cells *in vitro* by Rous sarcoma virus, *Virology* **8**, 209.

Ting, R. C., 1966, *In vitro* transformation of rat embryo cells by a murine sarcoma virus, *Virology* **28**, 783.

Toyoshima, K., and Vogt, P. K., 1969, Temperature-sensitive mutants of an avian sarcoma virus, *Virology* **39**, 930.

Toyoshima, K., Friis, R. R., and Vogt, P. K., 1970, The reproductive and cell-transforming capacities of avian sarcoma virus B77: Inactivation with UV light, *Virology* **42**, 163.

Travnicek, H., 1968, RNA with amino acid acceptor activity isolated from an oncogenic virus, *Biochim. Biophys. Acta* **166**, 757.

Travnicek, M., and Riman, J., 1970, Chromatographic differences between lysyl-tRNA's from avian tumor virus BAI strain A and virus-transformed cells, *Biochim. Biophys. Acta* **199**, 283.

Tronick, S. R., Scolnick, E. M., and Parks, W. P., 1972, Reversible inactivation of the deoxyribonucleic acid polymerase of Rauscher leukemia virus, *Virology* **10**, 885.

Ubertini, T., Noronha, F., Post, J. E., and Rickard, C. G., 1971, A fluorescent antibody technique for the detection of the group-specific antigen of feline leukemia virus in infected tissue-culture cells, *Virology* **44**, 219.

Valentine, A. F., and Bader, J. P., 1968, Production of virus by mammalian cells transformed by Rous sarcoma and murine sarcoma viruses, *J. Virol.* **2**, 224.

Varmus, H. E., Levinson, W. B., and Bishop, J. M., 1971, Extent of transcription by the RNA-dependent DNA polymerase of Rous sarcoma virus, *Nat. New Biol.* **233**, 19.

Varmus, H. E., Bishop, J. M., and Vogt, P. K., 1973, Appearance of virus-specific DNA in mammalian cells following transformation by Rous sarcoma virus, *J. Mol. Biol.* **74**, 613.

Verma, I. M., Temple, G. F., Fan, H., and Baltimore, D., 1971, A covalently linked RNA–DNA molecule as the initial product of the RNA tumor virus DNA polymerasee, *Nat. New Biol.* **233**, 131.

Verma, I. M., Meuth, N. L., and Baltimore, D., 1972, Covalent linkage between ribonucleic and primer and deoxyribonucleic acid product of the avian myeloblastosis virus deoxyribonucleic acid polymerase, *J. Virol.* **10**, 622.

Vigier, P., 1970, Persistance de la necessite d'une synthese d'ADN pour la replication du virus de Rous dans les cellules preinfectees par un virus apparente, *C. R. Hebd. Seances Acad. Sci. Ser. D Sci. Nat.* **270**, 1192.

Vigier, P., and Golde, A., 1964, Effects of actinomycin D and of mitomycin C on the development of Rous sarcoma virus, *Virology* **23**, 511.

Vogt, P. K., 1967a, Phenotypic mixing in the avian tumor virus group, *Virology* **32**, 708.

Vogt, P. K., 1967b, Enhancement of cellular transformation induced by avian sarcoma viruses, *Virology* **33**, 175.

Vogt, P. K., 1967c, A virus released by "nonproducing" Rous sarcoma cells, *Proc. Natl. Acad. Sci. USA* **58**, 801.

Vogt, P. K., 1971a, Spontaneous segregation of nontransforming viruses from cloned sarcoma viruses, *Virology* **46**, 939.

Vogt, P. K., 1971b, Genetically stable reassortment of markers during mixed infection with avian tumor viruses, *Virology* **46**, 947.

Vogt, P. K., and Duesberg, P. H., 1973, On the mechanism of recombination between avian RNA tumor viruses, *in* "Second ICN-UCLA Symposium on Molecular Biology" (C. F. Fox and W. S. Robinson, eds.), p. 505, Academic Press, New York.

Vogt, P. K., and Friis, R. R., 1971, An avian leukosis virus related to RSV(o): Properties and evidence for helper activity, *Virology* **43**, 223.

Vogt, P. K., and Ishizaki, R., 1965, Reciprocal patterns of genetic resistance to avian tumor viruses in two lines of chickens, *Virology* **26**, 664.

Vogt, P. K., and Ishizaki, R., 1966, Patterns of viral interference in the avian leukosis and sarcoma complex, *Virology* **30**, 368.

Vogt, P. K., and Rubin, H., 1962, The cytology of Rous sarcoma virus infection, *Cold Spring Harbor Symp. Quant. Biol.* **27**, 395.

Wang, L., and Duesberg, P. H., 1973, DNA polymerase of murine sarcoma-leukemia virus: Lack of detectable RNase H and low activity with viral RNA and natural DNA templates, *J. Virol.* **12**, 1512.

Warburg, O., 1956, On the origin of cancer cells, *Science (Wash., D.C.)* **123**, 309.

Ware, L. M., and Axelrod, A. A., 1972, Inherited resistance to N- and B-type murine leukemia viruses *in vitro*: Evidence that congenic mouse strains SIM and SIM-R differ at the *Fv-1* locus, *Virology* **50**, 339.

Waters, N. F., and Burmester, B. R., 1963, Mode of inheritance of resistance to induced erytheoblastosis in chickens, *Poultry Sci.* **42**, 95.

Watson, J. D., 1971, The structure and assembly of murine leukemia virus: Intracellular viral RNA, *Virology* **45**, 586.

Watson, K. K., Nowinski, R. C., Yaniv, A., and Spiegelman, S., 1972, Serological analysis of the deoxyribonucleic acid polymerase of avian oncornaviruses. I. Preparation and characterization of monospecific antiserum with purified deoxyribonucleic acid polymerase, *J. Virol.* **10**, 951.

Weinstein, I. B., Gebert, R., Stadler, U. C., Orenstein, J. M., and Axel, R., 1972, Type C virus from cell cultures of chemically induced rat hepatomas, *Science (Wash., D.C.)* **178**, 1098.

Weiss, R., 1967, Spontaneous virus production from "non-virus producing" Rous sarcoma cells, *Virology* **32**, 719.

Weiss, R. A., 1971, Cell transformation induced by Rous sarcoma virus: Analysis of density dependence, *Virology* **46**, 209.

Weiss, R. A., and Payne, L. N., 1971, The heritable nature of the factor in chicken cells which acts as a helper virus for Rous sarcoma virus, *Virology* **45**, 508.

Weiss, R. A., Friis, R. R., Katz, E., and Vogt, P. K., 1971, Induction of avian tumor viruses in normal cells by physical and chemical carcinogens, *Virology* **46**, 920.

Weiss, R. A., Mason, W. S., and Vogt, P. K., 1973, Genetic recombinants and heterozygotes derived endogenous and exogenous avian RNA tumor viruses, *Virology* **52**, 535.

Weissbach, A., Bolden, A., Muller, R., Hanafusa, H., and Hanafusa, T., 1972, Deoxyribonucleic acid polymerase activities in normal and leukovirus-infected chicken embryo cells, *J. Virol.* **10**, 321.

Wilson, R. G., and Bader, J. P., 1965, Viral ribonucleic acid polymerase: Chick embryo cells infected with vesicular stomatitis virus or Rous-associated virus, *Biochim. Biophys. Acta* **103**, 549.

Witte, O. N., Weissman, I. L., and Kaplan, H. S., 1973, Structural characteristics of some murine RNA tumor viruses studies by lactoperoxidase iodination, *Proc. Natl. Acad. Sci. USA* **70**, 36.

Wong, P. K. Y., and McCarter, J. A., 1973, Genetic studies of temperature-sensitive mutants of Moloney-murine leukemia virus, *Virology* **53**, 319.

Wyke, J. A., and Linial, M., 1973, Temperature-sensitive avian sarcoma viruses: A physiological comparison of twenty mutants, *Virology* **53**, 152.

Yoshii, S., and Vogt, P. K., 1970, A mutant of Rous sarcoma virus (type o) causing fusiform cell transformation, *Proc. Soc. Exp. Biol. Med.* **135**, 297.

Yoshikura, H., 1970, Radiological studies on the chronological relation between murine sarcoma virus infection and cell cycle, *J. Gen. Virol.* **8**, 113.

Yoshikura, H., 1972, Effect of 5-fluorouracil on ultraviolet inactivation of virus production by murine sarcoma-leukemia virus complex carrier cells, *Virology* **48**, 193.

Index